SYNCOPE:

Mechanisms and Management

Edited by

Blair P. Grubb, MD
Associate Professor of Medicine and Pediatrics
Director, Electrophysiology and Pacemaker Laboratories
The Medical College of Ohio
Toledo, Ohio

Brian Olshansky, MD
Professor of Medicine
Director, Cardiac Electrophysiology
Loyola University Medical Center
Maywood, Illinois

With the Editorial Assistance of
Shoei K. Stephen Huang, MD

Futura Publishing
Company, Inc.
Armonk, NY

Library of Congress Cataloging-in-Publication Data

Syncope : mechanisms and management / edited by Blair P. Grubb, Brian
   Olshansky; with the editorial assistance of Shoei K. Stephen Huang.
      p.   cm.
   Includes bibliographical references and index.
   ISBN 0-87993-683-5
      1. Syncope (Pathology)   I. Grubb, Blair P.   II. Olshansky, Brian.
   III. Huang, Shoei K.
      [DNLM: 1. Syncope.   WB 182 S9925   1997]
   RB150.L67S96   1997
   616′.047–dc21
   DNLM/DLC
   for Library of Congress   97-24424
                                                                          CIP

Copyright © 1998
Futura Publishing Company, Inc.

Published by
Futura Publishing Company, Inc.
135 Bedford Road
Armonk, New York 10504-0418

ISBN #: 0-87993-6-X

Printed in the United States of America.

This book is printed on acid-free paper.

Dedication

To Barbara Straus, MD,
Physician, teacher, mother, dancer, soul mate,
and source of all inspiration

And to Helen and Alex,
Who tolerated my frequent absences

-B.P.G.

To Darlene Marie Postacchini Olshansky—
My loving wife, friend, and advisor,
source of support, inspiration, and creativity

-B.O.

Contributors

Gohar Azhar, MBBS   Hebrew Rehabilitation Center for the Aged, Boston, MA

David Benditt, MD   Professor of Medicine, The University of Minnesota School of Medicine, Minneapolis, MN

Gerald J. Bloch, LLB   Attorney at Law, Milwaukee, WI

Hugh Calkins, MD   Associate Professor of Medicine, The Johns Hopkins Hospital, Baltimore, MD

Thomas Davis, MD   Assistant Professor of Neurology, Vanderbilt University School of Medicine, Nashville, TN

Blair P. Grubb, MD   Associate Professor of Medicine and Pediatrics, Director, Electrophysiology and Pacemaker Laboratories, The Medical College of Ohio, Toledo, OH

Mark Harvey, MD   Lecturer in Medicine, The University of Michigan Medical Center, Ann Arbor, MI

Shoei K. Stephen Huang, MD   Professor of Medicine, Director, Electrophysiology Laboratory, The University of Massachusetts Medical Center, Worcester, MA

Wishwa N. Kapoor, MD, MPH   Falk Professor of Medicine, University of Pittsburgh Medical Center, Pittsburgh, PA

George Klein, MD   Professor of Medicine, University of Western Ontario, Director, Division of Cardiology, University Hospital, London, Ontario, Canada

Daniel Kosinski, MD   Assistant Professor of Medicine, Director, Cardiac Autonomics Laboratory, The Medical College of Ohio, Toledo, OH

Andrew D. Krahn, MD   Assistant Professor of Medicine, University of Western Ontario, University Hospital, London, Ontario, Canada

Lewis A. Lipsitz, MD Associate Professor of Medicine, Harvard Medical School, Hebrew Rehabilitation Center for the Aged, Boston, MA

Fred Morady, MD Professor of Medicine, Director, Cardiac Electrophysiology, The University of Michigan Medical Center, Ann Arbor, MI

Brian Olshansky, MD Professor of Medicine, Director, Cardiac Electrophysiology, Loyola University Medical Center, Maywood, IL

David Robertson, MD Professor of Medicine, Pharmacology, and Neurology, Vanderbilt University School of Medicine, Director, Clinical Research Center, Vanderbilt University Medical Center, Nashville, TN

Bertrand Ross, MD Professor of Pediatrics, Eastern Virginia University School of Medicine Children's Hospital of the King's Daughters, Norfolk, VA

Peter Rowe, MD Associate Professor of Pediatrics, The Johns Hopkins Hospital, Baltimore, MD

Herbert Schulberg, PhD Professor of Psychiatry, Psychology, and Medicine, University of Pittsburgh Medical Center, Pittsburgh, PA

Richard Sutton, DScMed Cardiac Department, Royal Brompton and National Heart Hospital, London, United Kingdom

Edward R. Telfer, MD Assistant Professor of Medicine, Loyola University Medical Center, Maywood, IL

Alan B. Wagshal, MD Assistant Professor of Medicine, University of Massachusetts Medical Center, Worcester, MA

Raymond Yee, MD Associate Professor of Medicine, University of Western Ontario, Director, Arrhythmia Monitoring Unit, University Hospital, London, Ontario, Canada

Mark Zucker, MD, JD Assistant Professor of Medicine, University of Medicine and Dentistry of New Jersey, Director, Cardiothoracic Transplantation, Newark Beth Israel Medical Center, Newark, NJ

Foreword

Syncope is one of the most frequent and frustrating symptom complexes with which physicians have to cope. It has no gender predispositions and can occur at any age. The causes of this common symptom are multiple and the costs of trying to resolve the etiology of the problem are enormous, especially with use of presently available, highly technological approaches. It is in this light that Blair Grubb and Brian Olshansky have put forth *Syncope: Mechanisms and Management,* which is the first book to deal thoughtfully and comprehensively with this complex medical problem and provide useful guidelines for its management.

Clinicians of all disciplines must frequently grapple with the problem of syncope. It is an inescapable fact that this symptom remains one of the most common, yet misunderstood medical problems. Questions frequently arise concerning the proper approach to the patient, but clearly this one symptom complex challenges even the best physician's clinical acumen. The subtle diagnostic clues surrounding a syncopal event can provide a wealth of useful diagnostic information, which may ultimately lead to proper therapeutic management. Even so, multiple bewildering, therapeutic, and diagnostic decision-making issues complicate, rather than clarify, the management of syncope. These issues include the need for further evaluation of syncope, the type of evaluation used, the location of treatment (in hospital or out of hospital), and the concern of possible cardiac arrest. While no perfect diagnosis or therapeutic algorithm presently exists for this problem, this book serves as the first comprehensive text to address many of the serious issues involving syncope.

The book opens with an overview of the problem by Dr. Wishwa N. Kapoor, who was one of the first to demonstrate the seriousness of this symptom complex for patients in whom heart disease is an etiologic entity for syncope. The pathophysiological bases for this wide variety of etiologies are discussed in well-written, comprehensive chapters. The chapter by Olshansky that reviews an approach to the patient with syncope, the chapter that reviews the use of electrophysiological studies in patients with syncope, by Telfer and Olshansky, and the chapter by Krahn and coworkers, which discusses what to do about recurrent unexplained syncope when all else fails, offer the reader new insights and practical guidelines into the management of patients with syncope. Most of the other chapters provide critical and thorough review of the individual potential causes of syncope in a global sense. Additional chapters dealing with specific topics such as syncope in athletes, syncope in the elderly, and syncope in children and adolescents, provide excellent references for specific, yet highly controversial, topics. Finally, the social and legal issues related to syncope, which are often forgotten but highly relevant, are dealt with in a logical and practical manner.

This is a unique text that deals in practical terms with a major clinical and financial problem. Discussion of the role of the patient's history and physical examination in unraveling this complex problem and saving the expense of costly procedures is refreshing and should be mandatory reading for all clinicians.

In sum, *Syncope: Mechanisms and Management* is a text of remarkable clinical value. It provides a useful reference for physicians and subspecialists, including cardiologists, who are involved in the primary care of patients. The information in this book can provide cost-effective help, in terms of quality of life, for the management and outcome of hundreds and thousands of patients who experience syncope.

Mark E. Josephson, MD
Professor of Medicine
Harvard Medical School
Director, Thorndike Electrophysiology Institute and Arrhythmia Service

Preface

Syncope, the transient loss of consciousness and postural tone with spontaneous recovery, is a common malady that has afflicted patients and challenged medical practitioners from the beginnings of recorded history. Since the time of Hippocrates, physicians have struggled to understand the complex and diverse etiologies that may culminate in syncope. The extreme diversity of causes and the similarities in presentation make the task of diagnosis a challenging one. Combined with the ever-present knowledge that "today's syncope may be tomorrow's sudden death," the evaluation and management of the patient with recurrent, unexplained syncope may seem truly overwhelming. The practitioner, seeking guidance in the approach to the patient with recurrent syncope, has been forced to search throughout a widely scattered medical literature belonging to a variety of medical specialties. This situation has been compounded by the extremely rapid growth of knowledge and research into many of the causes of syncope.

The aim of this book is to bring together in one volume a comprehensive yet usable reference source on syncope. This collaboration has brought together the skills and perspectives of internists, pediatricians, gerontologists, neurologists, cardiologists, and psychiatrists. In each aspect, we have attempted to provide a useful and complete body of information that not only provides a summary of the published literature, but also gives the personal insights and experiences of each author. The book has been organized to make this diverse quantity of information easy to assimilate, with each section designed to stand alone while also being part of a coherent whole. When appropriate, different perspectives on the same disorder have been presented. With this, we hope to help form a solid foundation for further development in this rapidly expanding and increasingly complex field.

Blair P. Grubb
Toledo, Ohio

Brian Olshansky
Chicago, Illinois

Contents

Foreword   Mark E. Josephson, MD   vii

Preface   Blair P. Grubb, MD and Brian Olshansky, MD.   ix

Chapter 1. An Overview of the Evaluation and Management of Syncope
Wishwa N. Kapoor, MD, MPH   1

Chapter 2. Syncope: Overview and Approach to Management
Brian Olshansky, MD.   15

Chapter 3. Neurocardiogenic Syncope
Blair P. Grubb, MD.   73

Chapter 4. Dysautonomic (Orthostatic) Syncope
Blair P. Grubb, MD.   107

Chapter 5. Bradyarrhythmias as a Cause of Syncope
David G. Benditt, MD and Richard Sutton, DScMed   127

Chapter 6. Tachyarrhythmias as a Cause of Syncope
Mark N. Harvey, MD and Fred Morady, MD   167

Chapter 7. Use of Electrophysiological Studies in Syncope: Practical Aspects for Diagnosis and Treatment
Edward A. Telfer, MD and Brian Olshansky, MD   179

Chapter 8. Neurological and Related Causes of Syncope: The Importance of Recognition and Treatment
David Robertson, MD and Thomas L. Davis, MD   223

Chapter 9. Psychiatric Disorders in Patients With Syncope
Wishwa N. Kapoor, MD and Herbert C. Schulberg, PhD.   253

Chapter 10. Neurally Mediated Hypotension and the Chronic Fatigue Syndrome
Hugh Calkins, MD and Peter C. Rowe, MD   265

Chapter 11. Carotid Sinus Hypersensitivity
Alan B. Wagshal, MD and Shoei K. Stephen Huang, MD   281

Chapter 12. Miscellaneous Causes of Syncope
Daniel J. Kosinski, MD   297

Chapter 13. Syncope in the Child and Adolescent
Bertrand Ross, MD and Blair P. Grubb, MD   305

Chapter 14. Syncope in the Athlete
Daniel J. Kosinski, MD   317

Chapter 15. Syncope in the Elderly
Gohar Azhar, MBBS and Lewis A. Lipsitz, MD 337

Chapter 16. Recurrent Unexplained Syncope: When All Else Fails
Andrew D. Krahn, MD, George J. Klein, MD,
and Raymond Yee, MD 359

Chapter 17. Driving and Syncope
Brian Olshansky, MD and Blair P. Grubb, MD 371

Chapter 18. Syncope and the Law
Mark Jay Zucker, MD, JD, FACC and Gerald J. Bloch, LLB. 387

Index 405

Those who suffer from
frequent and severe fainting
often die suddenly

—Hippocrates
Aphorisms 2.41
1000 B.C.E.

Only if one knows the
causes of syncope will he
be able to recognize its
onset and combat the cause

—Maimonides
1135–1204 C.E.

Our rate of progress is such that
an individual human being, of ordinary
length of life, will be called upon to
face novel situations which find no
parallel in his past. The fixed person,
for the fixed duties, who in older
societies was such a godsend, in
the future will be a public danger

—Alfred North Whitehead
1861–1947 C.E.

He who saves a single life,
it is as if he had saved
an entire world ....

—The Talmud

Chapter 1

An Overview of the Evaluation and Management of Syncope

Wishwa N. Kapoor, MD, MPH

Syncope is defined as a sudden temporary loss of consciousness associated with a loss of postural tone, with spontaneous recovery that does not require electrical or chemical cardioversion. Syncope is a common symptom, accounting for 1% to 6% of hospital admissions and up to 3% of emergency room visits. Loss of consciousness is also common in healthy young adults (reported by 12% to 48%), although most do not seek medical attention. Syncope is a frequent symptom in the elderly; a 6% incidence and 23% previous lifetime episodes were found in one long-term care institution.[1]

The evaluation and management of syncope has dramatically changed over the past 15 years. Prior to 1980, the major contributions were made in descriptive studies of various etiologies, pathophysiology of vasovagal syncope, and natural history of various entities. In the early 1980s, several studies showed that the cause of syncope was often not established, and subgroups were identified with high mortality and sudden death rates.[2–5] These studies led to a search for newer diagnostic modalities in unexplained syncope. In the mid 1980s, a large number of studies on electrophysiological testing appeared. These led to a better understanding of the roles and limitations of tests in syncope.[6–25] Studies also showed that syncope in the elderly may involve complex interaction of comorbid diseases, physiological changes, and medications.[1,26] In the late 1980s and early 1990s, tilt table testing assumed an important role in the evaluation of

From Grubb BP, Olshansky B (eds.). *Syncope: Mechanisms and Management.* Armonk, NY: Futura Publishing Co., Inc.; © 1998.

syncope, showing that neurally mediated mechanism is a common etiology of unexplained syncope.[27-42]

The purpose of this review is to highlight what has been learned in the diagnosis and prognosis of syncope, and to discuss the likely direction of future research in this area.

How Often Are Causes Diagnosed?

Table 1 shows pooled estimates of causes in studies reporting on unselected patients with syncope.[2-5] These studies from the 1980s show that the cause of syncope was not established in 34% of patients (range 13% to 41%). With wider use of electrophysiological testing, tilt testing, event monitoring, attention to psychiatric issues, and recognition of multifactorial nature of syncope in the elderly, unexplained syncope is considerably rarer. Assuming that passive tilt testing is positive in 49% of patients with unexplained syncope with 10% false-positive rate (specificity 90%), the proportion of patients with unexplained syncope can be estimated to decrease to between 8% and 23%. The proportion of syncope patients with neurocardiogenic causes is estimated to increase to 36% to 57%, and overall causes assigned increase to 77% to 92%. The estimates are essentially the same if it is assumed that the test is done in conjunction with isoproterenol (approximately 64% of patients with

_____ **Table 1** _____

Causes of Syncope: Prevalence of Various Etiologies

Cause	Prevalence (Mean) %	Prevalence (Range) %
Reflex-medicated:		
Vasovagal	18	8–37
Situational	5	1–8
Carotid sinus	1	0–4
Orthostatic hypotension	8	4–10
Medications	3	1–7
Psychiatric	2	1–7
Neurological	10	3–32
Cardiac:		
Organic heart disease	4	1–8
Cardiac:		
Arrhythmias	14	4–38
Unknown	34	13–41

unexplained syncope with positive responses; specificity of 75%). These estimates suggest that neurocardiogenic syncope is the most common cause of syncope in unselected patients presenting to various medical centers and emergency departments. With appropriate use of diagnostic modalities, unexplained syncope is rare.

Prognosis After Syncope

A great deal has been learned about the prognosis after syncope, which has implications for the diagnostic evaluation. The findings on prognosis can be summarized as follows:

1. High-risk subgroups. The 1-year mortality of patients with cardiac causes of syncope is 18% to 33%,[2–5] which is higher than those in patients with noncardiac causes (0% to 12%) or in patients with unknown cause (6%). The incidence of sudden death in patients with cardiac causes is also markedly higher as compared to the other two groups.[2] Even when adjustments for differences in comorbidity are made, cardiac syncope is still an independent predictor of mortality and sudden death.[2]

2. Role of structural heart disease. Our recent studies show that underlying cardiac and noncardiac diseases are associated with increased mortality independent of syncope.[43] This implies that every attempt should be made to define the underlying structural heart disease in syncope patients and treat the cardiac diseases in order to have an impact on mortality and sudden death rates.

3. Outcome of neurocardiogenic syncope. Neurocardiogenic syncope has excellent long-term prognosis, but recurrences are common and a major reason for seeking medical care. Similarly, syncope associated with psychiatric disease has no increased mortality, but has 1-year recurrence rates of 26% to 50%.[44]

4. Recurrence rates. In patients presenting with syncope, recurrence rate is 34% over 3 years of follow-up.[45] Although recurrences are associated with fractures and soft-tissue injury in 12% of patients, they do not predict an increased risk of mortality or sudden death.[45]

5. The elderly. In a study of institutionalized individuals with a mean age of 87 years, a yearly incidence of 6% and recurrence rate of 30% was found in a 2-year prospective follow-up.[1, 26] There was no significant difference in mortality rate among patients with cardiac syncope, noncardiac syncope, or syncope of unknown etiology in this cohort. In another study of 210 community-dwelling elderly (mean age 71 years), patients with cardiac causes had higher mortality rate irrespective of whether they were elderly or young.[46] In patients with noncardiac causes or unknown causes of syncope, older age, a history of congestive heart failure, and male sex were important prognostic factors for mortality.[46]

Diagnostic Testing

Several studies show that history, physical examination, and ECG can be used to plan further diagnostic testing.

History, Physical Examination, and Baseline Laboratory Tests

The history and physical examination identify a potential cause of syncope in approximately 45% of patients.[2-5] Additionally, many other causes of syncope (eg, pulmonary hypertension, aortic stenosis, and pulmonary embolism) are usually suspected clinically and confirmed by specific testing. Suggestive findings of this type were present in 8% of additional patients in one study.[2] The details of history and physical examination are discussed elsewhere.

Initial laboratory blood tests are generally not abnormal and they generally do not lead to a diagnosis. Hypoglycemia, hyponatremia, hypocalcemia, or renal failure are found in 2% to 3% of patients, but these appear to be patients with seizures rather than syncope.[2-5] These abnormalities are often suspected clinically. Bleeding is generally diagnosed clinically and confirmed by a complete blood count or hemoccult tests.

Cardiovascular Testing

12-Lead ECG

Although ECG is often abnormal, causes of syncope are rarely assigned (<5% of patients) on the basis of ECG and rhythm strip.[2-5] An ECG is recommended in all patients with syncope because abnormalities found on ECG (such as bundle branch block) may guide further evaluation, or if a specific diagnosis is made the findings can be important in immediate decision making.

Prolonged Electrocardiographic Monitoring

It has become clear that results of ambulatory monitoring are often difficult to interpret in evaluating syncope because of the lack of a "gold standard" for diagnosis of arrhythmias and the rarity of symptoms during monitoring. The best way to assess the usefulness of ambulatory monitoring is to use presence or absence of symptoms during monitoring.[47] Approximately 4% of patients have symptoms concurrently with arrhythmias, and 17% have symptoms but no arrhythmias, thus potentially excluding arrhythmias as a cause of symptoms. In approximately 79% of patients there are no symptoms, but brief arrhythmias are found in 13%. In the absence of symptoms during monitoring, finding brief or no arrhythmias does not exclude arrhythmic syncope. Brief arrhythmias are nonspecific and can be found in asymptomatic healthy individuals. Additionally, absence of arrhythmias on monitoring does not exclude arrhythmic syncope because arrhythmias are episodic and may not be captured during monitoring. In patients with high pretest probability of arrhythmias such as brief sudden loss of consciousness without prodrome, patients with abnormal ECG, or those with structural heart disease, arrhythmias are still of concern and further testing is needed. Holter monitoring for 72 hours rather than for 24 hours does not yield greater numbers of symptomatic periods.[48] Ambulatory monitoring (for 24 hours) is recommended for patients with high pretest likelihood of arrhythmias, as defined above.

Long-term ambulatory loop event monitoring. Loop event monitors can be activated after a syncopal episode, and can record 2 to 5 minutes of rhythm strip prior to the activation and 30 to 60 seconds of the rhythm after the activation. Tracings can be transmitted via telephone and monitors can be worn for weeks to months. Studies of loop monitoring show that arrhythmias with symptoms are found in 8% to 20% of patients. In an additional 27 percent, there are symptoms without concurrent arrhythmias.[49] This test is recommended in patients with recurrent syncope when there is a high probability of a recurrent event during the monitoring period.

Electrophysiological Studies

Methodology and limitations of electrophysiological studies (EPS) will be discussed in detail elsewhere in this book. In patients with structural heart disease and/or abnormal ECG, the diagnostic yield of EPS is approximately 50%.[6–25] In patients without structural heart disease, the diagnostic yield is approximately 10%.[6–25] The structural heart diseases in these studies include coronary artery disease, congenital or valvular heart disease, and cardiomyopathy. Particularly important ECG findings include bundle branch block, prior myocardial infarction, and evidence of bypass tract. Bradyarrhythmias are much more likely to be diagnosed in patients with conduction disease on surface ECG, however, the sensitivity and specificity of EPS for detection of bradyarrhythmias is low.

It is recommended that patients with structural heart disease or abnormal ECG undergo electrophysiological testing if clinical assessment is suggestive of arrhythmic syncope and if noninvasive testing with Holter or loop monitoring have been nondiagnostic. In patients without structural heart disease or abnormal ECG, loop monitoring may be considered first for detection of arrhythmias if pretest likelihood of arrhythmias is high clinically.

Signal-Averaged ECG

Finding low-amplitude signals (late potentials) has a sensitivity of 73% to 89% and specificity of 89% to 100% for prediction of inducible sustained ventricular tachycardia by EPS.[50,51] This test has not been evaluated in unselected patients with unexplained syncope because most of the studies come from cardiovascular centers that patients have been referred to for electrophysiological testing. This test may be useful in deciding if there is a need for electrophysiological studies for diagnosis of ventricular tachycardia when these arrhythmias are the only concern. However, EPS is often performed for diagnosis of conduction system disease as well as of tachyarrhythmias. This test is not likely to be useful under such circumstances because complete assessment is needed.

Carotid Massage

In unselected studies of patients with syncope, carotid sinus syncope is rarely diagnosed. In the absence of symptom reproduction, carotid sinus syncope is likely when carotid sinus hypersensitivity is found and either 1) spontaneous episodes are related to activities that press or stretch the carotid sinus or 2) patient has recurrent syncope with a negative work-up.

Survival of patients with carotid sinus hypersensitivity is similar to that of the general population and is largely related to underlying diseases. Survival appears to be unrelated to pacemaker therapy.[52] Symptoms recur in 20% to 25% of untreated or medically treated patients with carotid sinus syndrome. However, syncope recurred in 57% of the nonpaced group versus 9% of the paced group in a prospective study of patients with severe carotid sinus syndrome (ie, patients with recurrent syncope, trauma, and reproduction of symptoms upon massage).[53]

Carotid massage is recommended when symptoms are suggestive of carotid sinus syncope and in elderly patients with unexplained syncope.

Echocardiogram

Echocardiography in the absence of clinical evidence of organic heart disease generally does not reveal unexpected findings that lead to an etiology for syncope.[54] The usefulness of echocardiogram in assessment of patients with known heart disease (eg, previous myocardial infarction or congestive heart failure) is not widely studied but is expected to be low. This test is not recommended for screening purposes in patients with syncope.

Exercise Testing

The yield of exercise testing in the diagnosis of the etiology of syncope is very low (less than 1%). Exercise testing is useful as an ancillary diagnostic test for evaluation of ischemic heart disease in patients with arrhythmic syncope, particularly ventricular tachycardia. In these patients, in addition to the treatment of ventricular arrhythmias, the management of underlying cardiac disease is critical. Exercise ECG is also recommended for the evaluation of symptoms with exercise and postexertional syncope.

Upright Tilt Testing

Maintaining the patient in an upright position for a brief duration on a tilt table has become a common means of testing for predisposition to vasovagal syncope. It is widely accepted that hypotension and/or bradycardia during upright tilt testing is equivalent to spontaneous vasovagal syncope. This is supported by the fact that the temporal sequence of blood pressure and heart rate changes during tilt testing is similar to spontaneous spells. In addition, catecholamine release immediately prior to tilt-induced syncope is similar to spontaneous vasovagal faint.

Two general types of testing procedures include upright tilt testing alone (passive testing) and tilt testing in conjunction with a chemical agent.[27-42] A vast majority of the reported studies employ passive testing or use isoproterenol after a brief period of passive tilt testing. Protocols using other agents (eg, edrophonium, intravenous or sublingual nitroglycerine) are not recommended for general use because of limited data on their performance characteristics. The protocols and their performance characteristics are discussed elsewhere in this book.

Approximately 50% of patients with unexplained syncope have a positive response to passive tilt testing.[42] With isoproterenol, overall positive responses are approximately 64%, two thirds of which occur during the isoproterenol phase.[42] With either type of testing, approximately two thirds of the responses appear to be cardioinhibitory (defined as bradycardia with or without associated hypotension) and the remaining are pure vasodepressor reactions (defined as hypotension without significant bradycardia). The higher proportion of positive responses with chemical stimulation is probably due to augmentation with isoproterenol, although the effect of angle and duration of testing and other variables in not entirely clear.[42]

Because there are no other "gold standards," the sensitivity of tilt testing can be calculated by testing patients with clinical diagnosis of vasovagal syncope. By use of this approach, the sensitivity of tilt testing is between 67% and 83%.[55] Specificity has generally been evaluated by performing upright tilt testing in subjects without prior syncope. With passive tilt testing, specificity has ranged between 0% and 100%, although an overall rate is approximately 90%.[42] The overall specificity of upright tilt testing with isoproterenol is approximately 75% and ranges from 35% to 100%.[42]

Upright tilt testing is recommended for patients with recurrent unexplained syncope in whom cardiac causes have been excluded or are not likely. Initial testing is recommended by use of a passive protocol for 45 to 60 minutes. In patients with negative passive tests and a high likelihood of neurally mediated syncope clinically (eg, young patients with concurrent autonomic symptoms), additional testing with isoproterenol is recommended. It is not possible to recommend any one protocol for this test. Women of child-bearing age should undergo a pregnancy test prior to tilt testing because hypotension should be avoided in these patients. Older patients (age >50) should also undergo stress testing prior to tilt testing because isoproterenol and precipitating hypotension is best avoided in patients with significant ischemic heart disease.

Neurological Testing

Generally, skull films, lumbar puncture, radionuclide brain scan, carotid Dopplers, and cerebral angiography do not yield diagnostic information for a cause of syncope in the absence of clinical findings that are suggestive of a specific neurological process.[2] Studies of EEG in syncope have shown that an epileptiform abnormality was found in 1% of patients; almost all of these were suspected clinically.[56] Head CT scans are rarely useful to assign an etiology, but are needed if subdural bleed due to head injury is suspected or in patients suspected to have a seizure as a cause of loss of consciousness.[2]

Psychiatric Assessment

Psychiatric illnesses must be considered as a cause of syncope, especially in young patients and those with multiple syncopal episodes who also have other nonspecific complaints.[44] The disorders that may cause syncope include generalized anxiety and panic disorders, major depression, somatization disorder, and alcohol and substance abuse. Screening instruments for these disorders are available and recommended. The high rate of recurrence of syncope in these patients makes detection of these illnesses especially important.

Approach to Diagnostic Testing

The clinical assessment and ECG comprise the initial step in the evaluation of patients with syncope. As noted in Figure 1, this assessment may

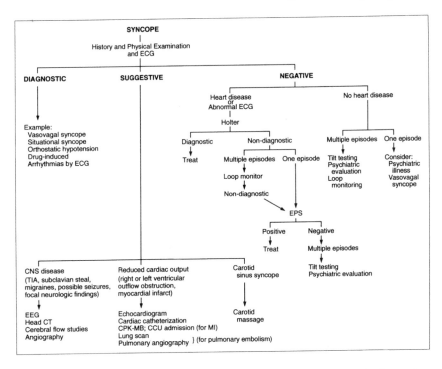

Figure 1. The clinical assessment and ECG comprise the initial step in the evaluation of patients with syncope.

lead to a diagnosis. Under such circumstances, treatment can be planned. The clinical assessment may not be diagnostic, but may provide suggestive evidence for specific entities [eg, signs of aortic stenosis or idiopathic hypertrophic subaortic stenosis (IHSS)]. These clues can be pursued with further testing to confirm or exclude these entities as the causes of syncope. A large group of patients will remain, in whom the initial clinical evaluation does not lead to a specific diagnosis and there are no suggestive findings as potential causes of syncope. An approach to the use of cardiovascular and neurological tests in these patients is shown in Figure 1. The central element in this approach is the presence or absence of structural heart disease and clinical presentation of the patient.

Future Directions

Studies over the past 15 years have greatly improved our understanding of the epidemiology, prognosis, evaluation, and management of syncope. These studies have led to the development of diagnostic tests that have enhanced the ability to assign a diagnosis in the vast majority of the patients. Some important issues for the future are:

1. Development of methods of risk stratification at presentation so streamlined and rapid testing can be performed;
2. Determining optimal methodology for the diagnostic evaluation of neurally mediated syncope;
3. Better understanding of the pathophysiology of neurally mediated syncope;
4. Controlled studies of the effectiveness of treatment of neurally mediated syncope;
5. Is prognosis of patients with abnormal EPS altered by aggressive treatment of arrhythmias and underlying structural heart disease?

A major issue for future studies is the development of methods for determining the sensitivity and specificity of most of the diagnostic testing, because "gold standards" for diagnosis are not available at this time. Greater understanding and improvement in the evaluation of syncope is likely to occur if we can develop methods of assessing performance characteristics of tests in syncope.

References

1. Lipsitz LA, Wei JY, Rowe JW. Syncope in an elderly, institutionalized population: Prevalence, incidence, and associated risk. *QJM* 1985;55:45–55.
2. Kapoor W. Evaluation and outcome of patients with syncope. *Medicine* 1990; 69:160–175.
3. Silverstein MD, Singer DE, Mulley A, et al. Patients with syncope admitted to medical intensive care units. *JAMA* 1982;248:1185–1189.
4. Martin GJ, Adams SL, Martin HG, et al. Prospective evaluation of syncope. *Ann Emerg Med* 1984;13:499–504.
5. Day SC, Cook EF, Funkenstein H, Goldman L. Evaluation and outcome of emergency room patients with transient loss of consciousness. *Am J Med* 1982;73:15–23.
6. DiMarco JP, Garan H, Harthorne JW, Ruskin JN. Intracardiac electrophysiology techniques in recurrent syncope of unknown cause. *Ann Intern Med* 1981;95:542–548.
7. Gulamhusein S, Naccarelli GV, Ko PT, et al. Value and limitations of clinical electrophysiologic study in assessment of patients with unexplained syncope. *Am J Med* 1982;73:700–705.
8. Hess DS, Morady F, Scheirman MM. Electrophysiological testing in the evaluation of patients with syncope of undetermined origin. *Am J Cardiol* 1982; 50:1309–1315.
9. Akhtar M, Shenasa M, Denker S, et al. Role of cardiac electrophysiologic studies in patients with unexplained recurrent syncope. *Pacing Clin Electrophysiol* 1983; 6:192–201.
10. Olshansky B, Mazuz M, Martins JB. Significance of inducible tachycardia in patients with syncope of unknown origin: A long-term follow-up. *J Am Coll Cardiol* 1985;5:216–233.
11. Doherty JU, Pembrook-Rogers D, Grogan EW, et al. Electrophysiologic evaluation and follow-up characteristics of patients with recurrent unexplained syncope and presyncope. *Am J Cardiol* 1985;55:703–708.

12. Teichman SL, Felder SD, Matos JA, et al. The value of electrophysiologic studies in syncope of undetermined origin: Report of 150 cases. *Am Heart J* 1985; 110:469–479.
13. Denes P, Vretz E, Ezri MD, Borbola J. Clinical predictors of electrophysiology findings in patients with syncope of unknown origin. *Arch Intern Med* 1988; 148:1922–1928.
14. Bass EB, Elson JJ, Fogoros RN, et al. Long-term prognosis of patients undergoing electrophysiologic studies for syncope of unknown origin. *Am J Cardiol* 1988;62:1186–1191.
15. Krol RB, Morady F, Flaker GC, et al. Electrophysiologic testing in patients with unexplained syncope: Clinical and noninvasive predictors of outcome. *J Am Coll Cardiol* 1987;10:358–363.
16. Kapoor WN, Hammill SC, Gersh BJ. Diagnosis and natural history of syncope and the role of invasive electrophysiologic testing. *Am J Cardiol* 1989;63:730–734.
17. Click RL, Gersh BJ, Sugrue DD, et al. Role of invasive electrophysiologic testing in patients with symptomatic bundle branch block. *Am J Cardiol* 1987;59(1):817–823.
18. Nelson SD, Kou WH, DeBuitleir M, et al. Value of programmed ventricular stimulation in presumed carotid sinus syndrome. *Am J Cardiol* 1987; 60(13):1073–1077.
19. McLaran CJ, Gersh BJ, Osborn MJ, et al. Increased vagal tone as an isolated finding in patients undergoing electrophysiologic testing for recurrent syncope: Response to long-term anticholinergic agents. *Br Heart J* 1986;55:53–57.
20. Hammill SC, Holmes DR, Wood DL, et al. Electrophysiologic testing in the upright position: Improved evaluation of patients with rhythm disturbances using a tilt table. *J Am Coll Cardiol* 1984;4:65–71.
21. Sugrue DD, Holmes DR, Gersh BJ, et al. Impact of intracardiac electrophysiologic testing on the management of elderly patients with recurrent or near syncope. *J Am Geriatr Soc* 1987;35:1079–1083.
22. Morady F, Scheinman MM. The role and limitations of electrophysiologic testing in patients with unexplained syncope. *Int J Cardiol* 1983;4:229–234.
23. Fujimura O, Yee R, Klein GJ, et al. The diagnostic sensitivity of electrophysiologic testing in patients with syncope caused by transient bradycardia. *N Engl J Med* 1989;321:1703.
24. DiMarco JP. Electrophysiologic studies in patients with unexplained syncope. *Circulation* 1987;75(suppl III):III-140–III-143.
25. McAnulty JH. Syncope of unknown origin: The role of electrophysiologic studies. *Circulation* 1987;75(suppl III):III-144–III-145.
26. Lipsitz LA, Pluchino FC, Wei JY, Rowe JW. Syncope in institutionalized elderly: The impact of multiple pathological conditions and situational stress. *J Chron Dis* 1986;39:619–630.
27. Mark AL. The Bezold-Jarisch reflex revisited: Clinical implications of inhibitory reflexed originating in the heart. *J Am Coll Cardiol* 1983;1:90–92.
28. Abboud FM. Ventricular syncope. *N Engl J Med* 1989;32:390–392.
29. Kenny RA, Ingram A, Bayliss J, Sutton R. Head-up tilt: A useful test for investigating unexplained syncope. *Lancet* 1986;1:1352–1355.
30. Fitzpatrick AP, Theodorakis G, Vardas P, Sutton R. Methodology of head-up tilt testing in patients with unexplained syncope. *J Am Coll Cardiol* 1991;17:125–130.
31. Strasberg B, Rechavia E, Sagie A, et al. The head-up tilt table test in patients with syncope of unknown origin. *Am Heart J* 1989;118(5 Pt 1):923–927.
32. Raviele A, Gasparini G, DiPede F, et al. Usefulness of head-up tilt test in evaluating patients with syncope of unknown origin and negative electrophysiologic study. *Am J Cardiol* 1990;65:1322–1327.

33. Abi-Samra FM, Maloney JD, Fouad-Tarazi FM, et al. The usefulness of head-up tilt testing and hemodynamic investigations in the work-up of syncope of unknown origin. *Pacing Clin Electrophysiol* 1987;10:406.
34. Brignole M, Menozzi C, Gianfranchi L, et al. Carotid sinus massage, eyeball compression, and head-up tilt test in patients with syncope of uncertain origin and in healthy control subjects. *Am Heart J* 1991;122:1664–1651.
35. Almquist A, Goldenberg IF, Milstein S, et al. Provocation of bradycardia and hypotension by isoproterenol and upright posture in patients with unexplained syncope. *N Engl J Med* 1989;320:346–351.
36. Sra JS, Anderson AJ, Sheikh SH, et al. Unexplained syncope evaluated by electrophysiologic studies and head-up tilt testing. *Ann Intern Med* 1991;114:1013–1019.
37. Grubb BP, Temesy-Armos P, Hahn H, Elliott L. Utility of upright tilt table testing in the evaluation and management of syncope of unknown origin. *Am J Med* 1991;90:6–10.
38. Pongigline G, Fish FA, Strasburger JF, et al. Heart rate and blood pressure response to upright tilt in young patients with unexplained syncope. *J Am Coll Cardiol* 1990;16:165–170.
39. Kapoor WN, Brant NL. Evaluation of syncope by upright tilt testing with isoproterenol: A nonspecific test. *Ann Int Med* 1992;116:358–363.
40. Waxman MB, Yao L, Cameron DA, et al. Isoproterenol induction of vasodepressor-type reaction in vasodepressor-prone patients. *Am J Cardiol* 1989;63(1):58–65.
41. Hackel A, Linzer M, Anderson N, Williams R. Cardiovascular and catecholamine responses to head-up tilt in the diagnosis of recurrent unexplained syncope in the elderly patients. *J Am Geriatr Soc* 1991;39:663–669.
42. Kapoor WN, Smith M, Miller NL. Upright tilt testing in evaluating syncope: A comprehensive literature review. *Am J Med* 1994;97:78–88.
43. Kapoor WN, Hanusa B. Is syncope a risk factor for poor outcomes? Comparison of patients with and without syncope. *Am J Med* 1996;100:646–655.
44. Kapoor WN, Fortunato M, Hanusa BH, Schulberg HC. Psychiatric illnesses in patients with syncope. *Am J Med* 1995:99;505–512.
45. Kapoor W, Peterson J, Wieand HS, Karpf M. Diagnostic and prognostic implications of recurrences in patients with syncope. *Am J Med* 1987;83:700–708.
46. Kapoor W, Snustad D, Peterson J, et al. Syncope in the elderly. *Am J Med* 1986;80:419–428.
47. DiMarco JP, Philbrick JT. Use of ambulatory electrocardiographic (Holter) monitoring. *Ann Intern Med* 1990;113:53–68.
48. Bass EB, Curtiss EI, Arena VC, et al. The duration of Holter monitoring in patients with syncope: Is 24 hours enough? *Arch Int Med* 1990;150:1073–1078.
49. Linzer M, Pritchett ELC, Pontinen M, et al. Incremental diagnostic yield of loop electrocardiographic recorders in unexplained syncope. *Am J Cardiol* 1990;66:214–219.
50. Steinberg JS, Prystowsky E, Freedman RA, et al. Use of the signal averaged electrocardiogram for predicting inducible ventricular tachycardia in patients with unexplained syncope: Relation to clinical variables in a multivariate analysis. *J Am Coll Cardiol* 1994;23:99–106.
51. Winters SL, Stewart D, Gomes JA. Signal averaging of the surface QRS complex predicts inducibility of ventricular tachycardia in patients with syncope of unknown origin: A prospective study. *J Am Coll Cardiol* 1987;10(4):775–781.
52. Brignole M, Oddone D, Cogorno S, et al. Long-term outcome in symptomatic carotid sinus hypersensitivity. *Am Heart J* 1992;123:687–692.

53. Brignole M, Menozzi C, Lolli G, et al. Long-term outcome of paced and nonpaced patients with severe carotid sinus syndrome. *Am J Cardiol* 1992; 69:1039–1043.
54. Recchia D, Barzilai B. Echocardiography in the evaluation of patients with syncope. *J Gen Intern Med* 1995;10:649–655.
55. Calkins H, Kadish A, Sousa J, et al. Comparison of responses to isoproterenol and epinephrine during head-up tilt in suspected vasodepressor syncope. *Am J Cardiol* 1991;67:207–209.
56. Davis TL, Freemoon FR. Electroencephalography should not be routine in the evaluation of syncope in adults. *Arch Intern Med* 1990;150:2027–2029.

Syncope:

Overview and Approach to Management

Brian Olshansky, MD

Introduction

Syncope is a common important medical problem caused by many conditions ranging from benign and self limiting to chronic, recurrent, and potentially fatal causes. Unfortunately, differentiating between benign and potentially malignant causes can be difficult and challenging. Even with knowledge of common syndromes and conditions that cause syncope, an effective approach to the problem requires the careful integration of clues provided in the patient's history and physical examination and keen clinical acumen. Management of this baffling problem can be frustrating, confusing, and often unrewarding. Treatment can be impossible to prescribe without a clear understanding of the cause.

Fortunately, experienced, astute clinicians can deliver effective care when careful attention is paid to detail. This chapter provides a general overview of the problem of syncope and offers guidelines for the approach to its management. Reference is given to other chapters in this book that provide more detail on specific topics.

Definitions

Syncope is often considered with several more vague symptoms that are manifestations of many clinical conditions. "Spells," transient confusion or weakness, dizziness, loss of memory, lightheadedness, near loss of consciousness ("presyncope" or "near syncope"), falling episodes, and

From Grubb BP, Olshansky B (eds.). *Syncope: Mechanisms and Management.* Armonk, NY: Futura Publishing Co., Inc.; © 1998.

coma are often confused with, and inappropriately labeled "true syncope." The distinction between sleeping, confusion, and fainting may not be completely clear. To make matters more difficult, an elderly patient, already confused, may fall and pass out with only vague recall of the event. This diverse collection of clinical presentations perplexes the patient and the physician. Episodes can be difficult to define even with careful observation.

True syncope is an abrupt but transient loss of consciousness associated with absence of postural tone, followed by rapid, usually complete recovery without the need for intervention to stop the episode. A prodrome may be present. While alarming, this *symptom* is nonspecific. It is generally triggered by a process that results in abrupt, transient (5 to 20 seconds) interruption of cerebral blood flow, specifically to the reticular activating system.

Collapse, associated with syncope, can be misinterpreted. In one study of 121 patients admitted to the emergency room with "collapse"as the admitting diagnosis, 19 had cardiac arrest, four were brought in dead and one was asleep.[1] Only 15 were ultimately diagnosed as having fainted. The final diagnosis in eight was still "collapse." Primary neurologic or metabolic derangements can also mimic but rarely cause true syncope.

The Importance of Syncope

The only difference between syncope and sudden death is that in one you wake up.[2]

Syncope can be the premonitory sign of a serious cardiac problem including cardiac arrest.   Generally, syncope is benign and self limited, but it can mimic a cardiac arrest and even be its precursor. Several causes of syncope, generally cardiac, are potentially fatal. When syncope is due to hemodynamic collapse from critical aortic stenosis, ventricular tachycardia, atrioventricular (AV) block, dissecting aortic aneurysm, or pulmonary embolus, an aggressive evaluation and treatment regimen is needed to forestall death. A potentially lethal cause should always be suspected, especially in elderly patients, or it will be missed. While less common, even younger individuals with syncope can be at risk for death.[3] For this age group, the long congenital QT interval syndrome, hypertrophic cardiomyopathy, and right ventricular dysplasia, among other causes, must be considered.

Syncope can have a major impact on lifestyle.   Patient reactions to syncope can vary from complete lack of recognition and concern to fear and difficulty returning to previous level of activities. Even if syncope is benign, it can have a major impact on quality of life and may change lifestyle dramatically, independent of physician concerns and recommendations. The degree of functional impairment from syncope can match that of other chronic diseases including rheumatoid arthritis, chronic back pain, or chronic obstructive lung disease.[4] Patients can have fear of recurrence and death. There can be imposed limitations on driving and work (see Chapter 17). Restrictions can be self imposed or imposed by the family, by the physician, or by legal constraints (see Chapter 18). Up to 76% of patients will change some activities of daily living, 64% will restrict their driving, and 39% will change their employment.[4] Seventy-three percent of patients become anxious or depressed, especially if a cause is not found and treated.[5,6]

Syncope can cause injuries. Injuries from syncope occur in 17% to 35% of patients.[7-11] When injuries occur, syncope is often suspected to be due to a serious, life-threatening, or cardiac cause, but data conflict.[11,12] Sudden *unexpected* loss of consciousness (sometimes referred to as "Stokes-Adams attacks") can have many causes. The circumstances that surround the episode and the absence of a prodrome cause most injuries. Injury itself does not necessarily indicate a life-threatening cause, an arrhythmic cause, or a nonarrythmic cardiac cause of syncope. While an arrhythmic cause is often suspected when serious injury results from syncope, little data support a more aggressive approach to evaluate or to treat syncope in injured patients. Minor injuries occur in 10% to 29%, fractures occur in 5% to 7% (more severe in the elderly) and traffic accidents in 1% to 5% of syncope patients.[9,13]

Syncope is expensive. Up to one million patients are evaluated for syncope annually in the United States. About 3% to 5% of emergency room visits are to evaluate syncope,[9,14-18] with 35% of these emergency room visits leading to hospital admission.[8] Between 1% and 6% of urgent hospital admissions are for syncope. The cost to evaluate and treat syncope exceeds $750 million per year. The cost for the average admission is more than $5500[14] and hospitalization is helpful in only 10% of patients admitted in whom the etiology was not clear by the admitting history, physical exam, and electrocardiogram. The cost expended to determine one syncope diagnosis in patients diagnosed in 1982 was $23,000[14] after a mean hospital stay of 9.1 days. When vasodepressor syncope is not recognized, evaluations can lead to tremendous expense.[19]

About 10% of falls in the elderly are due to syncope.[20] Serious injury is more frequent when syncope precedes the fall.[21] Falls occur in 20% of the population over 65 years old. The cost to treat falls in the elderly exceeds $7 billion annually in the United States.

Epidemiology

The frequency of syncope and its associated mortality varies with age, gender, and cause. In one large series, 60% of syncope patients were women,[9] but in Framingham, more younger syncope patients were women while more elderly syncope patients were men.[22] In Framingham, syncope had occurred in 3% of men and in 3.5% of women, based on biannual examinations,[22] with the highest frequency in the elderly. In the Framingham population, the annual incidence of syncope in those over 75 years old was 6% and the prevalence of syncope in the elderly was 5.6% compared to a low of 0.7% in the 35 to 44 year-old male population.[22] The elderly are most likely to have syncope, to be injured from syncope, to seek medical advice, and to be admitted to a hospital[23-25] (see Chapter 15).

Of 3000 US Air Force personnel surveyed[26] (mean age 29.1 years), 2.7% (82/3000) have had at least one episode of syncope. Other retrospective studies of healthy individuals suggest that up to 40% of the general population will experience syncope in their lifetime.[27,28] Wide variations in published data are due, in part, to variations in the population evaluated (outpatients, emergency room patients, hospitalized patients, the elderly), the definition of syncope, and the criteria for diagnosis (by examination or by questionnaire). It is likely that 20% to 30% of the population will pass out sometime in their lifetime.[9,16,29] Most individuals with syncope do not seek medical advice, but the actual percentage of those who do is unknown. It is suspected that most individuals who do not seek medical attention have a low recurrence rate and probably have an excellent long-term survival. Outpatients who are evaluated or never admitted for their episodes may also be at lower risk for recurrence and may have a benign long-term prognosis. Patients in these subgroups most likely have neurocardiogenic syncope or syncope with some other autonomically mediated cause.

Sixty to eighty-five percent of those who seek evaluation of syncope will not have a recurrence.[30] Despite widely different suspected causes (severe cardiovascular disease or not) and despite apparently effective treatment, the recurrence rate of syncope remains similar.[30] The fact that syncope is frequently an isolated occurrence can make it difficult to assess the need for treatment. An apparently therapeutic effect of any intervention may instead be related to the sporadic nature of the symptom and not to treatment of the underlying process of syncope[12,30,31] A report published in 1926[32] suggested that tonsillar enlargement caused tachycardia and syncope. Because syncope did not recur following tonsillectomy, tonsillectomy was assumed to prevent recurrent syncope. While this assumption is ludicrous, it is important to recognize the similarity of modern thinking on this topic.

Even without treatment, syncope can remain dormant for a protracted period or the patient can "respond" to the apparent effect of the evaluation itself. However, the goal of therapy, to reduce the frequency and severity of episodes, is achievable,. It appears that syncope is less likely to recur when its cause is diagnosed properly and treated effectively.[33–35]

The Differential Diagnosis

With so many potential causes of syncope, it is difficult, if not impossible, to provide a complete list of all common and uncommon causes (see Tables 1 and 2). New and creative ways to pass out are always developing[36] and syncope has its fads[37–40] (eg, "the mess trick": Valsalva during hyperventilation; this rarely causes syncope, but now mass fainting at rock concerts is possible). An older, retrospective study, reported by Wayne,[37] representing one of the largest collections of patients with syncope, still provides important insight into the most common causes of syncope. Between 1945 and 1957, from a total cohort of approximately 1000 syncope patients, data on 510 patients were evaluated.[37] The remaining patient charts were "unsatisfactory for analysis." In contrast to more recent data, a cause of syncope was diagnosed in nearly all (96%) of Wayne's patients (Figure 1).

___ **Table 1** _____

Common Causes of Syncope

Cardiovascular Disease	Noncardiovascular Disease	Other

Arrhythmic
  AV block with bradycardia
  Sinus pauses/bradycardia
  Ventricular tachycardia and
    structural heart disease
	Reflex mechanisms
	  Vasodepressor
	    "neurocardiogenic"
	  Micturition
	  Deglutition
		Syncope of unknown
		  origin
		  About 50% of all
		  syncope patients

Nonarrhythmic-hemodynamic
  Hypertrophic
    cardiomyopathy
  Aortic stenosis
	Orthostatic hypotension
	  Dysautonomia
	  Fluid depletion
	  Illness, bed rest
	  Drugs
		Undiagnosed
		  seizures
		
		Improperly diagnosed
		  syncope
		  confusional
		  states due to
		  hypoglycemia,

	Psychogenic
	  Hysterical
	  Panic disorder
	  Anxiety disorder
		stroke, etc.
		
		Drug-induced
		  Alcohol
		  Illicit drugs
		  Prescribed drugs
		    (esp. the elderly)

AV = atrioventricular.

_____ **Table 2** _____

Uncommon Causes of Syncope

Cardiovascular Disease	Noncardiovascular Disease

Arrhythmic etiology
  Supraventricular tachycardia
  The long QT interval syndrome
  Idiopathic ventricular tachycardia
  Myocardial infarction (and bradycardia/
    tachycardia)
	Reflexes
	  Post-tussive
	  Defecation
	  Glossopharyngeal
	  Postprandial
	  Carotid sinus hypersensitivity

Nonarrhythmic etiology
  Pulmonary embolus
  Pulmonary hypertension
  Dissecting aortic aneurysm
  Subclavian steal
  Atrial myxoma
  Cardiac tamponade
	Hyperventilation
	
	Migraine
	
	Carcinoid syndrome
	
	Systemic mastocytosis
	
	Metabolic
	  Hypoglycemia
	  Hypoxia
	
	Multivessel cerebrovascular disease

BREAKDOWN OF VARIOUS CAUSES OF SYNCOPE SEEN
IN 510 PATIENTS

Cause	No.
Vasovagal	298
Orthostatic hypotension	28
Epilepsy	26
Cerebral vascular disease	24
Unknown etiology	23
Postmicturition	17
Adams-Stokes syndrome	17
Hyperventilation	15
Hypersensitive carotid sinus	15
Tussive	13
Aortic stenosis	9
Paroxysmal tachycardia	8
Angina pectoris	4
Hysteria	4
Myocardial infarction	3
Pulmonary hypertension	2
Migraine	2
Hypertensive encephalopathy	2
Total	**510**

Wayne, 1961

Figure 1. Wayne's analysis of causes of syncope in 510 patients.

Common Causes of Syncope

Neurocardiogenic (Vasovagal) Syncope

A vasovagal episode was the most common cause of syncope in Wayne's study.[37] Vasovagal (neurocardiogenic) mechanisms account for or contribute to (in the presence of other clinical conditions) 50% to 80% of all syncopal episodes.[2,8,9,11,26,28,29,41,42,B] Neurocardiogenic syncope can be due to or provoked by several inciting, often noxious, stimuli. The specific stimulus can be difficult to characterize and may be highly individualized. Emotional stresses (danger, real or perceived, fear, or anxiety) are common triggers.[2] The responsible reflex that causes syncope can be "normal" and self limited. For example, vasovagal (neurocardiogenic) reflex can occur with severe volume loss due to diarrhea, and may never recur. Complete evaluation and long-term drug therapy is indicated only when episodes recur frequently and cannot be explained by a precipitating cause (see Chapters 3 and 4). Sometimes it is difficult to discover an initiating factor responsible for the complex vasovagal reflex, so the diagnosis is not clear. This may explain, in part, the wide variation in the diagnosis of vasovagal syncope between reports.

While generally benign, "a syndrome of 'malignant' vasovagal syncope" describes frequent and recurrent episodes without obvious prodrome and without apparent stimuli.[43] Testing the response to orthostatic stress (tilt table testing) can secure the diagnosis for individuals who have this symptom[44] (see Chapters 3 and 4). A more malignant and poorly understood vasovagal reflex may also cause death by asystole in some patients with severely impaired left ventricular function.[45]

Orthostatic Hypotension

The second most common cause of syncope in Wayne's study[37] was orthostatic hypotension (see Figure 1). This problem is often overlooked, underdiagnosed, and incompletely evaluated. Orthostatic hypotension[46-49,B] has many etiologies (see Chapter 4) but is generally due to a dysautonomic syndrome, drugs, volume depletion (eg, blood loss), or a combination of factors which, alone, would have no effect.

Peripheral autonomic denervation can be due to systemic diseases including diabetes and amyloidosis.[46] Specific disease states that can cause this condition include Addison's disease, porphyria, tabes dorsalis, syringomyelia, spinal cord transection, Guillian Barré syndrome, Riley- Day syndrome, surgically induced sympathectomy, pheochromocytoma, Bradbury-Eggleston syndrome,[50] and the Shy-Drager syndrome. Elderly patients frequently have difficulty with effective autoregulation of peripheral and cerebral blood flow and are highly susceptible to symptomatic orthostatic hypotension[23,49,51-56] The elderly tend to have slower heart rates at baseline.[54,57] Details on orthostatic hypotension are discussed in Chapters 4 and 8.

Medications can cause syncope by a variety of mechanisms, commonly including orthostatic hypotension.b Nearly 13% of syncopal and presyncopal spells in patients who presented to an ambulatory clinic were due to an adverse drug reaction.[58] Vasodilators (hydralazine, nitrates, angiotensin converting enzyme (ACE) inhibitors), α_1- and ß-adrenergic blockers and α_2-adrenergic stimulants, diuretics, tricyclic antidepressants and phenothiazines, and others can cause orthostatic hypotension.[58] Nitrates can also trigger an orthostatic hypotensive reaction due to a vagal or other autonomic response.[59,60] Nonsteroidal anti-inflammatory drugs may decrease peripheral vascular resistance and its response to orthostatic stress.[58,61] Hypokalemia can impair reactivity of vascular smooth muscle and limit increase in peripheral vascular resistance.

Orthostatic hypotension is commonly caused by volume depletion from blood loss or from use of diuretics.[56,B] Prolonged bed rest or chronic illness can provoke transient orthostatic hypotension in vulnerable patients such as the elderly or those with diabetes. Even normal individuals at prolonged bed rest, especially if volume depleted, may pass out abruptly on rising. Rarely, inherent circulating vasodilators present in carcinoid syndrome or in systemic mastocytosis can cause orthostatic hypotension.

The response to changes in position can be immediate or delayed. As part of the physical examination, orthostatic signs should always be obtained, but change in blood pressure from fluid depletion may be seen soon after standing, or for dysautonomic conditions, it may require several minutes of standing. An orthostatic change (lowering) in blood pressure, without a compensatory change (increase) in heart rate, suggests an autonomic neuropathy.

Arrhythmic Causes

Surprisingly, paroxysmal tachycardia and Stokes-Adams attacks were suspected as cause of syncope in only a few of Wayne's[37] patients (Figure1). Cardiac rhythm disturbances, bradycardias, and tachycardias, are now known to commonly cause syncope.[34] The arrhythmias can be benign (not associated with death) or malignant (associated with increased risk for death). In Wayne's report, techniques to detect cardiac arrhythmias were lacking.[37] Now, with more sophisticated diagnostic tools (prolonged monitoring techniques and electrophysiological tests), a primary arrhythmic etiology can be more easily identified. Common rhythm disturbances associated with syncope include: prolonged paroxysms of ventricular tachycardia, AV block associated with bradycardia, and marked sinus bradycardia ("sick sinus syndrome" and "tachy- brady syndrome").

Organic heart disease, especially in association with impaired left ventricular function, a bundle branch block, a long QT interval, or preexcitation (Wolff-Parkinson-White syndrome), should raise suspicions of an arrhythmic etiology for syncope. Arrhythmic syncope due to AV block (generally second- or third-degree) or ventricular tachycardia tends to have an abrupt onset with no prodrome ("Stokes-Adams attack," not specific for arrhythmic etiology for syncope), may have a malignant course (associated with cardiac arrest), and may be distinguishable from neurocardiogenic syncope.[62]

Supraventricular tachycardia (AV nodal reentry or AV reciprocating tachycardia), while generally benign, can occasionally cause syncope, but there is usually a history of palpitations or tachycardia.[63] Up to 15% of patients with supraventricular tachycardia will have syncope or near syncope due to the tachycardia.[64]

Atrial fibrillation rarely causes syncope unless the ventricular rate is excessively fast or slow. Slow rates tend to occur in the elderly due to autonomic changes[52-55,57] or AV nodal dysfunction, whereas fast rates can occur in younger patients with Wolff-Parkinson-White syndrome or with enhanced AV nodal conduction.[65]

There are special subgroups of arrhythmias that are important to consider. Short paroxysms of asymptomatic nonsustained ventricular tachycardia are problematic, and while sometimes ascribed to be the cause of syncope,[10] the two may be unrelated. Sinus arrest can cause syncope. While generally due to intrinsic sinus node disease (causing sick sinus syndrome or tachy-brady syndrome), it can be difficult to distinguish intrinsic sinus node disease from accentuated vagal tone. Ventricular bigeminy can be associated with hypotension and a slow pulse, but almost never with syncope. Ventricular pacing may cause dizziness and weakness, but it rarely causes loss of consciousness.[66] However, patients with pacemakers may have syncope from abrupt pacemaker failure or other unrelated causes, including malignant neurocardiogenic syncope.[66-68] Another special subgroup consists of patients who have implanted defibrillators. When a patient with an implanted cardioverter defibrillator (ICD) passes out, a recurrent ventricular arrhythmia must be suspected. Careful assessment of the functioning of the ICD is required.

Physiologically, tachycardias are less well-tolerated, hemodynamically, than bradycardias, whether or not AV synchrony is present. The abrupt onset of the arrhythmia can cause syncope.[69,70] Ventricular tachycardia is usually less well-tolerated than supraventricular tachycardia, even at the same heart rate, but hemodynamics worsen with increasing rate.[71] Syncope, however, is most directly related to an abrupt change in heart rate due to lack of effective reflex peripheral vascular vasoconstriction and presumably ineffective accommodation of cerebral blood flow.[32,69] For example, chronic sinus bradycardia is much less of a problem than is sinus rhythm with abrupt sinus arrest. Persistent atrial flutter or ventricular tachycardia is less likely to cause syncope than is a paroxysm of the same tachycardia, even at the same rate. It is common for the blood pressure to drop at the onset of tachycardia, causing syncope, but over several seconds, the blood pressure can rise and syncope can resolve, despite continuation of tachycardia,[72–74] due to reflex vasoconstriction and elevation in catecholamine levels. Ventricular function, body position and medications all influence the hemodynamic response to and presence of changes in heart rate, and the presence and length of syncope.[75] The presence of sustained ventricular tachycardia alone does not always explain syncope because it does not always cause syncope. In one series, only 15% of patients who presented to an emergency room with sustained ventricular tachycardia had syncope associated with tachycardia.[76]

An arrhythmia that is present at the time of syncope may be a secondary or unrelated phenomenon, and may not be explanatory. Treatment of the arrhythmia would therefore not treat syncope effectively. An example is a patient with a vasovagal spell who develops a "relative" bradycardia after hypotension and after syncope had started. Treating the bradycardia (with a pacemaker) would not be suspected to correct a primary peripheral hemodynamic or central nervous system problem, but each case must be considered individually.[77] In neurocardiogenic syncope, when bradycardia is a secondary issue, it is not surprising that its treatment may not help stop syncope recurrence.

> CASE: A 50 year-old avid bicyclist has recurrent syncope at rest (after exercise) with associated AV block and >8-second pauses, but the sinus rate does not slow. Carotid sinus massage is negative. A tilt table test is positive for hypotension and relative. On the treadmill, his heart rate exceeds 180 beats/minute. He refuses to stop exercising. The cause of his AV block is unclear, but may have been autonomically mediated. *Therapy:* A permanent dual-chamber pacemaker is placed, resulting in complete ending of symptoms.

> CASE: A 45 year-old woman has recurrent syncope and on a Holter monitor has 8-second pauses due to sinus arrest. A permanent pacemaker is placed, but she continues to pass out. A tilt table test is subsequently positive for hypotension and syncope despite pacing.

Seizures

Wayne[37] and others[78–81] noted that seizures can be mistaken for syncope. Generally, it is not difficult to distinguish seizures from syncope.[1A] When there is confusion, it is most likely that neurocardiogenic syncope is confused with seizures ("convulsive syncope"). A possible exception to this rule is akinetic seizures. These episodes are manifest by abrupt loss of consciousness and drop to the ground. They may be so violent that the patient appears to be thrown to the ground. As opposed to generalized seizures, at the end of an episode of akinetic seizures, the patient appears normal and has no postictal drowsiness. Although these seizures themselves are quite brief, their sudden and unpredictable nature may lead to injury. Myoclonic jerks may precede the attacks and the episodes tend to occur while going to sleep at night or on awakening in the morning. This type of seizure is most common in the 2 to 5 year pediatric age range, but older cases have been observed. The electroencephalogram is usually markedly abnormal, demonstrating either generalized or multifocal epileptiform discharges. This form of seizure is exceedingly difficult to treat. The usual antiseizure medications are often ineffective, although some patients may respond to valproic acid or a benzodiazepine. Some authors recommend section of the corpus callosum in patients with medically intractable seizures that result in repeated injury (this is controversial). Some patients have responded to a medium chain triglyceride (MCT 3 variant) of the ketogenic diet.

The incidence of seizure diagnoses as cause of syncope varies widely between reports.[8,11] Hofnagels[80] notes that only 31% of physicians caring for patients with "spells" could agree upon whether or not seizure was the cause. The distinction can be especially difficult if seizures are atypical or episodes are unwitnessed. This problem is compounded by the lack of sensitivity and specificity of the electroencephalogram as it is generally performed. An electroencephalogram by itself cannot be relied upon to diagnose a seizure disorder. Up to 50% of patients who have a seizure focus will have a negative electroencephalogram unless sleep deprivation is used or unless nasopharyngeal leads or deep brain stem leads are placed (See Chapter 8).[79,82-85] Also, up to 40% of asymptomatic elderly individuals will have asymptomatic electroencephalographic abnormalities. Seizures are likely to account for 10% to 15% of apparent syncopal episodes.[11,37] Patients with seizures rarely, however, have episodes with sudden onset and abrupt, rapid recovery. Instead, the postictal state is slow and lingering. The tilt table test may be useful to distinguish seizure from syncope.[78]

Alternatively, syncope with loss of cerebral blood flow can cause tonic-clonic movements and can mimic a seizure.[86] This apparent seizure activity is associated with slowing of the brain waves, not with epileptiform spikes on the electroencephalogram.

Micturition Syncope and Syncope Due to Other Autonomic Causes

Micturition syncope is one of several variations of autonomically mediated syncope, which include: deglutition syncope, carotid sinus hypersensitivity, post-tussive syncope, defecation syncope, and trumpet player's syncope.[16,26,37] The mechanism for this form of syncope is discussed elsewhere (see Chapters 8 and 12), but all, probably at least in part, are related to abrupt change in autonomic tone, intravascular volume, and changes in cerebrospinal fluid pressure. Micturition syncope, specifically, is due to an abrupt change in position combined with a strong vagal stimulus. Micturition syncope can occur in either sex. In contrast to previous studies suggesting a clear male predominance, Kapoor[87] reports that women have a higher incidence of syncope due to evening micturition.

While the exact mechanisms for these entities may not be identical, the autonomic nervous system appears critically involved in the initiation of the episode. Generally, all causes of syncope appear to involve a poorly tolerated hemodynamic response to specific autonomic cardiovascular reflexes. Autonomic reflexes are often critical in the initiation and termination of syncope, or else the presence of the preexisting problems would allow patients to lose consciousness continuously.

> CASE: A 52-year-old man with reactive airways disease and chronic aspiration due to gastroesophageal reflux has recurrent syncope after prolonged episodes of coughing. Syncope resolves after effective therapy for his pulmonary problems. *Diagnosis:* Post-tussive syncope.

> CASE: A 58-year-old man becomes asystolic during abdominal surgery during peritoneal manipulation. He gives a history of syncope when he drinks cold liquids and is noted to become asystolic (AV block and sinus arrest are both noted on different occasions) while drinking ice- water. Carotid massage causes seven seconds of symptomatic asystole. Temporary ventricular pacing during carotid massage is associated with hypotension but with dual chamber pacing, the blood pressure remains above 100 mm Hg systolic. *Diagnosis:* Deglutition syncope. *Therapy:* With permanent pacing, he remains asymptomatic for 7 years.

> CASE An 85-year-old man with history of coronary artery disease and history of benign prostatic hypertrophy has taken furosemide, digoxin, and captopril for mild congestive heart failure. He passes out suddenly when awakening to urinate. There is a 15 mm Hg drop in blood pressure with standing. *Diagnosis:* Micturition syncope. *Therapy:* Patient is warned to arise slowly before urinating in the evening and to sit when urinating.

Uncommon, but Important, Causes of Syncope

Cerebrovascular Disease

Cerebrovascular disease is an uncommon and probably overdiagnosed cause of syncope. Stroke and transient ischemic attacks tend to cause focal neurological deficits from which recovery is slow and incomplete. If posterior cerebral circulation is impaired, symptoms such as nausea or dizziness are more likely to occur than transient loss of consciousness. If the anterior circulation is impaired, a focal neurological defect will occur. Severe obstructive multivessel cerebrovascular disease can cause syncope but other neurological findings will likely occur first and will likely persist after syncope.

Myocardial Ischemia and Myocardial Infarction

Syncope is often suspected to be due myocardial infarction or ischemia, thus resulting in hospital admission to "rule out" myocardial infarction and assess ischemia. This process is usually unnecessary and unwarranted because myocardial infarction rarely causes syncope. Few patients in Wayne's report[37] had syncope due to a myocardial infarction. If myocardial infarction or ischemia is the cause of syncope, there are generally obvious clues from the patient's history and from the electrocardiogram. One potential cause of syncope is bradycardia and hypotension from the Bezold-Jarisch reflex, but other arrhythmic and nonarrhythmic causes are possible.[88]

Other Cardiac Causes of Syncope

Obstructive valvular lesions such as aortic stenosis and hypertrophic cardiomyopathy are well-recognized but relatively rare causes of syncope.[8,11,89-91] Other obstructive valvular lesions such as atrial myxoma and atrial ball valve thrombus are even rarer. Obstructive lesions such as aortic stenosis tend to cause an exaggerated and malignant form of an exercise-induced vasovagal response, leading to syncope and perhaps even death.[92] Other forms of syncope can be confused with obstructive hemodynamic problems.[93] The obstruction itself may not be the direct cause of collapse. When aortic stenosis causes syncope, the episodes tend to be markedly prolonged.

Metabolic Causes (see Chapter 12)

Syncope, characterized by abrupt onset and complete, brisk recovery, is rarely due to a toxic or metabolic cause. Hypoglycemia, hypoxia, meningitis, encephalitis, and sepsis can cause coma, stupor, and confusion, but rarely syncope.[94] Hypoxia can, however, influence vascular tone.[95] If a patient does not recall the history surrounding the event or if the event was unwitnessed, coma and syncope can be hard to distinguish. Neurally mediated (neurocardiogenic) syncope can mimic transient ischemic attacks.[96]

Neurological and Psychiatric Causes

There are several neurological and psychiatric causes of syncope that are discussed in detail in Chapters 8 and 9.[97,98]

> CASE: A 32-year-old woman is referred for a tilt table test for recurrent episodes of loss of consciousness associated with a prodrome of nausea and vomiting. Upon further questioning, the patient describes quadriparesis with near blindness after the episode while awake. *Diagnosis:* Migraine headaches.

Syncope of Unknown Etiology (SUO)

In Wayne's[37] original analysis, hardly any patients had syncope of unknown etiology. In contrast, most contemporary data would indicate that in nearly 50% of patients presenting with syncope (even evaluated by a meticulous history, physical examination, and proper diagnostic testing), no cause will be found, making this a critically important and large patient subgroup.[8-11] The marked discrepancy between different studies relates partly to the level of certainty tolerated for a diagnosis. Perhaps a low degree of accuracy was tolerated in Wayne's retrospective study. Differences may also result from selection bias relating to patient inclusion and exclusion and the physician's assumptions made in diagnosing the causes of syncope.

Thus, the assumed cause of syncope is often based on flawed methods and incorrect assumptions. It may only be possible to know the definite cause of syncope if the episode is witnessed with an electrocardiogram, arterial line, oximeter, and electroencephalogram attached to the patient. Even then, the causal mechanism may not be clear. Therefore, even in the best of circumstances, the diagnosis of syncope is often a leap of faith.

Various definitions for syncope of unknown origin exist, but perhaps the best accepted definition is: syncope without an apparent cause, despite a meticulous history and physical examination and monitoring but no involved diagnostic testing. In reality, *all* patients have syncope of unknown origin—even if testing shows possible causes—as long as the relationship between the abnormality and the episode is not proven. Because almost all diagnoses are presumptive, syncope of unknown etiology has been used to describe different types of patients. This is important when considering diagnostic evaluation and assessment of the prognosis of these patients. Those who undergo electrophysiological testing for syncope, for example, do not have a cause diagnosed, although an arrhythmic cause of syncope is usually suspected. If the test shows induced ventricular tachycardia, did ventricular tachycardia cause syncope or is the cause still unknown? If there are episodes of asymptomatic nonsustained ventricular tachycardia on Holter monitor, is this enough evidence to conclude that it caused syncope? Some investigators think so.[10] If all testing is unrevealing and the patient has no obvious underlying disease, it is likely that syncope under these circumstances is due to a neurocardiogenic or dysautonomic origin.

CASE: A 45-year-old woman develops abdominal pain and severe nausea and vomiting. She develops gross hematemasis and passes out at home. The paramedics are called. *Presumed Diagnosis:* Gastrointestinal bleed or vagal-induced bradycardia/hypotension. *Actual Diagnosis:* In the ambulance she is noted to have long runs of hemodynamically intolerable wide QRS complex tachycardia, causing recurrent syncope.

Classification

Based on a long differential diagnostic list of potential causes, it has become fashionable to subclassify the etiology of syncope into three broad categories: cardiovascular, noncardiovascular, and unknown.[8,10,11,91] Several contemporary reports lend support to this approach. Of patients who are admitted to hospitals or are seen in emergency rooms, a cardiovascular cause of syncope will be found in about 30%.[8,10,11] About 50% of patients with suspected cardiovascular disease will be diagnosed with an arrhythmia, although perhaps not as the cause of syncope.[10] There is a high sudden and total death rate, despite therapy, for patients with underlying cardiovascular disease, even if the presumed problem responsible is corrected.[10] The 5-year mortality in patients with syncope and a diagnosed cardiovascular cause approaches 50%, with a 30% incidence of death in the first year.[9,10] When a cardiovascular cause is diagnosed, treatment, including specific treatments of hemodynamically unstable and life- threatening arrhythmias, can improve the long-term outcome. Perhaps the treatment that prevents death also prevents recurrent syncope. This becomes difficult to determine, because in comparative trials, the recurrence rate of syncope is similar whether or not a cardiovascular cause is present and treated.[30]

A noncardiovascular cause will be found in 20% to 30% of patients.[9,10] Such causes include: neurological causes (see Chapter 8), vasodepressor syncope (see Chapter 3), and orthostatic hypotension (see Chapter 4). Although the mortality in patients with noncardiovascular causes of syncope is better, (>10% in 1 year, and 30% over a 5-year period), this type of syncope nonetheless represents a substantial risk to the welfare of the patient.[8,9]

In nearly half of the syncope patients, a cause is suspected but not diagnosed despite a complete but prudent evaluation.[9,10] These patients (with syncope of unknown origin) generally have a benign course, with a low (6% to <10%) 3-year risk and a modest (24%) 5-year risk of death[9,10] at one center, but it not all agree that syncope of unknown origin has such a benign prognosis.[99]

It appears to be helpful to consider the simple subclassification of syncope into one of three main causes: cardiovascular, noncardiovascular or of unknown origin. The advantage for patient categorization is that it allows clinical assessment of the prognostic meaning of syncope. Classification by patient age may also be helpful (Table 3). The elderly are at highest risk for death, with a 2-year mortality of 27% compared to 8% in the younger age group; but the presence of syncope has not been shown to influence mortality independently in the elderly.[23–25]

There are, nevertheless, several caveats concerning these classifications. The noncardiovascular group is not really all noncardiovascular. Vasodepressor syncope, often considered a noncardiovascular cause, is actu-

_____ **Table 3** _____

Common Causes of Syncope

Young (<35 years)	Middle-Aged (35–65 years)	Elderly (>65 years)
Neurocardiogenic	Neurocardiogenic	Multifactorial
Situational	Cardiac	Cardiac
Psychiatric	Arrhythmic	Mechanical/obstructive
(Undiagnosed seizures)	Mechanical/	Arrhythmic
(Long QT syndrome)	obstructive	Orthostatic hypotension
(WPW syndrome, other SVT)		Drug-induced
(Hypertrophy cardiomyopathy)		Neurally mediated
		(Neurocardiogenic)

( ) indicates less common, but important-potentially life threatening; WPW = Wolff-Parkinson-White; SVT = supraventricular tachycardia.

ally a cardiovascular reflex that could just as well be considered a cardiovascular cause of syncope. If this entity was considered a cardiovascular cause of syncope, the prognostic categorization would lose its meaning because most episodes of vasovagal syncope have benign prognoses. Pulmonary emboli and dissecting aortic aneurysm, often considered cardiovascular causes, can actually be considered noncardiac. If these were considered noncardiovascular, the prognostic value of this subclassification would change.[100]

Syncope is not always related to the cause of death. Syncope patients with dissecting aortic aneurysm, aortic stenosis, ventricular tachycardia, or pulmonary emboli have a high risk of dying even if syncope is not present. Also, syncope is not clearly an *independent* predictor of death.[A] It is not surprising that syncope patients with cardiovascular disease have a higher mortality than syncope patients without cardiovascular disease. The subgroups cardiovascular and noncardiovascular are not comparable by age of the patient, underlying disease, or prognosis otherwise. The long-term prognosis may be related more to the underlying cardiac disease than to syncope. To evaluate this further, Silverstein[101] stratified patients with and without syncope who were admitted to an intensive care unit. He found that the prognosis is independent of syncope, but depends on the severity of the underlying disease. Similarly, the Framingham study[22] does not indicate that patients with cardiovascular disease and with syncope are any more likely to die than are those with cardiovascular disease without syncope. Others have found similar results.[A] Even when the cause of syncope is found and treated in patients with cardiovascular disease, the mortality remains higher than in patients without known cardiovascular disease.[9,10]

Patients admitted to hospitals, especially if cardiovascular disease is diagnosed, tend to be sicker and older and tend to have a higher mortality independent of syncope or its cause. Syncope does not place an extremely elderly (or even young) patient at specifically higher risk for death than other individuals the same age.[24,25,53] Syncope is probably not a prognostic indicator for patients with the Wolff-Parkinson-White syndrome[102,103] or with hypertrophic cardiomyopathy,[104] even in younger patients.

Syncope with an arrhythmic or hemodynamic cardiac cause, however, can be associated with a high mortality. It is an especially important prognostic indicator if impaired left ventricular function, ventricular ectopy, and induced ventricular tachycardia at electrophysiological testing are all present.[12,28,33-35,105-114] Such patients have prognoses as poor as those who have had a cardiac arrest or sustained ventricular tachycardia.[115] Other examples of syncope with an arrhythmic or hemodynamic cause include syncope associated with the hereditary long QT interval syndrome (see Chapter 6), aortic stenosis, or an atrial myxoma. Treatment of these conditions can improve prognosis and prevent syncope recurrence. Similarly, repair of an aortic valve for aortic stenosis or removal of an atrial tumor will improve long-term prognosis and *may* treat the cause of syncope.[116] Treatment can alter mortality and syncope recurrence but this is disease-dependant. For example, an ICD may prevent cardiac arrest in a patient with the congenital long QT interval syndrome but not prevent syncope, while repair of an aortic valve may prevent syncope but still be associated with a significant cardiovascular mortality.

Recently, Middlekauff[117,118] and Tchou[119] found syncope to be an important prognostic predictor for a specific patient subgroup: those with impaired left ventricular function. In patients with advanced heart failure and syncope, the 1-year mortality is 45% compared to 12% in patients without syncope.[117,118] Patients with idiopathic dilated cardiomyopathy have a 56% 4-year mortality in contrast to a 4% 4-year mortality in patients with dilated cardiomyopathy who do not have syncope.[119] Using electrophysiological testing, several investigators have shown in separate studies that the survival rate in patients with induced ventricular tachycardia is improved if the tachycardia is treated properly.[34,35,115] Another report using electrophysiological testing showed that there is a 5% recurrence rate of syncope for treated patients versus 24% recurrence rate of syncope untreated.[33]

Martin et al[C] recently showed that risk straticication of syncope patients based on clinical variables is possible. Based on their study of 252 patients who presented to the emergency room with syncope, four clinical variables — abnormal ECG, history of ventricular arrhythmias, history of congestive heart failure, and age over 45 — predicted clinically important arryhthmias. There was a 37% 1-year mortality rate for patients with 3 of 4 clinical variables present compared to a 2% 1-year mortality rate for patients with none of the risk factors present.

The prognostic impact of syncope is clearly disease-specific, but prompt aggressive treatment of syncope patients with malignant ventricular arrhythmias is required and can be lifesaving. For other conditions, including various cardiovascular etiologies, the cause of death and syncope are not clearly directly linked. In this regard, categorization into cardiovascular, noncardiovascular, and unknown etiologies, while potentially useful, represents an oversimplification of an extraordinarily complex issue.

Initial Approach to the Patient with Syncope

The proper diagnostic and therapeutic approach requires careful analysis of the patient's symptoms and of the clinical findings. No specific battery of tests is ever indicated or is always useful. Extensive diagnostic evaluation is generally unnecessary, expensive, and risky. Repeated evaluation and hospital admission after an initial complete negative assessment is often unrewarding.

Since it is clearly impractical to wait to monitor all episodes of syncope in order to arrive at a diagnosis, with the present technology (although advances in technology are coming[120]; see Chapter 16), clinicians must base their decisions on historical features with the presumption that the description of the episode is accurate, complete, and based on common sense.[9,11,14,16,37,89,90,121-123] Diagnostic evaluation must be guided from the patient's history. The proper evaluation requires a balance of the judicious use of inpatient and outpatient diagnostic modalities. The expense and risk of the procedures and of hospitalization are intensified by the possibility of iatrogenic harm caused by diagnostic or therapeutic misadventures.

The location of the evaluation is important. In the emergency room, immediate decisions must be made especially concerning admission. For the hospitalized patient, diagnostic and therapeutic decisions concerning types of testing must be made early, and if necessary, further evaluation can be planned with the the goal of prompt discharge. Surprisingly few patients admitted with syncope without some kind of plan before admission will benefit from hospitalization. Arguably, patients admitted are their own subgroup and have a different, perhaps higher, risk for death. The outpatient with a vague or distant history of syncope can be evaluated more leisurely in contrast to the patient hospitalized in the intensive care unit with impaired left ventricular function. For each circumstance, the cause of and prognosis of syncope will differ. The approach to diagnosis and therapy will differ concomitantly.

Various clinical algorithms have been developed, but due to the diverse nature of syncope, it becomes impossible to implement an evaluation

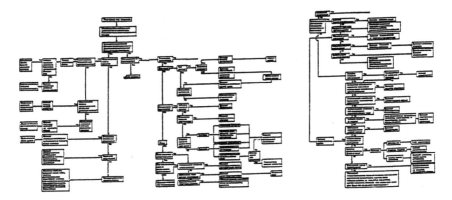

Figure 2. One algorithm for management of syncope. This may confuse more than help.

stratagem that will succeed in all circumstances and for all patients. Indeed, algorithms can confuse more than clarify (Figure 2).

The History

To evaluate syncope, sound clinical decisions are based on a carefully performed history with extreme attention to detail. The history, with its proper interpretation and a directed physical examination, is the only appropriate way to guide further diagnostic evaluation. The history and physical alone can be diagnostic in 25%-35% of patients[8,9,11,14,101,123] (Table 4). Of those for whom a cause is found, the history and physical alone are sufficient in 75%-85% of patients.[8] Symptoms and several historical features, summarized in Tables 5 and 6, can help direct further diagnostic procedures. Specific attention should be directed toward: 1) characteristic and length of the episode, 2) patient and witnessed accounts, 3) patient age, 4) concomitant (especially cardiac) disease, 5) associated temporally related symptoms (eg, neurological symptoms, angina, palpitations, and heart failure), 6) premonitory (prodromal) symptoms, 7) symptoms on awakening (postsyncope symptoms), 8) the circumstances, situations surrounding the episode, 9) exercise, body position, posture, and emotional state, 10) number, frequency, and timing of previous syncopal episodes, 11) medications, and 12) family history. As part of the initial assessment, early determination of the presence of heart disease is especially crucial because these patients are at highest risk for death.

Consider characteristics of the event itself, the patient, and the length of the episodes. One reason for discrepant outcomes for syncope patients relates to the nature of the episodes. Contrast an elderly man who has a

_____ **Table 4** _____

Evaluation of Syncope
How Often is the Cause Found by History and Physical?

	Patient Type	Patient Number	Diagnosis "Found"	History and Physical Helped
Kapoor	Admitted (SUO)	121	13	—
Day	ER	198	173	147
Silverstein	MICU	108	57	42
Kapoor	All comers	204	107	52
Eagle	Admitted	100	61	52
Martin	ER	170	106	90

SUO = syncope of unknown origin; ER = emergency room; MICU = medical intensive care unit.
History and Physical will provide clues to the diagnosis in 30%–75% of patients. Diagnosis based on history and physical may be (and often is) inaccurate. (Modified from Kapoor, American Journal of Cardiology, 1989).

series of syncopal attacks spaced by short episodes of recovery with a young woman with multiple episodes spaced over several years. Based on this information alone, the woman likely has neurocardiogenic syncope and the man has an arrhythmic or orthostatic cause. A patient who is witnessed collapsing and then noted to be pulseless and apneic and appears to require cardiopulmonary resuscitation is probably at higher risk for a malignant arrhythmia or a cardiac cause of syncope.

The patient may not remember events surrounding the episode, may have retrograde amnesia, or may be otherwise incapable of providing an adequate history.[124,125] Witnessed accounts, therefore, are of major importance, but while they are often heavily relied upon, they may be inaccurate. The pulse that appears to be absent may not have been properly taken (there are also several reasons why a patient may be—or may appear to be—pulseless). Inherent biases are always possible.

Try to define the episodes as completely as possible. The patient may remember very little of the episode, deny it, or remember it inaccurately. Always suspect that aspects of the history reported by the patient or by witnesses are incomplete or misinterpreted due to the startling nature of the symptom. Paramedics may ignore witnessed accounts and misinterpret the responses of an individual who appears healthy and alert and is talking by the time they arrive. The importance of a serious problem can be under- or overestimated.

Consider events that trigger the episodes. Emotions can trigger syncope by a variety of mechanisms,[2,126] but an emotional trigger raises the suspicion

_____ **Table 5** _____

History

Symptoms Related to Syncopal Spell

Symptom	Probable Cause
Nausea, diaphoresis, fear	Neurocardiogenic
Aura	Seizure
Palpitations	Tachycardia (nonspecific finding)
Exercise-related	Ventricular or supraventricular tachycardia, hypotension/bradycardia
Posture-related	Orthostatic hypotension, volume depletion, dysautonomia
Urination, defecation, eating, coughing	Vagal-induced hypotension, bradycardia
Diarrhea, vomiting	Hypovolemia, hypokalemic-induced arrhythmia, vagal-induced hypotension, bradycardia
Melena	Gastrointestinal bleed
Visual change, neurological abnormality	Stroke (unlikely presentation), seizure, migraine
Headaches	Migraine, intracerebral bleed
Chest pain	Ischemia-induced arrhythmia
Dyspnea	Pulmonary embolus, pneumothorax, hyperventilation (hysteria)
Abdominal pain	Aortic aneurysm, GI bleed, peritonitis acute abdomen, trauma
Back pain	Dissecting aneurysm, trauma
Flushing	Carcinoid syndrome
Prolonged syncope	Aortic stenosis, seizure, neurological or metabolic cause
Slow recovery	Seizure, drug, ethanol intoxication, hypoglycemia, sepsis
Injury	Arrhythmia, cardiac cause, neurocardiogenic
Confusion	Stroke, transient ischemic attack, intoxication, hypoglycemia
Prolonged weakness	Neurocardiogenic syncope
Skin color	Pallor—neurocardiogenic, Blue—cardiac, Red—carbon monoxide

of neurocardiogenic syncope. Chest pain can indicate the presence of ischemic heart disease or coronary vasospasm. An abrupt onset without premonitory symptoms may indicate a cardiac arrhythmia, but triggers can be misleading and in most cases they are nonspecific. Fatigue may be associated with neurocardiogenic syncope.[127]

Consider situations surrounding and preceding syncope. Syncope is often related to the situation in which it occurs. Vasovagal episodes are often provoked by noxious stimuli such as strong emotional outbursts, blood loss,

_____ **Table 6** _____

History
Important Data to Obtain

Witnesses	The entire event from multiple viewpoints
Situation	Was there a "trigger"?
Age elderly (>65)	Multifactorial—rule out heart disease. Consider medications
Age young (<40)	Neurocardiogenic most likely cause
Heart disease	Could indicate a poor long-term prognosis
Family history of sudden death	Increased predisposition for malignant arrhythmia or cardiac cause
Number of episodes	<3–possibly malignant and life-threatening >3–more likely to be benign and a continued problem
Previous evaluation	Obtain results from previous evaluation
Medications	Possible proarrhythmia, bradycardia, hypotension

or pain. Sometimes it is difficult, if not impossible, to discover the initiating factor. Slow recovery from symptoms is common in neurocardiogenic syncope, as it is after a seizure, but it is not common in orthostatic hypotension or after a long sinus pause. Consider that patients may try to explain circumstances such as motor vehicle accidents with syncope, when in fact, they did not pass out.

Consider specific aspects of the history. Upper extremity exercise preceding syncope suggests subclavian steal. Back pain raises the suspicion of a dissecting aortic aneurysm. Shortness of breath, a cardiac or pulmonary cause. Pulmonary emboli can cause syncope, but only with a large embolus. Associated tachypnea, cyanosis, hypotension, and acute right heart failure clarify the diagnosis. Similarly, the presence of angina may indicate the presence of an ischemically mediated arrhythmia.

Assess the relationship to meals, alcohol, and drugs. A large meal can cause peripheral vasodilation and hypotension and syncope by a vagal, or dysautonomic, mechanism.[51] When episodes begin with slow onset and gradual recovery, a toxic or metabolic cause such as hypoglycemia, hyperventilation, alcohol, or drugs (illicit or prescribed) should be considered. Alcohol and illicit drugs can cause syncope by several mechanisms including exacerbation of a supraventricular or ventricular tachyarrhythmia. Alcohol can also trigger syncope by abrupt change in hemodynamics and other mechanisms.[128-134] Alternatively, what might appear to be syncope from alcohol may instead be intoxication.

Consider the relation to exercise, position, posture, and events. If the episode begins after a coughing bout, consider post-tussive syncope. In this case, there is a Valsalva physiology, associated increased intracerebral pressure, and a vagal response. If the episodes occur after awakening to urinate, consider micturition syncope If the episode occurs during athletic competition or immediately at the end of exercise, it may be explained completely as a vasovagal response, but be careful not to ignore a potentially more severe underlying cause.[2,135-139] Even in a young patient, potentially malignant causes such as hypertrophic cardiomyopathy, congenital aortic valve disease, or even exercise-induced idiopathic right ventricular, left ventricular, or bidirectional ventricular tachycardia should be considered.[140,141] Exercise-induced supraventricular tachycardias, atrial flutter, and atrial fibrillation rarely cause syncope, but when they do there is usually a history of palpitations or tachycardia. Seizures are often associated with muscular jerks, incontinence, and tongue biting, and there may be postictal confusion or a preictal aura.

If there is syncope with an abrupt rise from a lying position, consider orthostatic hypotension. Even if there is no evidence on examination, orthostatic hypotension may be a possible cause of syncope if other precipitating contributors are factored in. Orthostatic hypotension should be suspected in the elderly and in diabetics if there is prolonged bed rest, and even when the patient is euvolemic. If the episodes occur after intense exposure to heat, consider heat syncope. If there is paresthesia, lip tingling, and anxiety, consider hyperventilation. If loud noises precede the episode, consider an autonomic mechanism or an arrhythmia due to long QT interval syndrome.[142]

Prodromal symptoms can help secure a diagnosis. Premonitory (prodromal) symptoms including diaphoresis, cold sweat, nausea, anxiety, dizziness, lightheadedness, impending doom, and pallor are common in vasovagal (neurocardiogenic) syncope. Yawning, pallor, nausea, visual blurring, darkening of the vision, sweating, and weakness are also consistent with vagal cause (neurocardiogenic syncope). If the episode is associated with a strong emotional reaction, nausea, diaphoresis, and sense of impeding doom, a neurocardiogenic cause is highly likely. These symptoms may also occur independent of syncope, but be neurocardiogenic in origin. If palpitations precede the episode, suspect an arrhythmic etiology. Unfortunately, palpitations are vague and nonspecific and do not diagnose a specific etiology. Palpitations may be of several types: sustained rapid, irregular, or pounding. Each type may provide some clues regarding a possible arrhythmic cause of syncope. By themselves palpations are unreliable but suggestive for further evaluation. An aura immediately preceding the episodes is consistent with a seizure. If the episode begins during exercise, consider aortic stenosis, hypertrophic cardiomyopathy, or an exercise-induced arrhythmia. If the episode begins after exercise, consider a strong vagal response to exercise.

Symptoms on awakening (postsyncopal symptoms) can be helpful. The recovery phase from the episodes can also provide important diagnostic clues. If there is confusion, headache, or dizziness, consider migraines, seizure, or other neurological cause.

Consider the number and frequency of episodes. The frequency of occurrence of syncope at initial presentation can be used to assess risk. Patients with recurrent episodes are unlikely to have a malignant arrhythmia as the cause, particularly if the episodes are distributed over several months to years. Patients with multiple syncope recurrences are at low risk for cardiac death. These episodes are most likely vasovagal, autonomically mediated, or due to a psychiatric cause (see Chapters 3, 4, and 9). In contrast, patients with isolated (<3) episodes of syncope or with a short history of recurrence are at risk for a cardiac death.[109,143] Even if only one episode is present, it can presage a cardiac arrest. Patients with new onset syncope, even if multiple episodes over a short time period, may have an underlying new cardiovascular cause of syncope that could be a serious premonitory sign.

Consider cardiac history. The most worrisome patient is the one with left ventricular dysfunction and coronary artery disease. If such a patient presents for evaluation for syncope and no other cause is obvious for syncope, immediate admission should be arranged for further inpatient evaluation. However, other forms of cardiac disease not even associated with left ventricular dysfunction can predict a malignant course. This includes patients with right ventricular dysplasia or a prolonged QT interval (congenital or drug-induced). Both may occur in young patients and both may lead to a malignant course.

Pay attention to associated temporally related symptoms. Angina in association with the episode suggests an ischemic etiology. Heart failure may suggest a hemodynamic or arrhythmic cause. A coughing bout suggests a pulmonary cause; jerking of the hand suggests a neurological etiology; melena suggests a gastrointestinal etiology, etc. The symptoms may not be obvious or directly related. This includes fever, causing hypotension by sepsis; constipation, causing straining; and a Valsalva maneuver, leading to hypotension and bradycardia.

Consider medications. Medications, particularly in the elderly, may be contributory to, if not causal for, syncope in a substantial number of patients. Changes in medications preceding syncope should be assessed. Check for antihypertensives, antiarrhythmic drugs, diuretics, and psychotropic drugs in particular. Check for electrolyte (such as potassium) abnormalities. A patient may have torsades de pointes if taking a class IA antiarrhythmic drug, especially if hypokalemia is present. Consider the additive effects of drugs. For example, digoxin and amiodarone may cause bradycardia or lead to digoxin toxicity.

Consider the family history of death or syncope. Syncope patients with a family history of the congenital long QT interval syndrome or right ventricular dysplasia have a higher risk of arrhythmic death, especially if other family members have died of the problem. Patients with hypertrophic cardiomyopathy or the Wolff-Parkinson- White syndrome who have a family history of sudden death related to the same presumed diagnosis also have a high risk of cardiac arrest. There may be a familial history of neurocardiogenic syncope.

As indicated in Table 3, the differential diagnosis for patients with syncope varies with age. While the middle aged (40-65), the elderly (65-80), and the very elderly (over 80) have incremental risk for mortality, the young and pediatric ages are also at risk for specific serious underlying causes. Based on these and other historical findings, the patient can be targeted for further diagnostic evaluation.

Physical Examination

The physical examination can provide important clues to support a diagnosis suspected from the patient's history. Attention should be directed to the vital signs, the cardiovascular examination, and the neurological examination (Table 7).

Obtain the patient's orthostatic vital signs. This includes blood pressure supine, sitting, and standing, initially and after several minutes, with attention to change in the heart rate and symptoms. An abrupt drop in blood pressure with standing, especially with reproduction of symptoms, suggests volume depletion as a potential cause. The heart rate should rise with standing in a volume-depleted patient. In patients with idiopathic orthostatic hypotension, diabetes, amyloidosis, and autonomic insufficiency, the blood pressure can drop over several minutes in the standing position and the heart rate may not change.

The respiratory rate and pattern may indicate a pulmonary cause. Hyperventilation may be present, and may be the cause of syncope.[144,145] Tachypnea may indicate pneumonia, pulmonary embolus, or congestive heart failure.

Carotid sinus massage can give insight into carotid sinus hypersensitivity (see Chapter 11). There are no firm standards for performing the carotid

____ **Table 7** ____

Physical Findings
Key Points

Finding	Implication
Heart rate—slow, fast	Arrhythmic cause for syncope, acute illness, GI bleed
Respiration rate— slow, fast	Hyper/hypoventilation, pneumothorax, heart failure
Carotid massage	Carotid hypersensitivity
Blood pressure	Orthostatic hypotension, drug-induced hypotension, volume depletion
Neck vein distension	Pulmonary embolus, congestive failure, cardiac causes
Skin pallor	Blood loss, neurocardiogenic cause
Carotid bruits	Concomitant heart disease. Unlikely primary cause for syncope
Heart murmur	Obstructive or other cardiac syncope
Left ventricular lift	Heart failure with cardiac syncope
S3 gallop	Heart failure with cardiac syncope
Rash	Anaphylaxis-causing syncope
Abdominal tenderness	Blood loss or hypotensive cause for syncope
Absent or variable pulses	Dissecting aneurysm, subclavian steal
Neurological findings	Seizure, stroke, transient ischemic attack
Stool guaiac	Blood loss

sinus massage and, not surprisingly, the results can therefore be highly variable (see Chapter 11). Even if it is positive (ie, a long sinus pause or prolonged AV block), as it is frequently in the elderly even without symptoms, other causes of syncope should be explored. A carotid massage is an integral part of the physical examination of the syncope patient, but the results cannot be relied upon as to the cause of syncope. It should be considered if there is a suggestive history, such as the onset of symptoms with neck compression from position or shaving.

An evaluation of the pulses can provide insight into the presence of a dissecting aneurysm or subclavian steal. The carotid impulse may reveal evidence for aortic stenosis but a carotid bruit does not provide a direct cause of syncope. It may indicate, however, the presence of other atherosclerotic lesions such as coronary artery disease (cardiac cause of syncope) or subclavian artery occlusion (subclavian steal-related syncope).

The cardiovascular examination is crucial. It may reveal murmurs consistent with hypertrophic cardiomyopathy, aortic stenosis, mitral valve prolapse, tricuspid regurgitation (then consider carcinoid syndrome), or pulmonary hypertension. If the baseline murmur is provoked by Valsalva maneuver, this may indicate that hypertrophic cardiomyopathy is present and is the cause of syncope. Evaluate the presence of S_4 and S_3 gallops, potential indicators of cardiac disease that may be responsible for syncope. An S_3 gallop could indicate the presence of congestive heart failure, but complete evaluation for congestive heart failure should be considered. Evidence for Eisenmenger's syndrome, pulmonic stenosis, prosthetic valve dysfunction, presence of a permanent pacemaker or implantable defibrillator, aortic stenosis, or a tumor plop (atrial myxoma) can provide further clues for the diagnosis of syncope.

The lung examination may reveal congestive heart failure. If CHF is present, suspect a potentially serious cardiac cause of syncope and consider the need for admission to the hospital for further evaluation. While a pulmonary embolus may be missed, a pneumothorax may be found.

An abdominal examination may reveal evidence for a gastrointestinal catastrophe. A vagal response to a ruptured viscous or a gastrointestinal bleed are among some possibilities. The abdominal examination may reveal tenderness consistent with an acute abdomen or an ulcer. The stool guaiac can reveal the presence of a gastrointestinal bleed.

The neurological evaluation may indicate focal or localizing signs or evidence for a systemic neurological proceed such as Parkinson's disease. Assess for evidence of a tremor, unilateral weakness, or visual changes. Changing neurological signs are also important. A new neurological deficit in a patient with syncope should be considered a premonitory sign for a cerebrovascular accident.

The complexion may indicate anemia or shift in blood flow.[146] Pallor occurring transiently during an episode may indicate neurocardiogenic syncope, yet if it persists after awakening, consider blood loss as the cause. Marked bradycardia can also cause a dusky or pale appearance. Bright red pallor may indicate carbon monoxide intoxication. Cyanosis can indicate a cardiopulmonary process such as a right to left shunt with Eisenmenger's physiology.

The physical and the patient's history remain the cornerstones for initial evaluation of syncope. This approach is cost-effective and may help prescribe other necessary (and help avoid unnecessary) diagnostic procedures. Unfortunately, for most patients the physical examination is negative and further evaluation may be needed to help understand the cause of syncope.

Diagnostic Testing

The proper diagnostic approach requires careful analysis of syncope in light of all available clinical findings. Diagnostic tests must be used sparingly. When used properly, they will increase the diagnostic yield compared to the history and physical alone. No specific test is always helpful and no specific battery of tests is ever indicated or always useful. All testing must be tailored to the patient based on the findings of the history and physical examinations and with knowledge of the sensitivity and specificity of each test to identify the cause of syncope. An abnormal test result does not necessarily indicate the cause of syncope and does not necessarily sanction a "wild goose chase." The presence of an abnormal tilt table test or the presence of inducible monomorphic ventricular tachycardia at electrophysiological testing must be interpreted carefully in light of the clinical situation.

Extensive and repeated diagnostic evaluations are generally unrewarding, expensive, painful, and possibly risky. Repeat evaluations in the hospital are discouraged unless new clues are uncovered. If the patient is evaluated for syncope but no cause can be diagnosed initially, further admissions are highly unlikely to result in a diagnosis or benefit the patient.

Even with appropriate diagnostic testing, a likely cause of syncope will not be found in many patients. Fortunately, most patients with an undiagnosed cause of syncope will not have a recurrence, but if they do, they tend to have a benign long-term prognosis. As part of a proper evaluation, it is important to know when to stop testing.

Occasionally, laboratory (blood) tests can identify the cause of syncope. However, a routine battery of blood tests is rarely productive. The hemoglobin count may provide a diagnosis of acute blood loss as a cause of syncope in about 5% of patients.[9] An SMA-6 has an even smaller diagnostic yield. It may help detect a seizure if metabolic acidosis is present.[147] An elevated blood urea nitrogen (BUN), creatinine, or sodium may indicate fluid depletion. An abnormal potassium value may indicate an arrhythmic cause of syncope. Oxygen desaturation may indicate a pulmonary embolus. As part of a general screening evaluation, it is probably useful and cost- effective to obtain a hemoglobin and perhaps an SMA-6, but it is not clear that even this evaluation is worthwhile. Drug levels (such as digoxin) should be tested, and other blood tests should be obtained based on the history.

All patients should have an electrocardiogram. An electrocardiogram is simple, inexpensive, and risk free, and it may provide helpful information in 5% to 10% of patients (Table 8). Twenty to fifty percent of patients will have an abnormal, but nondiagnostic, electrocardiogram. The presence of a bundle branch block in a syncope patient indicates the presence of His-Purkinje disease and may indicate the possibility of complete heart block.[148,149] Bundle branch block can also be an indication of organic heart disease. Up to 30% of patients with syncope and bundle branch block will have the induction of sustained monomorphic ventricular tachycardia at electrophysiological testing.[150–153] A patient with undiagnosed syncope and a bundle branch block, therefore, should be considered for an electro-

_____ **Table 8** _____

The Electrocardiogram
To Evaluate Syncope

Finding	Significance
Normal or Nonspecific	Common, does not rule out serious cause
Complete heart block	Pacemaker indicated
Second-degree heart block	Correlate with symptoms. Pacemaker may be indicated
First-degree heart block	No obvious significance in most cases
Delta waves	WPW pattern. Possible supraventricular tachycardia
Sinus bradycardia	Nonspecific—may indicate risk sinus syndrome
Myocardial infarction	Acute arrhythmia, hemodynamic problem Old—risk for death, arrhythmia
Epsilon waves	Right ventricular dysplasia
Bundle branch block	Possible heart block, or ventricular tachycardia
QT prolongation (>0.500)	Possible torsades de pointes
Ectopic beats	No known significance
Atrial fibrillation	May indicate underlying structural heart disease, arrhythmic cause
Supraventricular tachycardia	Rare. Likely cause for syncope
Ventricular tachycardia	Rare. Likely cause for syncope
Paced rhythm	Pacemaker malfunction

physiological test. The electrocardiogram can also show ventricular preexcitation (Wolff-Parkinson-White syndrome), ectopic beats, heart block, ventricular hypertrophy, atrial fibrillation, a myocardial infarction (new or old), a long QT interval (arguably, >0.500 seconds), or sustained ventricular tachycardia.

The signal-averaged electrocardiogram is not particularly useful in patients with syncope, but it may play a specific role in determining if a patient with intact left ventricular function but underlying coronary artery disease (with no bundle branch block) has a risk for ventricular tachycardia or for arrhythmic death and would otherwise benefit from electrophysiological testing.[154–156]

Use of an echocardiogram may be appropriate to evaluate ventricular function and valvular heart disease, but if the electrocardiogram is normal, there is no cardiac history, and there are no abnormalities found on the physical examination, an echocardiogram is not urgent. Younger patients without history of heart disease and with normal physical examination will be unlikely to benefit from an echocardiogram. Patients with suspected neurocardiogenic syncope do not need an echocardiogram. A chest x-ray may show cardiomegaly or pulmonary edema and should be obtained if there is other evidence on examination, but as a routine screen, it adds little but an increase in cost. No other tests are required as part of the initial evaluation.

What to Do After the Initial Evaluation

When to Hospitalize the Patient

A key aspect in the evaluation and treatment is to decide whether to, and when to, admit a patient who has had syncope. Based on the information collected as part of the history, physical, and initial evaluation, appropriate decisions can be made regarding hospitalization[157,158] (Table 9). This has become increasingly important in a time of managed medical care. With the costs of hospital admissions escalating, prudent admission criteria are required. Many hospitals are developing practice guidelines to care for patients with syncope (Chart 1).

There are some potential benefits of hospitalization. It can be can be useful to diagnose and treat the cause of syncope, to prevent death, injury, and symptoms, and to satisfy medical-legal requirements (the "standard of care"). However, most often, hospitalization is unnecessary and useless. It can be associated with iatrogenic complications for syncope patients. Despite hospitalization, syncope often remains undiagnosed. The prognosis and recurrence rates may not change. If a patient has previously been hospitalized, repeated hospitalizations for recurrent syncope are rarely productive; they are helpful in <15% of such patients. Clearly, considering the scope of the problem of syncope, the lack of benefit of admission, and the present medical environment, hospital admission for syncope should be considered carefully and used prudently.

The reasons given to hospitalize are: 1) To monitor the patient suspected of having a serious, poorly tolerated arrhythmia, 2) To perform tests not readily performed as an outpatient, 3) To formulate and undertake

_____ **Table 9** _____

Criteria for Hospitalization

Malignant arrhythmia or cardiovascular cause suspected
New neurologic abnormality present
Severe injury present
Multiple frequent episodes
Severe orthostatic hypotension
Uncontrolled "malignant" vasovagal syncope
Elderly patient
Treatment plans not possible as an outpatient

EVALUATION OF RECENT ONSET SYNCOPE

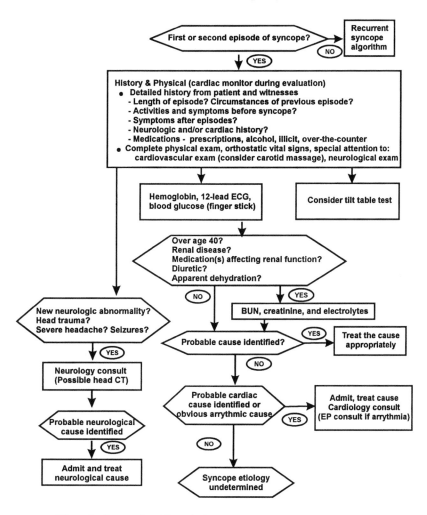

Chart 1. A sample of hospital practice guidelines for syncope.

specific treatment plans not possible as an outpatient (cardiac catheterization or electrophysiological testing when a life-threatening arrhythmia is suspected), 4) For medical-legal purposes, 5) When the patient is having multiple, closely spaced episodes, 6) When there is a new neurological abnormality or a suspected neurological cause, new seizure disorder, transient ischemic attack, or stroke, 7) When the patient is elderly, has been injured, or is at risk for serious injury, 8) When there is a severe abnormality on physical examination, 9) When any cardiovascular cause is suspected

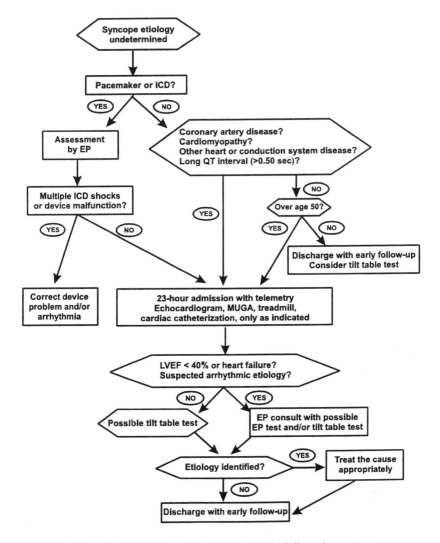

Chart 1b. A sample of hospital practice guidelines for syncope.

(due to an arrhythmia or due to a hemodynamic problem), 10) When there is symptomatic orthostatic hypotension, 11) For patients with suspected "malignant" vasovagal syncope or vasovagal syncope that is difficult to control and causes severe symptoms.

Often the reason to admit is to insure that the patient does not have frequent and recurrent symptoms, or is not on the verge of developing a more serious problem. If the risk at discharge from the emergency room is low, there is little reason to admit a patient (Charts 1 and 2). In addition

RECURRENT UNDIAGNOSED SYNCOPE

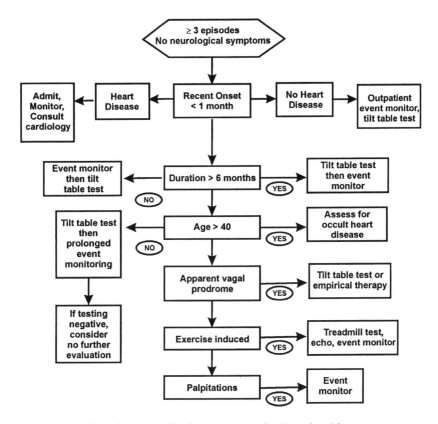

Chart 2. A sample of a syncope evaluation algorithm.

to protecting the patient from a life-threatening risk, expected results of hospitalization include finding the cause of syncope and initiating a treatment that cannot be performed on an outpatient basis. This can include treatment of a cardiac arrhythmia with drugs, surgery, or implanted devices. Patients who are suspected of having a new neurological event may benefit from close inpatient observation to note any worsening of their condition. Patient concerns also enter the decision for hospital admission.

When considering hospital admission, several additional factors must be appraised: patient age, cardiac risk factors, circumstances of the episodes, history from the patient and witnesses, underlying medical conditions, and results of physical examination. Hospitalization should be considered for formulation and undertaking of specific diagnostic and therapeutic plans that cannot be performed on an outpatient basis. The goals for hospitalization must be clear before admission because nondirected admissions for syncope are generally nonproductive. The prognosis and recurrence rate of syncope may not change with hospitalization. Patients who do not benefit from hospitalization include those with isolated episodes of syncope and no apparent heart disease; those with recurrent episodes but normal physical examination, echocardiogram, electrocardiogram, and no cardiac risk factors; and those who have undergone a previous complete evaluation. Repeat hospitalization to evaluate such patients is also unrewarding.

Mozes[159] found that prolonged inpatient monitoring was rarely productive. In his study, for patients hospitalized with syncope, a diagnostic evaluation leading to an appropriate therapeutic intervention was present in 24%, consistent with other reports. With admission based on the history, the physical, and the electrocardiogram, 85% of the hospitalizations could have been avoided.

In a study of 350 patients, clinical judgement was compared to "objective" diagnosis-related groups (DRG) criteria to evaluate the need for and benefit of hospitalization.[158] This study included patients with syncope. In this report, physicians' clinical judgement outperformed objective DRG data in identifying patients who needed and benefitted from acute-care hospitalization.

Medicode International Classification of Diseases, 9th Revision, Clinical Modification (ICD 9 CM) codes for syncope under: "780: general symptoms." Medicode ICD 9 CM "780.2: syncope and collapse" includes blackouts, fainting, vasovagal attacks, near or presyncope, but excludes carotid sinus syncope, heat syncope, neurocirculatory asthenia, orthostatic hypotension, or shock. ICD 9 CM 780.4 codes for "dizziness and giddiness" include "lightheadedness and vertigo." Sometimes syncope coding includes "DRG 427.89: cardiac dysrhythmia" and "427.9: cardiac dysrhythmia, unspecified." Over the course of 1 year at Loyola University Medical Center, 236 syncope patients were admitted with these diagnoses. The average length of stay was 3.7 days. Third-party payers applied less pressure for discharge during hospitalization as long as a treatment plan was in place, which is appropriate because in order for hospitalization to be worthwhile, a plan needs to be in place at the time of admission.

When to Consult a Specialist

Appropriately, patients often visit primary care physicians in an emergency room or in a clinical setting for initial episodes of syncope. While internists, emergency physicians, and family practitioners see the bulk of syncope patients, consultation may become necessary. A consultant should be considered after the complete initial evaluation has been undertaken and an etiology that requires disease-specific evaluation and treatment is suspected. The history and physical provide the best clues for the diagnosis and for the decision to call in consultants. The first step in evaluating syncope is *not* to call a neurology consult or an electrophysiology consult, although both can be helpful for specific patients. A neurology consult will rarely provide useful guidance unless there are no specific clues on the history or physical. An electrophysiologist will help to: 1) assess risk of an arrhythmic cause of syncope using electrophysiological testing, 2) provide information concerning the prognostic risk of syncope, 3) evaluate potential autonomic causes of syncope including neurocardiogenic causes, 4) perform tilt table testing and evaluate the results, and 5) manage (diagnose and treat) arrhythmic causes of syncope. Since the electrophysiologist can help manage patients with potential arrhythmic causes of syncope, he or she should be called early when there is organic heart disease, bundle branch block, or an arrhythmia history. A cardiologist should be called to help evaluate the patient with suspected cardiovascular disease as a cause of syncope. Such diseases include aortic valve disease, hypertrophic cardiomyopathy, other cardiomyopathies, or coronary artery disease.

A good consultant will help direct the evaluation of the syncope patient promptly, properly, and efficiently without encountering inappropriate testing. In this way, the consultant should actually improve the quality of care and lower the total costs. It is likely that electrophysiologists are not called often enough to see syncope patients. Neurologists are commonly called too early to help with the management, and should appropriately be called if there are neurological signs. Any neurological testing should be performed with the aid of a neurologist. Autonomic medicine is rapidly emerging as a separate medical speciality that deals with patients with neurocardiogenic and dysautonomic syncope that is difficult to treat.

Diagnostic Testing: When?

A variety of tests are used to evaluate syncope patients. Frequently, the following "complete work-up" is planned (Table 10): carotid Doppler examination, cardiac enzymes, prolonged in-hospital telemetric monitoring, echocardiogram, treadmill test, head computed axial tomography scan,

_____ **Table 10** _____

Initial Evaluation After Admission
Should These Be Routine?

Computed tomography scan
Carotid Doppler
Electroencephalogram
Cardiac enzymes
Neurology consult
Cardiac catheterization
Exercise test
NO!

and neurology consult. It is not clear where this "shotgun" approach originated, but it has no scientific basis and it is not advocated because it will almost never lead to a diagnostic cause of syncope.

The computed axial tomography (CT) and the MRI brain scans are almost never warranted, especially if there are no neurological findings. While an abnormality such as a tumor or cerebrovascular accident may be found, this may be concomitant (and perhaps asymptomatic) rather than a cause of syncope.

The electroencephalogram has been used as a screen in several reports that evaluate syncope.[34] The routine and undirected use of the electroencephalogram for undiagnosed syncope has not been helpful and cannot be recommended without other suggestive clinical information available.

Several diagnostic tests can help evaluate syncope, but it is important to consider the sensitivity, specificity, and diagnostic accuracy of any test used. An abnormality found does not necessarily indicate that it caused syncope. Induction of ventricular tachycardia at electrophysiological testing or a hypotensive bradycardia episode on a tilt table test is suggestive, but not indicative, of the cause of syncope. Any finding must be considered in light of all clinical findings and must be interpreted before using the results to initiate therapy. The test must be evaluated on its own merit and chosen based on the finding uncovered from the history and physical.

Tilt Table Testing

The tilt table test is used to evaluate neurocardiogenic causes of syncope; especially if the cause of syncope is otherwise not clear.[44,160,161] The tilt table test has been in use to evaluate syncope since before the 1950s.[26] It helps assess a reflex mechanism that is only now beginning to be understood.[162-166] Over the past decade, the use of and indications for tilt table testing have expanded tremendously. It has revolutionized evaluation and treatment of patients with suspected neurocardiogenic and dysautonomic syncope (see Chapters 3 and 4).

Not all patients with possible neurocardiogenic syncope require a tilt table test. If a patient has a clear history of neurocardiogenic syncope or has episodes related to a specific situation, the test may not be needed. Sensitivity and specificity issues may influence use of the tilt table test, but there is no other "gold standard" for evaluation of the presence of neurocardiogenic reflexes implicated as causes of syncope (the reflex itself may not be abnormal).[167] A negative test can occur, even in the presence of an obvious cause of neurocardiogenic syncope, and a positive test can occur when syncope is clearly due to other causes.[168] As with electrophysiological testing, a positive test (especially if "borderline positive") may potentially be misleading. Always consider that there may be other (or multiple) causes of syncope. This problem was well illustrated in the case of the basketball player, Reggie Lewis, who had syncope and a positive tilt table test, but died suddenly of ventricular fibrillation while playing basketball. When syncope appears to be clearly due to neurocardiogenic causes, treatment plans can potentially begin without a tilt table test (although some authors wish to determine exact response patterns during tilt table testing as a guide to therapy). Guidelines for tilt table testing have been published.[167] The tilt table test is best considered for patients with suspected neurocardiogenic syncope but in whom the cause is not obvious (see Chapters 3 and 4) or in patients with syncope of otherwise unknown origin.

Holter Monitoring

Holter monitoring is often ordered for syncope patients, but rarely does it diagnose a serious underlying arrhythmic cause; it rarely provides useful information unless the patient has an episode with the monitor attached. In several large studies using Holter monitoring, the correlation between arrhythmic abnormalities and symptoms, including syncope, was less than 5%.[169–173] If an asymptomatic abnormality is detected, it may not be the cause of syncope, and may it lead to further unnecessary diagnostic and perhaps therapeutic interventions.[174] Asymptomatic nonsustained ventricular tachycardia, premature ventricular beats, sinus pauses, or sinus bradycardia may have no specific meaning in this setting and may confuse, rather than reveal the cause of the syncope. The only reason to consider a Holter monitor is when a patient has multiple or frequent episodes of syncope or related symptoms over a short period of time (Figure 3). Prolonged Holter monitoring is an option for evaluation of select patients, but there are now better methods to monitor for arrhythmias long-term.

Endless-Loop Recorders, Event Recorders

Endless-loop recorders have emerged as highly prescribed and quite useful devices to manage syncope and assess its potential arrhythmic causes (Table 11).[175] The newer devices are technologically superior and smaller, with a larger battery capacity. They can be used to capture and save episodes even minutes after they have occurred. The newer devices can be attached to the patient for weeks or months at a time. A tape continuously records the electrocardiogram so that if a patient passes out, the episode can be saved by pushing a button on the recorder after awakening. Therefore, the episodes can be recorded and played back by the patient over the phone or by other knowledgeable individuals. This time interval recorded before the button is pushed is often programmable, but acceptably long compared to the length of routine syncope episodes. Little data are published on this highly promising technology, which is now used routinely to evaluate syncopal episodes. This technique is quite useful to cost-effectively diagnose a

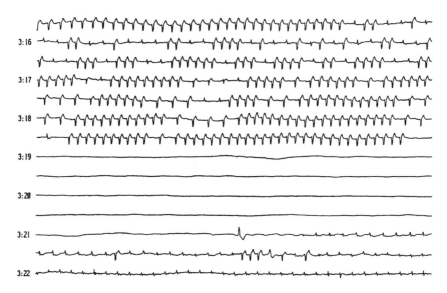

Figure 3. A Holter moniter performed on a patient with recurrent frequent episodes of syncope. The patient was admitted to the hospital and had a Holter monitor placed. The patient had more than 2 minutes of asystole.

potentially syncopal arrhythmia. Outpatient use of this device should be reserved for patients who are responsible and intelligent enough to learn to use the device and who are willing to do so. Implanted devices are now being developed and are already in use (see Chapter 16).

Electrophysiological Testing

Most arrhythmias that cause syncope are paroxysmal, infrequent and unpredictable. They can be difficult, if not impossible, to diagnose. Elec-

_____ **Table 11** _____

Holter Monitor vs. Endless Loop Recorders

To assess: AV block, sinus node dysfunction supraventricular/ventricular tachycardia

Holter:
    Advantage—For patients unable to comply with event recorder, or frequent episodes
    Disadvantage—Rare correlation of rhythm to symptoms for Holter

Endless Loop Recorder:
    Advantage—Long-term evaluation to correlate symptoms with rhythm.
    Disadvantage—Requires knowledge of how and when to use.

_____ **Table 12** _____

When to Perform Electrophysiological Testing

Coronary artery disease with left ventricular dysfunction*
Dilated cardiomyopathy
Valvular cardiomyopathy*
Bundle branch block*
Congestive heart failure, any cause*
Supraventricular tachycardia but not temporally associated syncope
Wolff-Parkinson-White Syndrome
Possible, for undiagnosed syncope multiple recurrence

* = cardiac catheterization, may need to be performed first, on a case by case basis.

trophysiological testing has emerged as a useful method to assess arrhythmic causes of syncope (Table 12) and to assess the risk for arrhythmic death. Various arrhythmias can be evaluated by electrophysiological testing, but the test has differing capabilities to assess each rhythm disturbance (Table 13). A compilation of electrophysiological test results are shown in Figure 4 and Table 14: Abnormal test results are seen in 7%-50% of patients selected for study.* This wide range of results reflects patient selection. The electrophysiological test is an invasive method used to try to initiate an arrhythmia by stimulation of the atria and ventricles (see Chapter 7). The goal is to try to uncover a clinically important arrhythmia that caused syncope.

The main use for electrophysiological testing in syncope patients is to evaluate monomorphic ventricular tachycardia. Electrophysiological testing can determine the cause of syncope and will also help determine the long-term prognosis. Induction of sustained monomorphic ventricular tachycardia is the most common abnormality seen in patients selected for electrophysiological testing, with an occurrence rate higher than would be expected in a matched nonsyncopal population with similar structural heart disease. Induction of sustained ventricular tachycardia likely indicates that it was the cause of syncope, but a negative test does not rule out ventricular tachycardia. Results are disease-specific. The electrophysiological test has the highest sensitivity and specificity to detect sustained monomorphic ventricular tachycardia and the cause of syncope in patients with coronary artery disease, who are not acutely ischemic. Another group with a high incidence of inducible ventricular tachycardia is patients with an

_____

*References 12, 31, 33, 35, 73, 76, 105-107, 111, 112, 151-153, 176-183.

_____ **Table 13** _____

Electrophysiological (EP) Testing
To Evaluate Syncope

Sustained ventricular tachycardia (also to assess risk for death)
Supraventricular tachycardia (rare finding at electrophysiology testing)
Bradycardia—fair → poor to evaluate the sinus node
Heart block—fair → poor to evaluate the AV node

CAVEATS:
    May not find the cause for syncope
    Not predictive for all populations
    Multiple abnormalities common
    Not clearly indicative for cause for syncope

underlying bundle branch block. Up to 30% of these patients will have ventricular tachycardia induced.

The ejection fraction can further dtetermine which patient will have an abnormal electrophysiological test. In one report,[109] 31 of 104 syncope patients had ventricular tachycardia induced at electrophysiological testing. Of patients with ejection fractions less than 0.40, ventricular tachycardia was induced in 35%, whereas of those with an ejection fraction over 0.40, only 3% had ventricular tachycardia induced. Patients with normal or near normal left ventricular ejection, even in the presence of structural heart disease, will likely have a normal electrophysiological test. The test is now not generally recommended as a firstline test for patients with a left ventricular ejection fraction greater than 0.40. Electrophysiological testing may

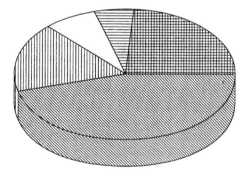

Figure 4. Electrophysiological Testing. Patients with syncpe of undetermined origin (12% of patients had multiple abnormalities). VT = ventricular tachycardia; SVT = supraventricular tachycardia; SND = sinus node disease; AVN/HP = atrioventricular node/His-Purkinje.

⊞ VT ☰ SVT ☐ SND ⊞ AVN/HP ▨ Normal

_____ Table 14 _____

Electrophysiological Testing for Syncope-Selected Studies

Study	All Patients	Positive Test	VT	SVT	SND	AVB	Other
Bass	70	37	31	3	0	3	0
Denes	89	53	13	13	15	58	0
DiMarco	25	17	9	0	1	3	4
Doherty	119	78	31	6	4	5	32
Gulamhusein	34	6	0	3	3	0	2
Hess	32	18	11	0	5	1	1
Kall	175	52	29	4	9	11	0
Krol	104	31	22	2	2	6	0
Morady	53	30	24	0	2	0	4
Olshansky	105	41	28	13	1	3	5
Reiffel	59	29	8	3	15	13	0
Teichman	105	112	36	16	19	69	20

VT = ventricular tachycardia; SVT = supraventricular tachycardia; SND = sinus node dysfunction; AVB = atrioventricular block.

be useful for such patients under the following ccircumstances: 1) if other testing is negative, 2) if syncope frequently recurs, 3) if there is a late potential on signal-averaged electrocardiogram, or 4) if there are prolonged episodes of nonsustained ventricular tachycardia on monitor. The Holter monitor, however, does not appear to be a useful method to assess which patient will benefit from an electrophysiological test.[34,169,182]

The electrophysiological test can miss a tachycardia that is responsible for syncope. Nonsustained ventricular tachycardia can cause syncope, but the sensitivity of the electrophysiological test to evaluate this rhythm is low. Electrophysiological testing can miss ventricular tachycardia in patients with dilated or valvular cardiomyopathy. The electrophysiological test cannot assess the "clinical arrhythmia" accurately for patients with polymorphic ventricular tachycardia, hypertrophic cardiomyopathy, or the long QT interval syndrome.

Occasionally, the electrophysiological test should be considered for patients with frequent episodes of syncope when no other cause can be found, even if the ejection fraction is intact. In such a patient with recurrent episodes, the tilt table test should be performed first. If negative, an electrophysiological test may be diagnostic, but a negative result would be expected in over 70% of these patients. One possible abnormality that may be found is an idiopathic monomorphic ventricular tachycardia that can be cured by radiofrequency ablation during the testing. Another is a poorly tolerated supraventricular tachycardia, which is even possible in patients without apparent structural heart disease. In one study of syncope patients, 13 of 105 had a supraventricular tachycardia induced (four of these patients also had ventricular tachycardia induced).[34] The incidence of supraventricular tachycardia induction varies between studies, but is relatively rare. Induction of supraventricular tachycardia is rare in previously asymptomatic patients and therefore, if induced and associated with hypotension, it should be considered a cause of syncope and treated, perhaps with radiofrequency ablative. The electrophysiological test is not adequate to assess atrial flutter or fibrillation adequately or to assess ability of the AV node to conduct very rapidly or very slowly under all conditions.

The use of the electrophysiological test to evaluate tachycardia in syncope patients appears warranted. Patients who have therapy guided by electrophysiological testing appear to have less syncope recurrence and risk of death (Table 15), although no prospective randomized trials have been performed. Olshansky has shown that when tachycardia was induced and a drug could have suppress it, 14% of patients had recurrent syncope or cardiac arrest if they took medications that appeared to be effective, versus 54% who were noncompliant with medications in a 25.8- month follow-up.[34] There are, however, studies suggesting that electrophysiological testing is useful in syncope patients.

Electrophysiological testing is fair at best to evaluate sinus bradycardias and AV block in syncope patients.[181,182,184] An abnormal sinus node recovery time is relatively specific for detection of sinus node disease, but its presence does not indicate that sinus node dysfunction caused syncope; also, sensitivity is low. If the sinus node recovery time is >3 seconds and there is no other apparent cause of syncope, sinus node dysfunction is the likely cause of syncope, and a pacemaker should be implanted. His-Purkinje conduction can be evaluated by the electrophysiological test, but rarely is an abnormal finding noted, and significant infra-Hisian block can be missed. An HV interval of >100 ms is a probable cause of syncope if no other cause

_____ **Table 15** _____

Electrophysiological Testing
Does Therapy Prevent Recurrent Syncope and Sudden Death?

Study	Patients	Follow-up	Syncope Effective Rx	Sudden Death Effective Rx	Syncope Ineffective Rx	Sudden Death Ineffective Rx
Bass	70	30	20	31	50	47
Kall	175	24	0	3	27	25
Olshansky	87	26	12% (14%)	0% (8%)	30% (54%)	16%

( ) indicates lack of compliance with therapy.

can be found. If there is a bundle branch block, pacing-induced infra-Hisian block can be seen. Procainamide or other class IA antiarrhythmic drugs can be used to "stress" the His-Purkinje system and determine the presence of pacing-induced infra-Hisian block.[185,186] Fujimura[181] found that only 2 of 13 patients had the correct diagnosis of infra-His block determined by electrophysiological testing. If present, infra-His block is the likely cause of syncope and a pacemaker should be implanted. Atrioventricular block in the AV node as cause of syncope cannot be evaluated accurately.

The electrophysiology results derived must be interpreted in light of the clinical situation and are not always helpful.[187] An induced arrhythmia may not be the cause of syncope, but may simply be a laboratory artifact.[188] Induction of ventricular fibrillation only has little, if any, clinical significance in syncope patients. Patients generally do not pass out from ventricular fibrillation; they die.[189] Induction of nonsustained, monomorphic ventricular tachycardia is similarly difficult to interpret.

At Loyola University Medical Center, 21% of primary electrophysiological tests have been performed to evaluate and diagnose a potential cause of syncope. The test has been performed in outpatients with history of syncope and is performed during acute hospitalization for recent episodes of syncope.

While electrophysiological testing is useful for a subset of syncope patients, there are several concerns: 1) not all arrhythmias are accurately diagnosed, 2) multiple "soft abnormalities" may be found, none of which may be responsible for syncope, 3) autonomic effects influencing a tachycardia may not be adequately evaluated, 4) sinus node and AV node dysfunction cannot be fully evaluated.

Other Testing

The echocardiogram is useful, but it cannot be recommended as an initial screen unless the history or physical examination warrants its use. Pericardial tamponade, valvular abnormities, aortic valve disease, and hypertrophic cardiomyopathy can all cause syncope and these abnormalities can be quantitated by the echocardiogram. The main reason to perform an echocardiogram without obvious physical findings is to assess the presence of left ventricular dysfunction or right ventricular enlargement (due to right ventricular dysplasia), which may suggest the presence of a ventricular arrhythmia. The test should be considered for evaluation of left ventricular function in patients over 50 years old, even if there is no history consistent with heart disease and even if the electrocardiogram is normal. It adds expense, but is safe and unlikely to lead to therapeutic misadventures.

The signal-averaged electrocardiogram is useful to detect risk of cardiac arrest and monomorphic ventricular tachycardia in syncope patients with apparent heart disease, and therefore it is useful in some patients with syncope. An abnormal result consists of the presence of a "late potential" or a prolonged QRS complex. The chance of finding the presence of ventricular tachycardia depends on the extent of the abnormalities observed For example, if three out of the three observed criteria (QRS duration, amplitude of the last 40 milliseconds of the QRS complex, and length of the low-amplitude signal at the end of the QRS complex) are abnormal, there is a greater chance of finding a ventricular tachycardia as the cause for syncope. This noninvasive test has its highest predictive accuracy when coronary artery disease is present. The most common use of the signal-averaged electrocardiogram is on patients who have coronary artery disease and syncope, but have preserved ventricular function (ejection fraction >0.40). If the ejection fraction is <0.40, proceeding directly to electrophysiological testing is recommended. The signal averaged electrocardiogram, however, may provide some adjunctive information for patients with coronary artery disease and ejection fraction <0.40 if the electrophysiological test is negative. The test may be falsely negative (and may miss risk for ventricular tachycardia) if there has been an inferior myocardial infarction. Also, the test lacks predictive accuracy for patients who do not have coronary artery disease. It may be falsely positive when a bundle branch block is present.

Cardiac catheterization is advocated for patients with suspected heart disease and syncope. The cardiac catheterization may find an underlying structural heart problem, but the test is not justified unless there is a history suggestive of a significant valvular problem or unless there is adequate suspicion for an ischemically mediated arrhythmia. The blanket use of cardiac catheterization in syncope patients, even when heart disease is diagnosed, is certainly not warranted; it is probably overused and can only be recommended on a case by case basis.

Treatment

Once a cause of syncope is identified, treatment should be *considered*. Treatment for all of the conditions mentioned is beyond the scope of this chapter and is discussed elsewhere. Not all patients who pass out require treatment, even if the cause is identified. For example, a patient who has an isolated vasovagal episode due to a specific situation unlikely to be reproduced will not require therapy.

> CASE: A 52-year-old woman has a viral syndrome associated with diarrhea, nausea, and vomiting. Fluid intake is inadequate. After abruptly standing up from bed, she develops nausea and lightheadedness. Several minutes later she becomes diaphoretic and collapses, waking up on the floor. After hydration and recovery from her viral infection, no further therapy is indicated.

Management of Recurrent Syncope with No Cause Identified

Proper evaluation of the syncope patient (before further evaluation is considered futile and excessive) depends on patient age, underlying medical conditions, and ensuing physical limitations imposed upon the patient. For patients with an unidentified cause of syncope, no specific therapy can be prescribed and no studies clearly document a valid, rational treatment plan. In many such patients, syncope will not recur or episodes will be rare, and nothing more must be done. The prognosis for patients with syncope of undetermined etiology by use of appropriate methods to evaluate the cause is relatively good in the short term. The recurrence rate of syncope can be up to 30%.[9,30]

For patients with recurrent syncope, reassessment may be necessary. Even after further extensive or repeated evaluation, however, in up to 85% of these patients, no cause of syncope is ever found. Repeat hospitalizations for monitoring, repeat tilt table testing, and repeat electrophysiological testing are, therefore, rarely indicated. Perhaps certain aspects of the history were not completely considered and should be revisited. It is likely that the cause of syncope in the majority of patients with syncope of unknown origin is an autonomically mediated cause; these patients are likely to have neurocardiogenic syncope. Always consider psychological causes as well (see Chapter 9). While such patients with undiagnosed syncope generally have a good prognosis,[9,10] specific patient subgroups fare poorly (patient with dilated cardiomyopathy, for example) and syncope recurrence is always possible. For some patients with recurrent debilitating episodes, a trial of empirical therapy may be warranted.

In the elderly the empirical placement of a pacemaker has been considered an option, but this remains highly controversial.[190–194] It has been shown with extensive monitoring that transient bradyarrhythmias can be diagnosed as the cause of syncope when no other causes can be found.[120] While some patients with undiagnosed syncope appear to benefit from pacing, it is always best to have good justification for a pacemaker. With newer techniques for monitoring, this should be possible in the near future.

Empirical therapy for syncope of unknown etiology is usually no better, and can be even worse than no therapy at all.[110,195,196] Moazez[110] found that the recurrence rate of syncope was even worse if empiric therapy was used. Therapy guided by the electrophysiological test may have helped prevent syncope recurrence.[110,196]

Patient Examples: Undiagnosed Syncope

Patient 1: 51-year-old NYHA Functional Class I woman with dilated cardiomyopathy, ejection fraction of 25%, and left bundle branch block plows her car into a truck, destroying it, after she passes out. When she awakens, she does not remember anything. History and physical are otherwise negative. On monitor, she has a three-beat run of ventricular tachycardia. An electrophysiological test is negative. She had passed out a year before but did not see a doctor. *Therapy:* An empiric implantable defibrillator is placed.

Patient 2: A 17-year-old woman has experienced over 10 episodes of syncope (once while driving a car), has no history of medical problems, a normal physical examination (except sinus bradycardia and occasional junctional rhythm), a normal electrocardiogram, and a normal tilt table test. She has seasonal asthma. An event monitor is not helpful. *Therapy:* Theophylline is started for presumed neurocardiogenic syncope and she remains asymptomatic for 3 years.

Patient 3: An 80-year-old male patient who lives in a nursing home falls frequently. He takes Procardia and Dyazide for hypertension. He collapses at the nursing home and brakes his right hip. Initially upon attachment of a monitor, he is found to be in atrial fibrillation with a rate of 50 and an associated blood pressure when awake of 165/70 without orthostatic signs. An echocardiogram shows left ventricular hypertrophy and intact left ventricular function. *Therapy:* A pacemaker is placed and he remains without symptoms.

Patient 4: A 39-year-old woman with history of mitral valve prolapse, passes out suddenly without warning on two occasions. She takes no medication. Physical reveals no orthostatic signs, a mid-systolic click is present. Electrocardiogram is normal. Echocardiogram shows mitral valve prolapse. A tilt table test is negative. An event monitor is given for 1 month, but she has no symptoms. *Therapy:* No further evaluation is performed and no therapy is given.

Patient 5: A 52-year-old hypertensive woman without known history collapses at home and goes to the emergency room with a rapid rate in atrial fibrillation, evidence for Wolff-Parkinson- White syndrome and a blood pressure of 90/60. She remains slightly lethargic even after DC cardioversion. Her sister states that she had the worst headache of her life before collapsing at home. CT scan reveals a subarachnoid bleed. *Therapy:* After resection of her berry aneurysm, and with no further therapy for Wolff-Parkinson-White syndrome, she recovers without incident.

A Protocol for Evaluation of Syncope

At Loyola University Medical Center, we have developed an evaluation schema to plan admission and evaluation for syncope patients (Charts 1A, 1B, and 2). After an initial history (including evaluation of prodrome, palpitations, cardiovascular disease, seizures, and medications) and physical examination (including orthostatic vital signs, a complete cardiac and neurological examination, and carotid massage) in the emergency room or other outpatient setting, an electrocardiogram, a hemoglobin and a blood glucose test, and cardiac monitoring (during evaluation in the emergency room) are obtained. If the patient is older than 40 years, taking a diuretic or a vasodilator, has evidence for dehydration or renal disease, then BUN, creatinine, and electrolytes are ordered. If there is history of a new neurological abnormality, head trauma, or a severe headache, a head-computed axial tomography scan is considered in conjunction with a neurology consult. Otherwise, a CT scan is not ordered. If no specific etiology of syncope is identified, attention is directed to categorization by age and underlying medical conditions. Is there pacemaker or implanted defibrillator present, which may have malfunctioned? Did the implanted defibrillator discharge? Is there a long QT or corrected QT interval either continuously or intermittently (>0.500 seconds)? Is there a bundle branch block? Is there a known or suspected heart condition? If the answer to any of these question is yes, the patient is admitted. If there is an implanted defibrillator or a pacemaker, it is interrogated immediately, even before admission. If the patient is older than 50, but the answer to the above questions is no, the patient is either discharged with early follow-up by the following physical or an internist or is admitted for a 23-hour ("outpatient") admission with a beside cardiac monitor. In the hospital, an electrophysiology consult is obtained if there is a history of heart disease, impaired left ventricular function, bundle branch block, pacemaker, or implantable cardioverter defibrillator. Testing directed at the specific cause of syncope is planned and performed in the hospital or on an outpatient basis. If no cause is identified, the patient is discharged, often with an event monitor. A tilt table test is considered.

A valid universal algorithmic approach to syncope is shown in Figure 5. Such an approach can be applied to the great majority of patients who have syncope. Specific intricacies of each patient's problems must be considered.These intricacies may further direct proper diagnostic approaches and therapeutic strategies.

Summary and Conclusions

This chapter reviews an initial approach to patients who present with syncope. It is not meant to be inclusive. Throughout the chapter, the reader is referred to other chapters for more in depth coverage of the many topics presented.

Syncope is a common manifestation of many disease processes. In a minority of cases, the problem is recurrent and handicapping. Patients with syncope and heart disease, particularly when there is impaired left ventricular function, bundle branch block, evidence of congestive heart failure, or a positive family history of syncope and heart disease, appear to be at particularly high risk for death and require an aggressive initial approach.

Syncope

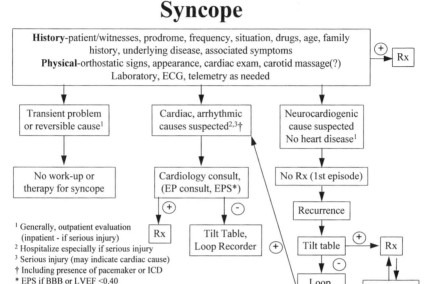

Figure 5. A universal algorithmic approach to syncope.

Patients who benefit most from hospitalization include those with suspected cardiac disease, the elderly, those with serious injuries, and those with new neurological findings.

Diagnostic tests should be used sparingly, directed by a carefully performed history and physical examination. No series of tests is universally applicable. Extensive undirected testing and repeat hospital admissions are usually unrewarding and expensive.

Over the past two decades, there have been advances in our abilities to properly evaluate the syncope patient. The tilt table test, the endless-loop recorder, and the electrophysiological test are among these advances. Chronically implanted electrocardiographic monitors are being developed (see Chapter 16).

The initial management is best directed by the savvy clinician who can discern clues from the history and physical examination to direct further diagnostic evaluation when needed. Up to one half of the patients with syncope still remain undiagnosed, an indication that while we have come a long way, we still have a long way to go.

Acknowledgment The author wishes to thank Dr. Richard Carroll for his comments and suggestions.

References

1. McLaren AJ, Lear J, Daniels RG. Collapse in an accident and emergency department. *J R Soc Med* 1994;87:138–139.
1a. Wiederholt WG. Seizure disorders. In: Wiederholt WG (ed). *Neurology for Nonneurologists.* Philadelphia PA: W.B. Saunders Co.; 1995:211–231.
2. Engel GL. Psychologic stress, vasodepressor syncope, and sudden death. *Ann Intern Med* 1978;89:403–412.
3. Liberthson R. Sudden death from cardiac causes in children and young adults. *N Engl J Med* 1996;334:1039–1044.
4. Linzer M, Potinen M, Gold DT, et al. Impairment of physical and psychosocial function in recurrent syncope. *J Clin Epidemiol* 1991;44:1037–1043.
5. Linzer M, Gold DT, Pontinen M, et al. Recurrent syncope as a chronic disease. *J Gen Intern Med* 1994;9:181–186.
6. Linzer M, Varia I, Pontinen M, et al. Medically unexplained syncope: Relationship to psychiatric illness. *Am J Med* 1992;92(1A):18S–25S.
7. Hori S. Diagnosis of patients with syncope in emergency room. *Keio J Med* 1994;43:185–191.
8. Day SC, Cook EF, Funkenstein H, et al. Evaluation and outcome of emergency room patients with transient loss of consciousness. *Am J Med* 1982;73:15–23.
9. Kapoor WN. Evaluation and outcome of patients with syncope. *Medicine* 1990;69:160–175.
10. Kapoor WN, Karpf M, Wieand S, et al. A prospective evaluation and follow-up of patients with syncope. *N Engl J Med* 1983;309:197–308.
11. Eagle KA, Black HR, Cook EF, et al. Evaluation of prognostic classifications for patients with syncope. *Am J Med* 1985;79:455–460.
12. Morady F, Shen EN, Schwartz A, et al. Long-term follow-up of patients with recurrent unexplained syncope evaluated by electrophysiological testing. *J Am Coll Cardiol* 1983;2:1053–1059.
13. Blanc JJ, Genet L, Forneiro I, et al. Short loss of consciousness: Etiology and diagnostic approach. Results of a prospective study. *Presse Med* 1989;18:923–826.
14. Kapoor WN, Karpf M, Maher Y, et al. Syncope of unknown origin: The need for more cost-effective approach to its diagnostic evaluation. *JAMA* 1982; 247:2687–2691.
15. Kapoor WN. How do you evaluate the patient with syncope? *Cardiovasc Med* 1985;10:51–54.
16. Manolis AS, Linzer M, Salem D. Syncope: Current diagnostic evaluation and management. *Ann Int Med* 1990;112:850–863.
17. Manolis AS. The clinical spectrum and diagnosis of syncope. *Herz* 1993;18:143–154.
18. Kapoor WN. Evaluation and management of the patient with syncope. *JAMA* 1992;268:2553–2559.
19. Calkins H, Byrne M, et-Atassi R, et al. The economic burden of unrecognized vasodepressor syncope. *Am J Med* 1993;95:473–479.
20. Campbell AJ, Reinken J, Allan BC, et al. Falls in old age: A study of frequency and related clinical factors. *Age Ageing* 1981;10:264–270.
21. Nevitt MC, Cummings SR, Hudes ES. Risk factors for injurious falls: A prospective study. *J Gerontol* 1991;46:M164–M170.
22. Savage DD, Corwin L, McGee DL, et al. Epidemiologic features of isolated syncope: The Framingham study. *Stroke* 1985;16:626–628.
23. Lipsitz LA. Syncope in the elderly. *Ann Intern Med* 1983;99:92–104.

24. Lipsitz LA, Wei JY, Rowe JW. Syncope in an elderly, institutionalized population: Prevalence, incidence, and associated risk. *QJM* 1985;55:45–54.
25. Kapoor WN, Snustad D, Peterson JA, et al. Syncope in the elderly. *Am J Med* 1986;80:419–428.
26. Dermkasian G, Lamb LE. Syncope in a population of healthy young adults. *JAMA* 1958;168:1200–1207.
27. Murdock BD. Loss of consciousness in healthy South African men. *S Afr Med J* 1980;57:771–74.
28. Williams RL Allen PD. Loss of consciousness. *Aerospace Med* 1962;33:545–51.
29. Schaal SF, Nelson SD, Boudoulas H. et al. Syncope. *Curr Probl Cardiol* 1992;17:205–264.
30. Kapoor WN, Peterson JR, Wieand HS, et al. The diagnostic and prognostic implications of recurrences in patients with syncope. *Am J Med* 1987;83:700–708.
31. Hess DS, Morady F, Scheinman MM. Electrophysiological testing in the evaluation of patients with syncope of undetermined origin. *Am J Cardiol* 1982;50:1309–1315.
32. Barnes AR. Cerebral manifestations of paroxysmal tachycardia. *Am J Med Sci* 1926;171:489–495.
33. Denniss AR, Ross DL, Richards DA, et al. Electrophysiological studies in patients with unexplained syncope. *Int J Cardiol* 1992;35:211–217.
34. Olshansky B, Mazuz M, Martins JB. Significance of inducible tachycardia in patients with syncope of unknown origin: A long-term follow-up. *J Am Coll Cardiol* 1985;5:216–223.
35. Kall JG, Olshansky B, Wilber D. Sudden death and recurrent syncope in patients presenting with syncope of unknown origin: Predictive value of electrophysiological testing. *Pacing Clin Electrophysiol* 1991;14:387A.
36. Esber EJ, Davis WR, Mullen KD, et al. Toothpick in ano: An unusual cause of syncope. *Am J Gastroenterol* 1994;89:941–942.
37. Wayne HH. Syncope: Physiologicalal considerations and an analysis of the clinical characteristics in 510 patients. *Am J Med* 1961;30:418–438.
38. Hecker JGC. *Die Tanzwuth, eine Volkrankheit im Mittelalter, Vol. 1* Berlin, Germany: T.C.F. Enslin; 1832;1–92.
39. Lempert T, Bauer M. Mass fainting at rock concerts. *N Eng J Med* 1995;332:1721.
40. Morens DM. Mass fainting at medieval rock concerts. *N Eng J Med* 1995;333:1361.
41. Kapoor WN, Karpf M, Levey GS. Issues in evaluating patients with syncope. *Ann Intern Med* 1984;100:755–757.
42. Wright KE Jr, McIntosh HD. Syncope: A review of pathophysiological mechanisms. *Prog Cardiovasc Dis* 1971;13:580–594.
43. Maloney JD, Jaeger FJ, Fouad-Tarazi FM, et al. Malignant vasovagal syncope: Prolonged asystole provoked by head-up tilt. *Cleve Clin J Med* 1988;55;542–548.
44. Fitzpatrick A, Sutton R. Tilting toward a diagnosis in recurrent unexplained syncope. *Lancet* 1989;1:658–660.
45. Luu M, Stevenson WG, Stevenson LW, et al. Diverse mechanisms of unexpected cardiac arrest in advanced heart failure. *Circulation* 1989;80:1675–1680.
46. Thomas JE, Schirger A, Fealey RD, et al. Orthostatic hypotension. *Mayo Clin Proc* 1981;56:117–125.
47. Ibrahim MM, Tarazi RC, Dustan HP. Orthostatic hypotension: Mechanisms and management. *Am Heart J* 1975;90:513–570.
48. Bradshaw MJ, Edwards RTM. Postural hypotension pathophysiology and management. *QJM* 1986;60:643–657.

49. Hickler RB. Orthostatic hypotension and syncope. *N Eng J Med* 1977; 296:336–337.
50. Bradbury S, Eggleston C. Postural hypotension. *Am Heart J* 1925;1:73–86.
51. Lipsitz LA, Nyquist RP, Wei JY, et al. Postprandial reduction in blood pressure in the elderly. *N Engl J Med* 1983;309:81–83.
52. Wehrmacher WH. Syncope among the aging population. *Am J Geriatr Cardiol* 1993;1:50–57.
53. Whiteside-Yim C. Syncope in the elderly: A clinical approach. *Geriatrics* 1987;42:37–41.
54. McIntosh HD. Evaluating elderly patients with syncope. *Cardiovascular Reviews & Reports* 1988;9:54–58.
55. Collins KJ, Exton-Smith AN, James MH, et al. Functional changes in autonomic nervous responses with ageing. *Age & Ageing* 1980;9:17–24.
56. Noble RJ. Syncope. *Cardiovascular Clinics* 1981;12:119–130.
57. Camm AJ, Evans KE, Ward DE, et al. The rhythm of the heart in active elderly subjects. *Am Heart J* 1980;99:598–603.
58. Hanlon JT, Linzer M, MacMillan JP, et al. Syncope and presyncope associated with probable adverse drug reactions. *Arch Int Med* 1990;150:2309–2312.
59. Raviele A, Gasparini G, Di Pede F, et al. Nitroglycerin infusion during upright tilt: A new test for the diagnosis of vasovagal syncope. *Am Heart J* 1994;124:103–111.
60. Ma SX, Schmid P, Long JP. Noradrenergic mechanisms and the cardiovascular actions of nitroglycerin. *Life Sci* 1994;55:1595–1603.
61. Richards CJ, Mark AL, Van Orden DE, et al. Effects of indomethacin on the vascular abnormalities of Bartter's syndrome. *Circulation* 1978 58:554–549.
62. Calkins H, Shyr Y, Frumin H, et al. The value of the clinical history in the differentiation of syncope due to ventricular tachycardia, atrioventricular block and neurocardiogenic syncope. *Am J Med* 1995;98:365–373.
63. Leitch JW, Klein GJ, Yee R, et al. Syncope associated with supraventricular tachycardia: An expression of tachycardia rate or vasomotor response? *Circulation* 1992;85:1064–1071.
64. Dhala A, Bremner S, Blanck Z, et al. Impairment of driving abilities in patients with supraventricular tachycardia. *Am J Cardiol* 1995;75:516–518.
65. Benditt DG, Klein GJ, Kriett JM, et al. Enhanced atrioventricular nodal conduction in man: Electrophysiological effects of pharmacologic autonomic blockade. *Circulation* 1984;69:1088–1095.
66. Fitzpatrick AP, Travill CM, Vardas PE, et al. Recurrent symptoms after ventricular pacing in unexplained syncope. *Pacing Clin Electrophysiol* 1990;13:619–624.
67. Morley CA, Perrins EJ, Grant, P et al. Carotid sinus syncope treated by pacing: Analysis of persistent symptoms and role of atrioventricular sequential pacing. *Br Heart J* 1982;47:411–418.
68. Sgarbossa EB, Pinski SL, Jaeger FJ, et al. Incidence and predictors of syncope in paced patients with sick sinus syndrome. *Pacing Clin Electrophysiol* 1992;15:2055–2060.
69. Esmein, Donzelot. Le forme syncopale a tachycardie paroxystique. *La Press Médicale* 1914; 27:489–490.
70. Ross RT. *Syncope*. London, England: W.B. Saunders Company; 1988:41–59.
71. Hamer AWF, Rubin SA, Peter T, et al. Factors that predict syncope during ventricular tachycardia in patients. *Am Heart J* 1984;107:997–1005.
72. Waxman MB, Cameron DA. The reflex effects of tachycardias on autonomic tone. *Ann NY Acad Sci* 1990;601:378–393.
73. Waxman MB, Wald RW, Carmeron D. Interactions between the autonomic nervous system and tachycardias in man. *Cardiol Clin* 1983;1:143–185.

74. Waxman MB, Sharma AD, Cameron DA, et al. Reflex mechanisms responsible for early spontaneous termination of paroxysmal supraventricular tachycardia. *Am J Cardiol* 1982;49:259–272.
75. Daoud EG, Dimitrijevic R, Morady F. Syncope mediated by posturally induced ventricular tachycardia. *Ann Int Med* 1995;123:431–432.
76. Morady, F, Shen EN, Bhandari A, et al. Clinical symptoms in patients with sustained ventricular tachycardia. *West J Med* 1985;142:341–344.
77. Sra JS, Akhtar M. Cardiac pacing during neurocardiogenic (vasovagal) syncope. *J Cardiovasc Electrophysiol* 1995;6:751–760.
78. Grubb BP, Gerard G, Roush K, et al. Differentiation of convulsive syncope and epilepsy with head-up tilt testing. *Ann Int Med* 1991;115:871–876.
79. Hofnagels WA, Padberg GW, Overweg J, et al. Syncope or seizure? The diagnostic value of the EEG and hyperventilation test in transient loss of consciousness. *J Neurol Neurosurg Psychiatry* 1991;54:953–956.
80. Hofnagels WA, Padberg GW, Overweg J, et al. Syncope or seizure? A matter of opinion. *Clin Neurol Neurosurg* 1992;94:153–156.
81. Hofnagels WA, Padberg GW, Overweg J, et al. Transient loss of consciousness: The value of the history for distinguishing seizure from syncope. *J Neurol* 1991;238:39–41.
82. Samuel M, Duncan JS. Use of the hand held video camcorder in the evaluation of seizures. *J Neurol Neurosurg Psychiatry* 1994;57:1417–1418.
83. Van Ness PC. Invasive electroencephalography in the evaluation of supplementary motor area seizure. *Adv in Neurol* 1996;70:319–340.
84. Verity CM. The place of the EEG and imaging in the management of seizures. *Arch Dis Child* 1995;73:557–562.
85. Swoboda KJ, Drislane FW. Seizure disorder: Syndromes, diagnosis, and management. *Compr Ther* 1994;20:67–73.
86. Aminoff MJ, Scheiman MM, Griffin JC, et al. Electrocerebral accompaniments of syncope associated with malignant ventricular arrhythmias. *Ann Int Med* 1988;108:791–796.
87. Kapoor WN, Peterson JR, Karpf M. Micturition syncope: A reappraisal. *JAMA* 1985;253:796–798.
88. Mark AL. The Bezold-Jarisch reflex revisited: Clinical implications of inhibitory reflexes originating in the heart. *J Am Coll Cardiol* 1983;1:90–102.
89. Benditt DG. Syncope. *Cardiovasc Med* 1995;1404–1421.
90. Chang-Sing P, Peter T. Syncope: Evaluation and management. *Cardiol Clin* 1991;9:641–651.
91. Farrehi PM, Santinga JT, Eagle KA. Syncope: Diagnosis of cardiac and noncardiac causes. *Geriatrics* 1995;50:24–30.
92. Mark AL, Kioschos JM, Abboub FM, et al. Abnormal vascular response to exercise in patients with aortic stenosis. *J Clin Invest* 1973;52:1138–1146.
93. White CW, Zimmerman TJ, Ahmad M. Idiopathic hypertrophic subaortic stenosis presenting as cough syncope. *Chest* 1975;62:250–53.
94. Weisberg LA. Differential diagnosis of coma: A step-by-step strategy. *J Critical Illness* 1989;4:97–108.
95. Heistad DD, Abboud FM, Mark AL, et al. Impaired reflex vasoconstriction in chronically hypoxemic patients. *J Clin Invest* 1972;51:331–337.
96. Grubb BP, Samiol D, Temsey-Armos P, et al. Episodic periods of neurally mediated hypotension and bradycardia mimicking transient ischemic attacks in the elderly: Identification with head-up tilt-table testing. *Cardiol Elderly* 1993;1:221–225.
97. Shihabuddin L, Shehadeh A, Agle D. Syncope as a conversion mechanism. *Psychosomatics* 1994;35:496–498.

98. Kapoor WN, Fortunato M, Hanusa BH, et al. Psychiatric illnesses in patients with syncope. *Am J Med* 1995;99:505–512.
99. Eagle KA, Black HR. Evaluation of patients with syncope.[letter] *N Engl J Med* 1983;309:1650.
100. Johnson RL. Evaluation of patients with syncope.[letter] *N Engl J Med* 1983;309:1650.
101. Silverstein MD, Singer DE, Mulley AG, et al. Patients with syncope admitted to medical intensive care units. *JAMA* 1982;248:1185–1189.
102. Yee R, Klein GJ. Syncope in Wolff-Parkinson-White syndrome: Incidence and electrophysiological correlates. *Pacing Clin Electrophysiol* 1984;7:381–388.
103. Auricchio A, Klein H, Trappe HJ, et al. Lack of prognostic value of syncope in patients with Wolff-Parkinson-White syndrome. *J Am Coll Cardiol* 1991;17:153–158.
104. Nienaber CA, Hiller S, Spielmann RP, et al. Syncope in hypertrophic cardiomyopathy: Multivariate analysis of prognostic determinants. *J Am Coll Cardiol* 1990;15:948–955.
105. Bachinsky WB, Linzer M, Weld L, et al. Usefulness of clinical characteristics in predicting the outcome of electrophysiological studies in unexplained syncope. *Am J Cardiol* 1992;69:1044–1049.
106. Bass EB, Elson JJ, Fogoros RN, et al. Long-term prognosis of patients undergoing electrophysiological studies for syncope of unknown origin. *Am J Cardiol* 1988;62:1186–1191.
107. Denes P, Uretz E, Ezri MD, et al. Clinical predicator of electrophysiological findings in patients with syncope of unknown origin. *Arch Intern Med* 1988;148:1922–1928.
108. Kapoor WN, Hammill SC, Gersh BJ. Diagnosis and natural history of syncope and the role of invasive electrophysiology testing. *Am J Cardiol* 1989;63:730–734.
109. Krol RB, Morady F, Flaker GC, et al. Electrophysiological testing in patients with unexplained syncope: Clinical and noninvasive predictors of outcome. *J Am Coll Cardiol* 1987;10:358–363.
110. Moazez F, Peter T, Simonson J, et al. Syncope of unknown origin: Clinical, noninvasive and electrophysiological determinants of arrhythmia induction and symptom recurrence during long-term follow-up. *Am Heart J* 1991;121:81–88.
111. Prystowsky EN, Knilans TK, Evans JJ. Diagnostic evaluation and treatment strategies for patients at risk for serious cardiac arrhythmias, Part 1: Syncope of unknown origin. *Mod Concepts Cardiovasc Dis* 1991;1991:49–54.
112. Teichman SL, Felder SD, Matos JA, et al. The value of electrophysiological studies in syncope of undetermined origin: Report of 150 cases. *Am Heart J* 1985;110:469–478.
113. DiMarco JP, Garan H, Harthorne JW, et al. Intracardiac electrophysiology techniques in recurrent syncope of unknown cause. *Ann Intern Med* 1981;95:542–548.
114. Morady F. The evaluation of syncope with electrophysiology studies. *Cardiol Clin* 1986;4:515–526.
115. Olshansky B, Hahn E, Hartz V and the ESVEM Investigators. Is Syncope in the ESVEM trial a marker of cardiac arrest of all-cause mortality? *Circulation* 1994;90:I-456.
116. Wilmshurst PT, Willicombe RP, Webb-Peploe MM. Effects of aortic valve replacement on syncope in patients with aortic stenosis. *Br Heart J* 1993;70:542–543.
117. Middlekauff HR, Stevenson WG, Saxon LA. Prognosis after syncope: Impact of left ventricular function. *Am Heart J* 1993;125:121–127.

118. Middlekauff HR, Stevenson WG, Stevenson, LW, et al. Syncope in advanced heart failure: High risk of sudden death regardless of origin of syncope. *J Am Coll Cardiol* 1993;21:110–116.

119. Tchou P, Krebs AC, Sra J, et al. Syncope: A warning sign of sudden death in idiopathic dilated cardiomyopathy patients. *J Am Coll Cardiol* 1991;17:196A.

120. Krahn AD, Klein GJ, Norris C, et al. The etiology of syncope in patients with negative tilt table and electrophysiological testing. *Circulation* 1995;92:1819–1824.

121. Haddad RM, Sellar TD. Syncope as a symptom: A practical approach to etiologic diagnosis. *Postgrad Med* 1986;79:48–62.

122. Noble RJ. The patient with syncope. *JAMA* 1977;237:1372–1376.

123. Martin GJ, Adams SL, Martin HG, et al. Prospective evaluation of syncope. *Ann Emerg Med* 1984;13:499–504.

124. Kenny RA. Syncope. History may be inaccurate in elderly people.[letter] *Br Med J* 1994;309:474.

125. Sutton R, Nathan A, Perrins J, et al. Syncope: A good history is not enough.[letter] *Br Med J* 1994;309:474–475.

126. Taggart P, Carruthers M, Somerville W. Some effects of emotion on the normal and abnormal heart. In: *Current Problems in Cardiology*. Chicago IL: Year Book Medical Publishers, Inc; 1983:2–29.

127. Rowe PC, Bou-Holagah I, Kan JS, et al. Is neurally mediated hypotension an unrecognized cause of chronic fatigue? *Lancet* 1995;345:623–624.

128. Tsutsui M, Matsuguchi T, Tsutsui H, et al. Alcohol-induced sinus bradycardia and hypotension in patients with syncope. *Jpn Heart J* 1992;33:875–879.

129. Kirkman E, Marshall HW, Banks JR, et al. Ethanol augments the baroreflex-inhibitory effects of sciatic nerve stimulation in the anaesthetized dog. *Exp Physiol* 1994;79:81–91.

130. Kettunen RV, Timijarvi J, Heikkila J, et al. The acute dose-dependent effects of ethanol on canine myocardial perfusion. *Alcohol* 1994;11:351–354.

131. Chaudhuri KR, Maule S, Thomaides T, et al. Alcohol ingestion lowers supine blood pressure, causes splanchnic vasodilation and worsens postural hypotension in primary autonomic failure. *J Neurol* 1994;241:145–152.

132. Brackett Dr, Gauvin DV, Lerner MR, et al. Dose- and time-dependent cardiovascular responses inducted by ethanol. *J Pharmacol Exp Ther* 1994;268:78–84.

133. Lu CY, Wang DX, Yu SB. Effects of acute ingestion of ethanol on hemodynamics and hypoxic pulmonary vasoconstriction in dogs: Role of leukotrienes. *J Tongji Med Univ* 1992;12:253–256.

134. Freedland ES, McMicken DB. Alcohol-related seizures, Part I: Pathophysiology, differential diagnosis, and evaluation. *J Emerg Med* 1993;11:463–473.

135. Byrne JM, Marais HJ, Cheek GA. Exercise-induced complete heart block in a patient with chronic bifascicular block. *J Electrocardiol* 1994;27:339–342.

136. Oswald S, Brooks R, O'Nunain SS, et al. Asystole after exercise in healthy persons. *Ann Intern Med* 1994;120:1008–1011.

137. Sakaguchi S, Shultz JJ, Shultz J, et al. Syncope associated with exercise, a manifestation of neurally mediated syncope. *Am J Cardiol* 1995;75:476–481.

138. Williams CC, Bernhardt DT. Syncope in athletes. *Sports Med* 1995;19:223–234.

139. Calkins H, Seifert M, Morady F. Clinical presentation and long-term follow-up of athletes with exercise-induced vasodepressor syncope. *Am Heart J* 1995;139:1159–1164.

140. Leenhardt A, Lucet V, Dejoy I, et al. Catecholaminergic polymorphic ventricular tachycardia in children: A 7-year follow-up of 21 patients. *Circulation* 1995;91:1512–1519.

141. Freed, MD. Advances in the diagnosis and therapy of syncope and palpitations in children. *Curr Opin Pediatr* 1994;6:368–372.
142. Nakajima T, Misu K, Iwasawa K, et al. Auditory stimuli as a major cause of syncope in a patient with idiopathic long QT syndrome. *Jpn Circ J* 1995;59:241–246.
143. Kushner JA, Kou WA, Kadish AH, et al. Natural history with unexplained syncope and a non-diagnostic electrophysiological study. *J Am Coll Cardiol* 1989;14:391–396.
144. Evans RW. Neurological aspects of hyperventilation syndrome. *Semin Neurol* 1995;15:115–125.
145. Nixon GF. Hyperventilation and cardiac symptoms. *Intern Med* 1989;10:67–84.
146. Aita JF. Etiology of syncope in 100 patients with associated pale facial appearance. *Nebr Med J* 1993;1:182–183.
147. Martin GJ, Adams SL, Martin HG. Evaluation of patients with syncope.[letter] *N Engl J Med* 1983;309:1650.
148. Dhingra RC, Denes P, Wu D, et al. Syncope in patients with chronic bifascicular block: Significance, causative mechanisms and clinical implications. *Ann Intern Med* 1974;81:302–306.
149. McAnulty JH, Rahimtoola SH, Murphy E, et al. Natural history of "high-risk" bundle- branch block: Final report of a prospective study. *N Engl J Med* 1982;307:137–143.
150. Morady F, Higgins J, Peters RW, et al. Electrophysiological testing in bundle branch block and unexplained syncope. *Am J Cardiol* 1984;54:587–591.
151. Click RL, Gersh BJ, Sugrue DD, et al. Role of invasive electrophysiological testing in patients with symptomatic bundle branch block. *Am J Cardiol* 1987;59:817–823.
152. Ezri M, Lerman BB, Marchlinski FE, et al. Electrophysiological evaluation of syncope in patients with bifascicular block. *Am Heart J* 1983;106:693–697.
153. Englund A, Bergfeldt L, Rehnqvist N, et al. Diagnostic value of programmed ventricular stimulation in patients with bifascicular block: A prospective study of patients with and without syncope. *J Am Coll Cardiol* 1995;26:1508–1515.
154. Gang ES, Peter T, Rosenthal PT, et al. Detection of late potentials on the surface electrocardiogram in unexplained syncope. *Am J Cardiol* 1986;58:1014–1020.
155. Winters SL, Stewart D, Targonski A, et al. Signal averaging of the surface QRS complex predicts inducibility of ventricular tachycardia in patients with syncope of unknown origin: A prospective study. *J Am Coll Cardiol* 1987;10:775–781.
156. Kuchar DL, Thornburn CW, Sammel NL. Signal-averaged electrocardiogram for evaluation or recurrent syncope. *Am J Cardiol* 1986;58:949–953.
157. Ben-Chetrit E, Flugelman M, Eliakim M. Syncope: A retrospective study of 101 hospitalized patients. *Isr J Med Sci* 1985;21:950–953.
158. Graff L, Mucci D, Radford MJ. Decision to hospitalize: Objective diagnosis related group criteria versus clinical judgement. *Ann Emerg Med* 1988;17:943–952.
159. Mozes B, Confino-Cohen R, Halkin H. Cost-effectiveness of in-hospital evaluation of patients with syncope. *Isr J Med Sci* 1988;24:302–306.
160. Kenny RA, Bayliss J, Ingram A, et al. Head-up tilt: A useful test for investigating unexplained syncope. *Lancet* 1986;1:1352–1354.
161. Almquist A, Goldenberg IF, Milstein S, et al. Provocation of bradycardia and hypotension by isoproterenol and upright posture in patients with unexplained syncope. *N Engl J Med* 1989;320:346–352.

162. Abboud FM. Ventricular syncope: Is the heart a sensory organ? *N Engl J Med* 1989;320:390–392.

163. Rea RF, Thames MD. Neural control mechanisms and vasovagal syncope. *J Cardiovasc Electrophys* 1993;4:587–595.

164. Kosinski DJ, Wolfe DA, Grubb BP. Neurocardiogenic syncope: A review of pathophysiology, diagnosis, and treatment. *Cardiovascular Reviews & Reports* 1993;21–23.

165. Samoil D, Grubb BP. Vasovagal (neurally mediated) syncope: Pathophysiology, diagnosis, and therapeutic approach. *Eur JCPE* 1992;4:234–241.

166. Wiley TM, O'Donoghue S, Platia EV, et al. Neurocardiogenic syncope: Evaluation and management. *Cardiovascular Reviews & Reports* 1993;14:12–25.

167. Benditt DG, Ferguson DW, Grubb BP, et al. Tilt table testing for assessing syncope: ACC expert consensus document. *J Am Coll Cardiol* 1996;28:263–275.

168. Kapoor WN, Brant N. Evaluation of syncope by upright tilt testing with isoproterenol: A nonspecific test. *Ann Intern Med* 1992;116:358–363.

169. Boudoulas H, Geleris P, Schaal SF, et al. Comparison between electrophysiological studies and ambulatory monitoring in patients with syncope. *J Electrocardiol* 1983;16:91–96.

170. Clark PI, Glasser SP, Spoto E. Arrhythmias detected by ambulatory monitoring: Lack of correlation with symptoms of dizziness and syncope. *Chest* 1980; 77:722–725.

171. Gibson TC, Heitzman MR. Diagnostic efficacy of 24-hour electrocardiographic monitoring for syncope. *Am J Cardiol* 1984;53:1013–1017.

172. Lacroix D, Dubuc M, Kus T, et al. Evaluation of arrhythmic causes of syncope: Correlation between Holter monitoring, electrophysiological testing, and body surface mapping. *Am Heart J* 1991;122:1346–1354.

173. Zeldis SM, Levine BJ, Michelson EL, et al. Cardiovascular complaints: Correlation with cardiac arrhythmias on 24-hour electrocardiographic monitoring. *Chest* 1980;78:456–462.

174. Gordon M, Huang M, Gryfe CI. An evaluation of falls, syncope and dizziness by prolonged ambulatory cardiographic monitoring in a geriatric institutional setting. *J Am Geriatr Soc* 1982;30:6–12.

175. Linzer M, Prystowsky EN, Brunetti LL, et al. Recurrent syncope of unknown origin diagnosed by ambulatory continuous loop ECG recording. *Am Heart J* 1988;116:1632–1634.

176. Akhtar M, Shenasa M, Denker S, et al. Role of cardiac electrophysiological studies in patients with unexplained recurrent syncope. *Pacing Clin Electrophysiol* 1983;6:192–201.

177. Denes P, Ezri, M. The role of electrophysiological studies in the management of patients with unexplained syncope. *Pacing Clin Electrophysiol* 1985;8:424–435.

178. DiMarco JP. Electrophysiological studies in patients with unexplained syncope. *Circulation* 1987;75:III140–III145.

179. Doherty JU, Pembrook-Rogers D, Grogan EW, et al. Electrophysiological evaluation and follow-up characteristics of patients with recurrent unexplained syncope and presyncope. *Am J Cardiol* 1985;55:703–708.

180. Fisher JD. Role of electrophysiological testing in the diagnosis and treatment of patients with known and suspected bradycardias and tachycardias. *Prog Cardiovasc Dis* 1981;24:25–90.

181. Fujimura O, Yee R, Klein GJ, et al. The diagnostic sensitivity of electrophysiological testing in patients with syncope caused by transient bradycardia. *N Engl J Med* 1989;321:1703–1707.

182. Reiffel JA, Wang P, Bower R, et al. Electrophysiological testing in patients with recurrent syncope: Are results predicted by prior ambulatory monitoring? *Am Heart J* 1985;110:1146–1153.
183. Gulamhusein S, Naccarelli GB, Ko PT, et al. Value and limitations of clinical electrophysiological study in assessment of patients with unexplained syncope. *Am J Med* 1985;73:700–705.
184. Gann D, Tolentino A, Samet P. Electrophysiological evaluation of elderly patients with sinus bradycardia: A long-term follow-up study. *Ann Intern Med* 1979;90:24–29.
185. Wilber DW, Kall J, Olshansky B, Scanlon P. Pacing-induced infra-His block in patients with syncope of unknown origin: Incidence and clinical significance. *Pacing Clin Electrophysiol* 1990;13:562A.
186. Kaul U, Dev V, Narula J, et al. Evaluation of patients with bundle branch block and "unexplained" syncope: A study based on comprehensive electrophysiological testing and ajmaline stress. *Pacing Clin Electrophysiol* 1988;11:289–297.
187. Klein GJ, Gersh BJ, Yee R. Electrophysiological testing: The final court of appeal for diagnosis of syncope? *Circulation* 1995;92:1332–1335.
188. Aonuma K, Iesaka Y, Gosselin AJ, et al. Cardiac syncope: An exhibiting dichotomy beteewn clinical impression and electrophysioloigc evaluation. *Pacing Clin Electrophysiol* 1986;9:178–187.
189. Masrani K, Cowley C, Bekheit S, et al. Recurrent syncope for over a decade due to idiopathic ventricular fibrillation. *Chest* 1994;106:1601–1603.
190. Rattes MF, Klein GJ, Sharma AD, et al. Efficacy of empirical cardiac pacing in syncope of unknown cause. *Can Med Assoc J* 1989;140:381–385.
191. Proyclemer A, Facchin D, Sternotti G, et al. Value of pacemaker treatment in patients with syncope of unknown origin. *New Trends Arrhyt* 1990;6:323–332.
192. Kwoh CK, Beck JR, Pauker SG, et al. Repeated syncope with negative diagnostic evaluation. *Med Decis Making* 1984;4:351–377.
193. Shaw DB, Kekwick CA, Veale D, Whistance TW. Unexplained syncope: A diagnostic pacemaker? *Pacing Clin Electrophysiol* 1983;6:720–725.
194. Fisher M, Cotter L. Recurrent syncope of unknown origin: Value of permanent pacemaker insertion. *Int J Cardiol* 1995;51:93–97.
195. Raviele A, Gasparini G, Di Pede F et al. Usefulness of head-up tilt test in evaluating patients with syncope of unknown origin and negative electrophysiologicalal study. *Am J Cardiol* 1990;65:1322–1327.
196. Muller T, Roy D, Talajic, et al. Electrophysiologic evaluation and outcome of patients with syncope of unknown origin. *Eur Heart J* 1991;12:139–143.
  a. Kapoor WN, Hanusa BH. Is syncope a risk factor for poor outcomes? Comparison of patients with and without syncope. *Am J Med* 1996;100:646–655.
  b. Benditt DG, Remole S, Milstein S, Bailin. Syncope: Casues, clinical evaluation and current therapy. *Ann Rev Med* 1992;43:283–300.
  c. Martin TP, Hanusa BH, Kapoor WN. Risk stratification of patients with syncope. *Ann Emerg Med* 1997;29:459–466.

Neurocardiogenic Syncope

Blair P. Grubb, MD

Introduction

The term neurocardiogenic syncope (also called vasovagal or neurally mediated syncope) is used to describe episodes of transient centrally mediated hypotension and bradycardia that ultimately lead to loss of consciousness. Neurocardiogenic syncope may take many forms, ranging from the common faint to a sudden dramatic loss of consciousness indistinguishable from Stokes-Adams attacks, and possibly even to sudden death. Often, the individuals who suffer from these disorders exhibit no evidence of underlying structural heart disease or of abnormalities in the cardiac conducting system.

Until relatively recently, patients with recurrent unexplained syncope were routinely subjected to a long and expensive battery of tests that often included glucose tolerance testing, Holter monitoring, cranial computed tomography, electroencephalography, exercise tolerance testing, and electrophysiological studies.[1] Yet despite these extensive evaluations (that cost up to $16,000 per patient), in up to 50% of patients, a diagnosis was never arrived at.[2,3] Linzer and colleagues[4] report that the degree of functional impairment suffered by these individuals with recurrent unexplained syncope is not dissimilar to that observed in chronic debilitating disorders such as rheumatoid arthritis. Recurrent syncopal episodes also placed the patient at risk for bodily trauma secondary to falls, and syncope while driving a motor vehicle could have disastrous consequences.[5] In the elderly, a single syncopal episode may result in injuries sufficiently profound that the patient may require permanent nursing home placement, at a tremendous cost to the individual and to society as a whole.

From Grubb BP, Olshansky B (eds.). *Syncope: Mechanisms and Management.* Armonk, NY: Futura Publishing Co., Inc.; © 1998.

A number of investigators had, for some time, postulated that transient episodes of centrally mediated hypotension and bradycardia could be responsible for many of these episodes. However, until recently, there was no effective means of reproducing these episodes and thereby confirming the diagnosis. In addition, many aspects of these disorders were shrouded in mystery due to the relative inability to consistently observe spontaneous events.

To uncover an individual's predisposition to these episodes of centrally mediated hypotension and bradycardia, investigators proposed that a strong orthostatic stimulus such as prolonged upright posture be used. Since the landmark study in 1986 by Kenny et al,[6] numerous centers around the world have reported that head upright tilt table testing appears to be a safe and effective means of revealing an individual's predisposition to neurocardiogenic events. At the same time, the ability to provoke these episodes in a controlled setting has afforded a unique opportunity to directly observe and record the events that occur during syncope, allowing for a marked enhancement in our knowledge of this disorder.[7] This chapter deals with our current understanding of the pathophysiology of neurocardiogenic syncope, its clinical manifestations, and the use of tilt table testing in diagnosis, as well as potential therapeutic options available for the treatment of these disorders.

Pathophysiology of Neurocardiogenic Syncope

Fainting has been observed in all peoples throughout history, and speculations as to its origins are centuries old. John Hunter,[8] in 1773, observed patients who would faint during phlebotomy (a common practice at the time) and suggested that vasodilation may play an important role. In 1888, a brilliant report by Foster[9] noted that during spontaneous syncopal spells, profound bradycardia sometimes occurred, which he felt lowered cerebral blood flow to a level inadequate to maintain consciousness. In 1932 Sir Thomas Lewis[10] observed that although the bradycardia associated with syncope could be reversed by the administration of atropine, hypotension and loss of consciousness would still occur. The concurrence of both a vasodilatory and bradycardic component led to his use of the neurological "vasovagal" to describe this phenomenon.

Starting in the 1940s, physiologists began to explore the human body's response to changes in position, with later investigators focusing on the body's response to the stresses of aviation and the microgravity environment of space travel. During this period, head upright tilt table testing came into use in order to provide a controlled setting in which the body's responses to incremental changes in position could be carefully observed and recorded.[11] Based on these observations it has become well established that in the normal subject, the assumption of upright posture leads to a gravity-mediated displacement of blood downward, with pooling in the lower extremities. This has been found to be accompanied by a compensatory increase in both heart rate and peripheral vascular resistance.[12] Recent investigations have confirmed these observations. Mehdirad et al[13] performed echocardiography during tilt table testing on 17 subjects. They noted no differences in left ventricular volume or cardiac output between subjects at rest. After upright tilt, significant changes began to appear at 10 minutes. Subjects who went on to develop syncope also went on to develop marked decrease in left ventricular end-systolic and end-diastolic volumes when compared to nonsyncopal subjects, an observation consistent with peripheral venous pooling. Similar findings are reported by El-Bedawi and Hainsworth[14,15] by use of a combination of head-up tilt and lower body negative pressure on a series of patients. Here tilt table testing produced a decrease in cardiac output of approximately 1.4 L/min, again suggesting peripheral sequestration of blood.

The reduction in blood pressure produced by this downward displacement of blood is sensed by arterial baroreceptors, which are scattered throughout the vasculature but located principally in the aortic arch and carotid sinus.[16] These receptors send afferent signals to the medulla, where they communicate with the nucleus ambiguous and dorsal motor nucleus of the vagus nerve (governing parasympathetic activity) and the costal ventromedial and ventrolateral medulla (governing sympathetic activity).[17] During increased arterial pressure, there is a greater degree of stretch on these receptors with an increase in receptor afferent transmission, leading to a centrally mediated decrease in sympathetic tone with a subsequent reduction in heart rate. Reductions in arterial blood pressure have the opposite effect. The heart itself functions as a part of this baroreflex activity by virtue of the presence of mechanoreceptors (or C-fibers), consisting of unmyelinated fibers found in the atria, ventricles (particularly in the inferoposterior aspect of the left ventricle), and the pulmonary artery.[18] Although C-fibers seem to respond to either stretch or pressure, stretch activations appear to be more important. These fibers send afferent projections centrally to the dorsal vagal nucleus of the brain stem. As with arterial baroreceptors, a decrease in C-fiber output results in a reflex increase in sympathetic stimulation. Therefore, the normal response to upright posture is an increase in heart rate, an increase in diastolic pressure, and an unchanged or slightly decreased systolic blood pressure.[12]

Although the exact processes involved in the production of neurocardiogenic syncope remain the subject of considerable debate, some basic mechanisms have been elaborated.[7] To date, most investigators have felt that excessive venous pooling associated with upright posture results in central hypovolemia, causing an abrupt fall in venous return to the heart. This sudden reduction in ventricular volume is thought to result in extremely vigorous ventricular contractions, which in turn cause the activation of a large number of C-fibers that would normally respond to mechanical stretch. The resultant surge in afferent neural traffic to the medulla is thought to mimic the conditions seen during hypertension, thereby resulting in an apparent "paradoxic" sympathetic withdrawal with bradycardia and hypotension. Studies by use of echocardiography during tilt have tended to support this contention.[19]

Some investigators, however, have voiced reservations concerning the aforementioned hypothesis. In animal studies, surgical denervation of the heart did not prevent sudden sympathetic withdrawal during sudden blood volume reduction.[20] In addition, both Fitzpatrick et al[22] and Lightfoot et al[21] report neurocardiogenic hypotension and bradycardia during orthostatic stress in patients who had received orthotopic heart transplants. Since mechanoreceptor C-fibers have also been identified in the atria and pulmonary arteries, these observations do not exclude their contribution to neurocardiogenic syncope. Waxman et al[23] and Rudas et al[24] also point out that vagal afferent reinnervation of the donor hearts may have occurred. Vasodilators have also been reported to provoke syncope in transplant recipients.[25]

In considering the aforementioned observations, it is important to realize that activation of ventricular mechanoreceptors is not the only mechanism that has been shown to provoke neurocardiogenic syncope. Using a cat model, Lofring[26] found that direct electrical stimulation of the anterior cingulate gyrus of the limbic system can trigger a vasovagal response. In humans, syncope is well known to be provoked by strong emotion or by a stimulus such as the sight of blood. Temporal lobe epilepsy has been shown to provoke vasovagal episodes.[27] These observations suggest that higher neural centers may also participate in the provocation of neurocardiogenic syncope.

An alternative hypothesis concerning the mechanism of neurocardiogenic syncope was recently advanced by Dickenson.[28] Previous observations have demonstrated that when the intraluminal pressure within the carotid artery falls to near zero, the rate of discharge of the carotid sinus baroreceptors increases.[29] Dickenson postulates that a similar process may occur in the atria and great veins; when the fall in intrathoracic pressure exceeds atrial and venous filling pressure, the venoarterial stretch receptors exhibit a comparable "collapse firing." This sudden increase in afferent nerve traffic could thereby elicit a similar type of "paradoxic" sympathetic withdrawal. Evidence supporting this theory has come from a study of eight heart-lung transplant patients (in whom afferent nerve projections have been severed), none of whom had vasovagal reactions during tilt.[30] However this observation may have resulted from the use of a less aggressive tilt protocol than that of other studies.

The term "vasovagal" was initially applied to the process of fainting because of the perception that parasympathetic activity was felt to predominate.[10] Although parasympathetic activity does appear to increase somewhat during syncope (and is responsible for the observed bradycardia), the principal phenomenon responsible for loss of consciousness is vasodilation resulting in hypotension.[31] Several studies have reported that while the administration of atropine or cardiac pacing will eliminate bradycardia, it will seldom prevent syncope.[10,32]

The first detailed investigations into the neurophysiological mechanisms involved in neurocardiogenic syncope are reported by Öberg and Thorén.[33] They used an open-chest cat preparation and caused sudden hemorrhagic hypovolemia. A marked initial tachycardia was found to be an essential component of ventricular C-fiber stimulation. Later Wallin and Sundlöff[34] were able to record peripheral autonomic nervous system activity during neurocardiogenic syncope from peroneal nerve fascicles by use of microelectrodes.[34] Sympathetic activity was initially noted to increase, followed by a dramatic decrease at the onset of syncope. Sra et al[35] have demonstrated that during the initial phases of upright tilt-induced syncope, both norepinephrine and epinephrine increase. Consistent with the previous observations, at the onset of syncope plasma epinephrine levels were noted to increase while norepinephrine levels fell. Lewis et al[36] also report that peripheral sympathetic inhibition was demonstrated prior to syncope induced by either head-up tilt or lower-body negative pressure.

Therefore, the initial fall in central blood volume due to peripheral venous pooling provokes a reflex increase in sympathetic output with resultant tachycardia and vasoconstrictions, in an apparent effort to maintain normal hemodynamics. Yet this very increase in sympathetic tone may both sensitize and facilitate activation of the cardiac mechanoreceptors that have been implicated in the production of vasovagal events.[37] The paroxysmal increase in neural traffic seen during vigorous ventricular contraction (or from C-fiber activation by myocardial ischemia and reperfusion) leads to a sudden centrally mediated sympathetic withdrawal with peripheral sympathetic inhibition followed by vasodilation.[38] There may also be some aspect of decreased α-receptor responsiveness or increased β-receptor responsiveness involved.[18,31]

The central mechanisms that contribute to the production of neurocardiogenic syncope are still unclear, but have been the subject of several recent investigations. Studies on the hemodynamic and neuroendocrine responses to acute hypovolemia in conscious mammals (a condition most investigators feel is roughly analogous to neurocardiogenic syncope) have tended to focus on the contributions of two substances: endogenous opioids and serotonin.[7] By use of a rat model, evidence has been generated that suggests that the vasodepressor response to hemorrhage appears to be centrally mediated by endogenous opiates.[31] Inhibition of renal sympathetic nerve activity occurs if opiate receptor antagonists are given during hypotensive hemorrhage in rabbits.[39] It has also been reported that the intracisternal administration of naloxone (an opiate receptor antagonist) can block the vasodilatory response seen during acute hemorrhage in rabbits.[40] Ferguson et al[41] report that in humans, naloxone augments the cardiopulmonary baroreflex activation of sympathetic activity. In addition, two studies have found significant increases in plasma β-endorphin levels prior to tilt-induced syncope.[42,43] Unfortunately in humans, opiate antagonists have not been reported to prevent vasodepressor syncope during lower-body negative pressure; however this may, in part, be due to the fact that the dosages of naloxone used were proportionally many times lower than those used during animal studies.[44,45]

Serotonin (5-hydroxytryptamine or 5-HT) is a biologic amine widely distributed throughout the nervous system.[46] Serotonin has long been recognized to play an important role in blood pressure regulation.[47] The application of serotonin directly to the brain (through the lateral ventricle) results in inhibition of efferent sympathetic activity, whereas the direct administration of serotonin into the nucleus tractus solitari causes parasympathetic stimulation and bradycardia as well as sympathetic withdrawal.[48,49] Abboud[50] reports that the administration of intracerebroventricular serotonin induces hypotension, inhibition of renal sympathetic nerve activity, and excitation of adrenal sympathetic nerve activity. In normal volunteers, the administration of $5HT_1$ receptor-activating compounds results in profound sympathetic blockage.[51] Serotonin has also been shown to be an important modulator of the responses seen during acute hemorrhage. Using a cat model, Elam et al[52] found that depletion of serotonin stores blunts the vasodilatory response to hemorrhage. Other studies have found that the administration of the serotonin receptor blocker methysergide during acute blood loss produces a marked pressor effect. Hasser[53] reports that methysergide can increase blood pressure when administered to conscious animals made hypotensive during acute hemorrhage. Based on these and other observations, Morgan[54] suggests that sympathoinhibitory mechanisms in the central nervous system may be stimulated during acute hemorrhage.

Data confirming the role of serotonergic activity in neurocardiogenic syncope are provided by Theodorakis et al.[55] Based on the fact that changes in central serotonergic activity influence the release of prolactin and cortisol, they measured the serum content of these hormones in 28 patients with recurrent syncope who underwent tilt table testing. Nine patients experienced syncope during the test while 19 did not. Cortisol and prolactin levels were significantly increased only in tilt-positive patients. Interestingly, they note that the patterns of release of these hormones during syncope appeared quite similar to those caused by drugs that activate central serotonergic neurons (clomipramine and fenfluramine), suggesting an important role for serotonin in neurocardiogenic syncope.

There are at least 14 distinct types of serotonin receptors in the central nervous system, with different receptors postulated to govern various functions. Matzen et al[56] evaluated the effects of various specific serotonin receptor blockers during upright tilt-induced syncope. They found that methysergide (a $5HT_1 + _2$ receptor antagonist) and ondansetron (a $5HT_3$ receptor antagonist) attenuate the sympathetic response to head-up tilt as reflected in the blunting in the aforementioned increases in plasma catecholamine levels.

Grubb and associates[57] have found that the use of serotonin reuptake inhibitors can be an effective treatment in patients suffering from severe recurrent neurocardiogenic syncope. These agents, as opposed to the tricyclic antidepressant compounds, are characterized by highly selective serotonin reuptake inhibition with little or no affinity for adrenergic, cholinergic, or histamine receptors. As extracellular serotonin levels increase, 5HT neuronal release is attenuated and impulse transmission velocity increases, both contributing to a progressive decrease in postsynaptic receptor density ("downregulation").[46] This downregulation in postsynaptic receptor density is thought to blunt the potential responses to rapid shifts in central serotonin levels and thereby reduce the ability for such surges to result in abrupt sympathetic withdrawal.

Recent studies also suggest a role for nitric oxide in the regulation of sympathetic tone, however at present there is insufficient data to fully comment on this possibility.[58] The potential role of the responses of the cerebral vasculature during neurocardiogenic syncope has also been explored. It was previously believed that cerebral autoregulation of cerebral blood flow occurred solely at the local arteriolar level in response to arterial pressure changes: arteriolar vasoconstriction during peripheral blood pressure increases and vasodilation following systemic pressure decreases. However, recent studies by Grubb et al,[59] Janosik et al,[60] Gomez et al,[61] and Njemanze[62] using transcranial Doppler ultrasonography have generated considerable evidence that during upright tilt-induced neurocardiogenic syncope, a paradoxic intense cerebral vasoconstriction (rather than the expected vasodilation) occurs in the face of increasing hypotension. Kaminer et al[63] also demonstrate significant abnormalities in cerebral hemodynamics in children during head-up tilt-induced syncope.[62] These apparently "paradoxic" changes would suggest that sudden alterations in cerebral vascular resistance (arteriolar vasoconstriction) might play a significant role in the production of neurocardiogenic syncope. Fredman et al[64] and Gomez et al[61] both recently reported that syncope may occur on the basis of cerebral vascular changes alone. Further studies will be necessary to better clarify this phenomenon.

Clinical Aspects of Neurocardiogenic Syncope

As mentioned in the introduction, neurocardiogenic syncope may have a wide variety of presentations. Indeed there seem to exist a number of triggers that may all ultimately result in neurocardiogenically mediated hypotension and bradycardia. The postprandial state, upright posture, vigorous exercise in warm environments, sodium restriction or diuretic use, and emotional or stressful situations are a few of the important triggers to consider. Alcohol is well recognized to increase predisposition to these events. Rapid changes in time zones during air travel (jet lag) also seem to exacerbate these tendencies.

There are typically three identifiable phases to an event: presyncope or aura, the actual loss of consciousness, and the postsyncopal period. Patients with the more classic forms of vasovagal syncope will often give a longstanding history of recurrent events ("easy fainters"). The situations that provoke fainting in this group are those that are most likely to cause fear, emotional distress, anxiety, and anticipation (the very events that are most likely to result in increased sympathetic nervous system stimulation). A somewhat similar response is seen in some animal species when they are placed in life-threatening situations in which neither "fight" nor "flight" is possible. These animals have then been observed to experience loss of sympathetic tone, leading to vasodilation, bradycardia, and resultant loss of motion; in effect they "play dead."[65]

During the aura phase, the typical warning phenomena often include weakness, diaphoresis, epigastric discomfort, dizziness/vertigo, visual blurring, palpitations, headache, nausea, and vomiting. These prodromal symptoms may last anywhere from less than 1 second to several minutes, giving the patient who recognizes them an opportunity to lie down and ward off (or lessen the severity of) an event. Linzer et al[66] have analyzed the frequency of presyncopal symptoms in a large number of patients, finding that the most common were dizziness (44%), weakness (44%), blurred vision (33%), sweating (33%), nausea (29%), and abdominal discomfort (11%).

The actual loss of consciousness is usually not remembered by the patient. Observers who witness a syncopal episode will often report that the patient appeared pale or ashen in color, with cold skin and profuse sweating, dilated pupils, and rarely urinary (or even fecal) incontinence.[67] The sign that often seems to make the greatest impression on observers is the appearance of tonic and/or clonic movements. The appearance of convulsions indicates that the cerebral anoxic threshold has been reached, allowing an acute "decortication" to occur. These movements usually (but not always) begin after loss of consciousness with a tonic contraction of extended legs, extended arms in adduction, and elevation and backward throw of the head (opisthotonos).[68] These are in contrast to the sequence of decreasing frequency and increasing amplitude that are characteristic of the tonic/clonic grand mal seizures of epilepsy. The loss of consciousness itself is usually short, with rapid recovery and little, if any, postictal period of confusion. Although mentally clear, during the postsyncopal period, patients may complain of nervousness, nausea, headache, or dizziness.[69]

While the aforementioned description holds for many patients with neurocardiogenic syncopal episodes, it is important to realize that many patients will have atypical presentations as well. Some patients (particularly many older ones) will give no history of any prodrome whatsoever, describing a "drop attack" that may mimic Adams-Stokes syncope secondary to atrioventricular block. The abruptness of these episodes may lead to severe injury due to the trauma associated with falling. This is of particular concern in older patients, where falls are an important cause of both morbidity and mortality. Even though the majority of patients are unconscious for a brief period of time (seconds), in some patients the period of loss of consciousness may be prolonged, lasting up to 15 minutes. In occasional patients, the convulsive movements seen during the syncopal episode may be remarkably similar to those of an epileptic seizure, and episodes may be associated with incontinence or a prolonged postictal period.[70]

There are patients in whom the sudden vagally mediated fall in blood pressure and heart rate will be sufficient to produce symptoms of cerebral hypoperfusion, but will not be sufficient to produce full loss of consciousness. These individuals will often present with complaints of severe dizziness, lightheadedness, vertigo, and disequilibrium, and are frequently referred to an otolaryngologist for evaluation.[71] In elderly patients, neurocardiogenic hypotension may cause periods of focal neurological dysfunction that can appear remarkably similar to transient ischemic attacks.[72] Patients may experience disorientation, dysarthria, and even visual field cuts.

Controversy exists over whether neurocardiogenic syncope may be lethal. In Europe, the term "malignant" is applied to episodes of neurocardiogenic syncope that occur without warning and result in bodily injury.[73] In North America the term "malignant" is applied to episodes of neurocardiogenic syncope associated with prolonged cardiac asystole.[74] Both spontaneous and tilt-induced episodes of neurocardiogenic asystole have lasted as long as 73 seconds, and there is at least one reported episode of sustained polymorphic ventricular tachycardia induced during upright tilt.[75] Episodes of near-fatal cardiac asystole have occurred during tilt table testing.[76] Engle[77] and others have postulated that prolonged asystole may degenerate into ventricular fibrillation and death, particularly in those individuals with preexistent coronary disease and myocardial dysfunction.[77] At The Medical College of Ohio, we have seen several patients who were resuscitated from apparent sudden death episodes, in whom the only abnormality found (despite extensive evaluations) was reproducible neurocardiogenic asystole.

In general, younger patients, adolescents in particular, tend to have more classic presentations while atypical presentations are more frequent in older patients. In adolescents, there is often a history of a rapid growth spurt in the period just preceding the first syncopal episode. It is not uncommon for these tendencies to run in families. Often, even frequent and severe syncopal spells that begin in adolescence will spontaneously abate by the time the patient reaches his mid-twenties. In young women there is a definite tendency for these episodes to be more frequent around the time of the menstrual cycle, in particular during the premenstrual period. Patients who suffered from recurrent syncope during adolescence, which later resolved, may begin to experience recurrences during or immediately following pregnancy.

Linzer et al[78] describe an increased incidence of neuropsychiatric disorders in patients suffering from recurrent neurocardiogenic syncope. The three most common disorders are major depression, somatization disorder, and panic disorders, (the latter being more common among female patients). Patients with recurrent neurocardiogenic syncope have also been noted to have an increased incidence of neurosomatic disorders such as chronic vascular headaches or migraine headaches as well as functional gastrointestinal conditions such as peptic ulcer disease, unstable bowel syndrome, and indigestion. Recent reports provide evidence for a link between neurocardiogenic hypotension and chronic fatigue syndrome.[79] Indeed, one of the more common complaints of the patients with neurocardiogenic syncope at our institution is fatigue.

Clinical reproduction of the syncopal or near syncopal event is important in establishing the diagnosis and the responses to therapy. Over the years, a number of maneuvers were used to trigger vagal reactions. These included carotid sinus compression, Weber and Valsalva maneuvers, hyperventilation, and ocular compression. However, these techniques were ultimately abandoned due to their relatively low sensitivity and weak correlation with clinical events.

Head-Upright Tilt Table Testing

Until relatively recently, the diagnosis of neurocardiogenic syncope was made principally by history and a process of exclusion, mainly because there was no effective laboratory technique for reproducing episodes and thereby confirming the diagnosis. To address this difficulty, it was reasoned that a potent orthostatic stimulus, such as prolonged upright posture, could be used to produce a state of maximal venous pooling, thus provoking the previously described responses in susceptible individuals. As mentioned previously, tilt tables were first used by physiologists to study compensatory changes produced during movement from the supine to the head-upright position. During the course of these studies, it was noted that a small proportion of the subjects studied developed hypotension and bradycardia of a degree sufficient to result in fainting.[80] Despite these observations, tilt table testing was not used as a potential diagnostic modality for neurocardiogenic syncope until the groundbreaking report by Kenny et al[6] report in 1986. Since then, a number of reports have appeared, attesting to the utility of the test to reproduce syncopal episodes in patients who are prone to neurocardiogenic hypotension and bradycardia.

Several observations can be cited to support the concept that a "positive head-up tilt table test" is for the most part equivalent to spontaneously occurring episodes.[81] Principal among these observations is the fact that both spontaneous and tilt-induced syncopal episodes are associated with virtually identical signs, as well symptoms such as nausea, lightheadedness, pallor, diaphoresis, and loss of postural tone. In addition, the temporal sequence of heart rate and blood pressure changes noted during tilt-induced syncope are for the most part the same as those reported during spontaneous episodes. The plasma catecholamine changes alluded to previously are similar in both spontaneous and tilt-induced episodes, with rapid surges in plasma epinephrine occurring prior to loss of consciousness. Finally, tilt table testing has been able to reproduce spontaneously occurring episodes of asystole in patients with negative electrophysiological studies, (see Figure 4).[74]

Two principal methods of tilt table testing have evolved, both of which are simple, safe, and inexpensive. The first uses a passive tilt for a period of 45 minutes at an angle between 60° and 80°. No provocative pharmacological agents are used. The second method frequently uses a shorter period of upright tilt in association with a variety of provocative agents to facilitate the induction of syncope. A number of agents have been used, including isoproterenol, nitroglycerin, edrophonium, and adenosine.

Early studies indicated that the use of a tilt angle less than 60° is associated with a loss of sensitivity, while angles of 80° or more are believed to produce a loss of specificity.[83] Initial studies using tilt table testing revealed that the test only rarely provoked syncope in normal subjects. Shvartz et al[83,84] note only three syncopal episodes among a total of 36 subjects tilted at an angle of 70° for 20 minutes, while Vogt et al[85] note only two episodes of syncope during 64 tilts at 70° among nine healthy male volunteers.[83-85] Fitzpatrick et al[82] note only two (7%) episodes of syncope among 27 normal control subjects tilted at 60° for 60 minutes, while only five (15%) of 34 patients with syncope known to be due to conduction system disease had positive tests.[82] The use of a 60° tilt for 60 minutes has become known as the Westminster protocol, and has an apparent specificity of 91% and a positive yield of 27% to 75% with a mean of about 50%.[86]

The response to head-up tilt, of patients with a history of recurrent syncope thought to be neurocardiogenic in nature is quite different. The initial report by Kenny et al[6] found that 10 of 15 patients (67%) suffering from unexplained syncope had a positive response after a mean of 29±19 minutes upright. Strasberg et al[87] studied 40 patients with recurrent unexplained syncope (as well as 10 normal controls) with a 60° tilt for 60 minutes. Syncope that was the same as that experienced clinically was produced in 15 patients (38%) after a mean tilt time of 42±12 minutes. Similar results were obtained by Raviele et al[88] in 30 patients with unexplained syncope, also using a 60° tilt for 60 minutes. Fifteen patients (50%) had syncope similar to the clinical episodes provoked, whereas eight concomitant controls were asymptomatic. A larger study by Abi-Samra et al[89] reports reproduction of syncope similar to that experienced clinically in 63 of 154 patients undergoing tilt table testing.

Following observations that endogenous catecholamine levels increase prior to syncope, some investigators postulate that the infusion of the catecholamine-like substance isoproterenol may increase the sensitivity of the test. This concept was first evaluated by Almquist et al.[90] In this study, only 5 of 24 patients with recurrent idiopathic syncope had positive responses during the initial baseline tilt. However, after retilt with a concomitant isoproterenol infusion, an additional nine patients had positive responses. Comparable results are reported by Grubb et al.[91] and Pongiglione.[92] Sheldon et al[93] have used a single upright tilt with a concomitant isoproterenol infusion of 5 μg/min for 10 minutes, with similar outcomes.[93] However, Kapoor[94] et al raise questions as to whether the potential increase in sensitivity seen with isoproterenol use may result in a decrease in sensitivity.

Several recent studies have sought to address this point. Morillo et al[95] evaluated 120 patients with recurrent syncope, 30 healthy controls, and 30 patients with documented syncope not related to a vasodepressor reaction. Each underwent a 60° head-up tilt for 15 minutes, followed by an infusion of isoproterenol sufficient to increase the heart rate by 25%. The false-positive rate in both the control group and the documented syncope group was 6.6%. The initial tilt was positive in 30 (25%) of the 120 patients, with an additional 43 (36%) demonstrating positive responses during isoproterenol infusion. Overall, "sensitivity," specificity, and reproducibility were 61%, 93%, and 86% respectively.

A more comprehensive evaluation was undertaken by Natale et al.[96] Here 150 normal subjects were randomized into 2 groups of 75 each. One group was further randomized to a 60, a 70, and an 80° tilt followed by a second tilt with an isoproterenol infusion that increased the heart rate by 20%. The second group underwent tilt at 70° with either a low dose, 3 μg/min, or 5 μg/min isoproterenol infusion. They found that tilt table testing at a 60° or 70° angle with or without low dose isoproterenol provided a specificity of approximately 88% to 92%. They also reported that higher angles of tilt or higher dosages of isoproterenol were less specific.

Over the last several years the tilt protocol we have used has undergone considerable evolution. Based on the aforementioned observations and those of our own group, we presently use a two-stage tilt table protocol. Studies are performed in the morning after an overnight fast and an intravenous line is established. After a 15-minute rest period, the patient is positioned on a tilt table with footboard support and inclined to an angle of 70° for a period of 45 minutes. (Figure 1) Heart rate and rhythm are monitored continuously via a defibrillator monitor, and blood pressures are taken using a sphygmomanometer every 3 minutes. Cardiopulmonary resuscitation equipment is present and a registered nurse and a physician are present. If symptomatic hypotension and bradycardia occur, reproducing the patient's symptoms, the patient is then lowered to the supine position and the test ended. If no syncope occurs during this initial phase, the patient is lowered to the supine position and an intravenous infusion of isoproterenol is started. The dose is then titrated to increase the heart rate to 20% to 25% above the initial supine value. Upright tilt is then performed as previously described. Isoproterenol infusions are not used in the presence of known severe coronary artery disease or hypertrophic cardiomyopathy.

The exact sensitivity of head-upright tilt table testing is difficult to ascertain due to a lack of a "gold standard" against which to compare it. Reported estimates of the accuracy of tilt table testing range between 30% and 80%.[81] However, it should be kept in mind that the exact specificity of tilt table is, to a great extent, dependent on the physiological processes that result in neurocardiogenic syncope. The sequence of reflex events alluded to previously appears to be a normal (albeit paradoxic) response that could potentially be produced in most (if not all) people, given the right amount of stimulation. Therefore, tilt table testing cannot be thought to identify an underlying pathology, rather it determines an exaggerated susceptibility to this normal reflex. The actual specificity might thus be underestimated

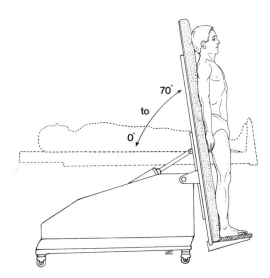

Figure 1. A 70° tilt table test. After 15 minutes of rest, the patient is positioned on a tilt table and inclined to an angle of 70° for 45 minutes.

because healthy asymptomatic subjects who have positive tilt tests may be more susceptible than other individuals and could potentially experience clinical syncopal episodes. A study by Grubb et al[97] found that a control subject with tilt-induced syncope later experienced a spontaneous neuro-cardiogenic clinical syncope.

There are various positive response patterns seen during head-up tilt table testing. We tend to group these into four groups. (Figures 2 and 3) The first is the "classic vasovagal" (or neurocardiogenic) described in detail previously, which is characterized by the sudden onset of hypotension with or without coexistent bradycardia. In between episodes of syncope these patients appear perfectly healthy and normal, with few if any other complaints. For the most part, these patients tend to be younger (although we have observed this response in virtually all age groups). A second pattern has been termed a "dysautonomic response," characterized by gradual parallel declines in systolic and diastolic blood pressure, leading to loss of consciousness. This pattern has been reported to be associated with low levels of circulating catecholamines. These patients are often noted to have other signs of autonomic dysfunction such as abnormal sweating and thermoregulatory control as well as orthostatic hypotension, and syncope itself is but one manifestation of a general state of autonomic failure (primary autonomic failure).[98] As opposed to patients with the more classic vasovagal form, these patients never really feel "well" and are much more disabled by their illness. We call the third pattern a psychogenic or psychosomatic response. These patients experience syncope during tilt table testing with no ascertainable alteration in heart rate, blood pressure, electroencephalographic, or transcranial blood flow patterns.[99] This group of patients

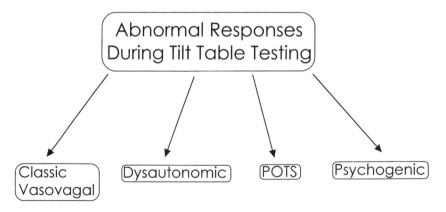

Figure 2. Positive response patterns to head-up tilt table testing are divided into four groups. POTS = postural orthostatic tachycardia syndrome.

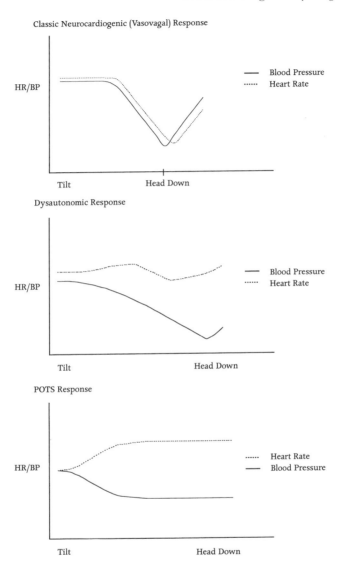

Figure 3. Blood pressure and heart rate patterns observed in abnormal responses to tilt table testing. POTS = postural orthostatic tachycardia syndrome.

usually suffers from underlying psychiatric disturbances that range from somatoform disorders (or conversion reactions) to anxiety disorders and major depression. Interestingly, serum catecholamines in these patients are quite high prior to, during, and after syncope (in contrast to the low

levels seen in dysautonomic patients and the abrupt decline in catecholamines seen in the classic vasovagal pattern).

We have recently realized that a fourth tilt pattern exists. We have
termed this tilt pattern the Postural Orthostatic Tachycardia Syndrome
(POTS).[100] This pattern is characterized by an increase in heart rate of at
least 30 beats per minute (or a maximum heart rate of 120 beats per minute) within the first 10 minutes upright during the baseline tilt. The tachycardia is not associated with profound hypotension. Several investigators
have reported that these patients demonstrate a mild form of autonomic
dysfunction in which a deficiency in peripheral vascular function (peripheral blood pooling) results in an excessive compensatory postural tachycardia. These patients also demonstrate exaggerated heart rate responses
to the infusion of isoproterenol. Streeten[101] postulates that this may represent the earliest and most sensitive sign of autonomic dysfunction. In this
group of patients, near syncope tends to occur more frequently than does
full syncope. Many of these patients will complain of exercise intolerance,
dizziness, and chronic disabling fatigue. Many times these patients are referred for evaluation of a persistent sinus tachycardia. Approximately 50%
of these patients will report the onset of symptoms following a severe viral
illness, suggesting a possible autoimmune etiology.

An alternative classification system has been developed by Sutton et
al, which basically divides responses into cardioinhibitory, vasodepressor
and mixed types.[102] The cardioinhibitory response was further divided into
those where the arterial pressure falls before heart rate, and those where
the fall in heart rate appears to pull the pressure down with it.

The reproducibility of tilt table testing has been assessed by several
studies. With use of prolonged passive head-up tilt alone, the reproducibility of a positive test is 62% to 77% over a period of 3 to 7 days.[103,104]
When using isoproterenol infusions with tilt table testing, the clinical reproducibility is reported to range between 67% to 88% when performed
over periods of 30 minutes to 2 weeks.[105,106] Interestingly, the reproducibility of negative tests is 85% to 100% over the same period. Overall the
results of the first test are 80% reproducible on subsequent testing, suggesting that there may be little to be achieved by performing a second tilt
on a patient suffering from recurrent unexplained syncope who has an
initial normal test result.

Indications For Tilt Table Testing

An expert writing committee of the American College of Cardiology
has developed a set of suggested indications for head-upright tilt table testing.[107] Indications were divided into four groups: I. Generally agreed upon
indications; II. Accepted indications where some disagreement exists; III.
Emerging indications for tilt table testing; and IV. Contraindications.

Class I: General Agreement that Tilt-Table Testing is Indicated

A. The evaluation of recurrent syncope, or a single syncopal event accompanied by physical injury, motor vehicle accident, or occurring in a "high-risk" setting (eg, commercial vehicle driver, machine operator, pilot, commercial painter, surgeon, window washer, competitive athlete) and presumed to be, but not conclusively known to be (by medical history or other evidence), vasovagal in origin.

   1. Patients in whom there is no history of or overt evidence for organic cardiovascular disease, and in whom the historical aspects are suggestive of vasovagal episodes (ie, episodes tend to occur while standing or sitting, or are associated with prodromal symptoms such as dizziness, diaphoresis, nausea, weakness, or a "flushed feeling").

   2. Patients in whom organic cardiovascular disease is present, but in whom historical aspects are suggestive of vasovagal episodes (see above), and in whom other causes of syncope have not been identified by appropriate testing (including conventional electrophysiological study).

B. The evaluation of unexplained syncope in settings as described in subsection A above.

   1. Patients without a history of or overt evidence for organic cardiovascular disease, and in whom vasovagal syncope may be a potential cause.

   2. In patients with concomitant cardiovascular disease after appropriate testing to rule out the potential causes of syncope.

   3. Patients in whom peripheral neuropathies or dysautonomias may contribute to symptomatic hypotension.

C. The further evaluation of patients in whom an alternative specific cause of syncope has been established by physiological recordings, either during a spontaneous event or by demonstration of reproduction of symptoms during electrophysiological/hemodynamic study (eg, asystole, high grade AV block), but in whom the demonstration of susceptibility to hypotension/bradycardia of a neurally mediated origin may affect treatment plans (eg, use of education, reassurance, or pharmacological therapy instead of or in conjunction with implantable pacemaker therapy).

D. Evaluation of recurrent exercise-induced syncope when a thorough history and physical examination, 12-lead ECG, echocardiogram, and formal exercise tolerance testing demonstrate no evidence of organic heart disease.

Class II: Differences of Opinion Exist Regarding the Utility of Tilt Table Testing

A. Differentiating convulsive syncope from epilepsy in patients with recurrent unexplained loss of consciousness with associated tonic-clonic activity in the setting of repeated normal electroencephalograms (EEG) and failure to respond to anti-seizure medications. Tilt table testing is further supported if other aspects of the episodes suggest vasovagal syncope such as a provocative situation or environment, occurrence in standing or sitting positions, or prodromal symptoms, as described earlier.

B. Evaluating patients (especially the elderly) in whom recurrent falls remain unexplained, and in whom a history of premonitory symptoms compatible with vasovagal symptoms is not obtained.

C. Recurrent "near syncopal" spells or "dizziness" presumed to be neurocardiogenic in origin, in whom clinical aspects otherwise conform to those in Class I subsections A1 or A2.

D. The evaluation of unexplained syncope in settings as described in patients in whom peripheral neuropathies or dysautonomias may contribute to symptomatic hypotension (2).

E. Follow-up evaluation of therapy to prevent syncope recurrences.
   1. Tilt table testing may be helpful in assessing the ability of a particular therapy (pharmacological, physical maneuvers, etc.) to prevent syncope.
   2. Tilt table testing may be helpful in determining whether temporary dual-chamber cardiac pacing will be useful in preventing or lessening symptoms in patients with neurally mediated bradycardia or asystole prior to permanent dual-chamber pacemaker implantation.

Class III: Potentially Emerging Indications for Tilt Table Testing

A. Recurrent idiopathic vertigo in patients in whom clinical aspects (see Class IA) suggest the possibility of a neurally mediated hypotension-bradycardia as a cause, and in whom extensive evaluation has failed to disclose an otolaryngologic source.

B. Recurrent transient ischemic attacks. Some older patients may experience episodic neurocardiogenic hypotension and bradycardia of sufficient degree to cause transient neurological dysfunction but not full syncope. Patients should be considered for tilt table testing if clinical settings are suggestive of a neurally mediated origin (see Class IA). Such testing would be especially warranted if Doppler ultrasonography, carotid angiography, and transesophageal echocardiography have failed to disclose an etiology.

C. Chronic fatigue syndrome. Preliminary observations suggest that some individuals suffering from chronic fatigue syndrome may exhibit neurally mediated hypotension/bradycardia and that head-up tilt table testing may help to identify a subgroup of these patients in whom therapy directed at the neurocardiogenic disorder may be of benefit.

D. Sudden infant death syndrome (SIDS). Preliminary data suggest that neurally mediated hypotension/bradycardia may play a role in some SIDS deaths. Initial results suggest that severe bradycardic episodes may be reproduced in SIDS survivors using upright tilt table testing.

Tilt Table Testing Is Not Indicated

A. Single syncopal episode, without injury and not in a high-risk setting (see Class IA), in which clinical features (see Class IA) support a diagnosis of vasovagal syncope.

B. Syncope in which an alternative specific cause has been established by physiological recordings either during a spontaneous event or by demonstration of reproduction of symptoms during electrophysiological/hemodynamic study, and in which the potential additional demonstration of a neurally mediated contribution to the etiology would not alter treatment plans (see Class IC).

Class IV: Relative Contraindications to Tilt Table Testing

A. Syncope with clinically severe aortic stenosis or obstructive cardiomyopathy.

B. Syncope in the presence of critical mitral stenosis.

C. Syncope in the setting of known critical proximal coronary artery stenosis.

Therapeutic Approaches

The therapeutic approach to any patient who suffers from recurrent neurocardiogenic syncope must be individualized. In many of these patients, syncope occurs infrequently and only under exceptional circumstances. Therefore, the cornerstone of any therapy is the education of the patient as to the nature of the disorder and counseling to avoid any known predisposing factors (such as extreme heat or dehydration). Drugs that could potentially enhance a person's predisposition to syncope should be identified and, if possible, discontinued. Agents such as alcohol, angiotensin converting enzyme (ACE) inhibitors, hydralazine, some calcium channel blockers, and benzodiazepam may all worsen the tendency toward syncope [most probably due to the vasodilatory effect enhancing the tendency to peripheral venous pooling (see Table 1)]. Patients should also be advised to lie down at the onset of any premonitory symptoms and not remain standing or sitting. If another person is present during a spontaneous syncopal episode, he or she should place the affected individual supine (with the feet elevated and the head down) until a stable blood pressure and pulse rate returns. A common error is to attempt to have the patient try to sit up moments after he or she has regained consciousness; this will only provoke another episode. Once the patient has regained consciousness in the supine position, it is best to allow at least 5 to 10 minutes to elapse before allowing him or her to sit up. Patients who begin to experience warning signs will often experience a strong urge to get up and walk (probably reflecting an unconscious desire to increase venous return through skeletal muscle contraction), thereby increasing the degree of orthostatic stress and precipitating a syncopal event. When given a choice between falling down or lying down, most informed patients will chose the latter.

For some individuals however, the prodromal phase is either quite brief or absent altogether (a finding more common in older patients).[86] Patients in whom syncope is sudden, recurrent, and without warning will usually require some type of prophylactic therapy (especially those who experience repeated bodily injury resulting from a syncopal event). However, before beginning any form of treatment, it must be kept in mind that drug therapy for these disorders (like most chronic illnesses) is palliative rather than curative in nature. Thus, even well-controlled patients may, on occasion, experience recurrences due to exceptional stress or noncompliance.

A wide range of therapies has been used to help prevent further syncopal episodes (see Table 2). The most widely used agents to date have

_____ Table 1 _____

Agents That May Exacerbate Syncope

Alcohol
Angiotensin Converting Enzyme Inhibitors
Calcium Channel Blockers
Methyldopa
Reserpine
Barbituates
Prazosin
Anesthetics
β Blockers
Hydralazine
Diuretics

_____ **Table 2** _____

Potential Therapies for Neurocardiogenic Syncope

Treatment	Use/Dosage	Side Effects/Problems
Elastic support hose	30–40 mm Hg ankle counterpressure	difficult to put on, uncomfortable, hot
β blockers (atenolol)	50–100 mg/day	presyncope, fatigue, bradycardia, impotence
Fludrocortisone	0.1 mg twice daily	hypokalemia, bloating, headaches, hypertension
Disopyramide	200 mg CR twice daily	urinary retention, confusion, dry mouth, proarrhythmia
Theophylline	200 mg CR twice daily	nausea, arrhythmic insomnia, tremor
Fluoxetine	20 mg PO daily	nausea, diarrhea, insomnia, diminished libido
Sertraline	50–100 mg PO daily	nausea, diarrhea, insomnia
Nefazadone	100–150 mg PO BID	nausea, diarrhea
Methylphenidate	5–15 mg PO TID, last dose, before 7 p.m.	CNS stimulation, nausea, insomnia, hypertension
Midodrine	5–10 mg PO Q 2–4 hr up to 40 mg a day	nausea, hypertension, scalp pruritus
Permanent cardiac pacing	DDD mode	invasive, expensive

been the β_1-adrenergic blockers.[108,109] These agents were presumed to exert their effects via their negative inotropic actions, which are thought to diminish the degree of cardiac mechanoreceptor activation. However, two recent studies by Hjorth and colleagues[110,111] have demonstrated that β-blockers have powerful central serotonin-blocking activities (principally at the $5HT_1$ A & B receptors) that may somehow contribute to their therapeutic effects. It is important to remember that β-blocking agents may occasionally worsen the tendency toward syncope rather than reduce it (resulting in a phenomenon that we have called "Prosyncope").[112] Transdermal scopolamine is reported to be helpful in some individuals, however the product is no longer available on the US market. Milstein et al[113] report that disopyramide, an agent possessing negative inotropic, anticholinergic, and direct peripheral vasoconstrictive effects, was useful in preventing recurrent neurocardiogenic syncope. However, Morillo et al[114] report that the efficacy of disopyramide is no better than placebo. Fludrocortisone, a mineral corticoid agent, is often quite useful. Although it was initially believed that its principal effect was an increase in blood volume, fludrocortisone also appears to increase the sensitivity of blood vessels to the vasoconstrictive effects of norepinephrine.[115] In our experience, it has been most effective in younger patients, for whom it can be used as monotherapy. In older patients it is often a useful adjuvant therapy. Some patients will become severely hypokalemic or hypomagnesemic on fludrocortisone and may require potassium or magnesium supplementation. Nelson et al[116] report that oral theophylline therapy, which has a peripheral antiadenosine effect, is helpful to some patients. Mild vasoconstrictive agents such as ergotamine and etilefrine have been used, and Campbell et al report[117] that pseudoephedrine can be an effective treatment in pediatric patients. Although it is initially effective, our experience has been that tachyphylaxis results are relatively seen with long-term use. Susmano et al[118] have successfully used dextroamphetamine to increase peripheral vascular resistance by means of a receptor stimulation. Although it is useful, the drug has a number of side effects and a high potential for abuse. This lead our group[119] to explore the use of the chemically similar agent, methylphenidate (Ritalin) in patients who are refractory to other therapies. We found it to be a reasonably well-tolerated and quite effective therapy in this otherwise refractory group. The newly released sympathomimetic agent, midodrine is a direct-acting α-adrenergic agonist that is quite similar to methylphenidate. The drug causes vasoconstriction in arterioles and venous capacitance vessels without stimulating the cardiac or central nervous system. The response rates seem to be roughly equivalent to those seen with methylphenidate.

Based on the aforementioned role of serotonin in the pathophysiological processes that result in neurocardiogenic syncope, the use of serotonin-altering drugs as a potential therapy has also been explored.[46] The serotonin reuptake inhibitors prevent reuptake of serotonin at the synaptic cleft, thereby increasing intrasynaptic serotonin concentrations and producing a downregulation in postsynaptic serotonin receptor density. Both fluoxetine hydrochloride and sertraline hydrochloride are reported to be effective therapies for patients who are refractory to or intolerant of other agents, with response rates of roughly 50%.[120,121] In a recent randomized trial of sertraline versus atenolol and disopyramide in recurrent neurocardiogenic syncope, Williamson et al[122] found that the efficacy of sertraline in preventing recurrences was comparable to the other agents (interestingly patient tolerance was best with sertraline).

For patients in whom there are known situations that can provoke syncope (the sight of blood or a needle for example), biofeedback has been very successfully used to help "desensitize" the individual to the psychological trigger, thereby blunting its effect.[123] Elastic support hose may be helpful for some patients, but they tend to be uncomfortable and difficult to put on. When support hose are used, at least 30 mm Hg counterpressure should be provided to achieve any real effect, and the hose should be waist high.

As previously mentioned, during an episode of syncope some patients will demonstrate significant bradycardia or asystole (Figure 4). There is perhaps, no other treatment modality that is more controversial than the role of permanent pacemaker insertion. The first reports on the use of permanent pacing for neurocardiogenic syncope demonstrated that VVI mode pacing is almost always ineffective and may actually aggravate syncope because of retrograde ventriculoatrial conduction.[124] In their original paper on tilt table testing, Kenny et al[6] also reported the successful use of dual-chamber cardiac pacing for neurocardiogenic syncope. Later, Fitzpatrick and Sutton[125] reported the results of pacing in 20 tilt-positive patients with induced symptomatic bradycardia (<60 beats/min). Syncope

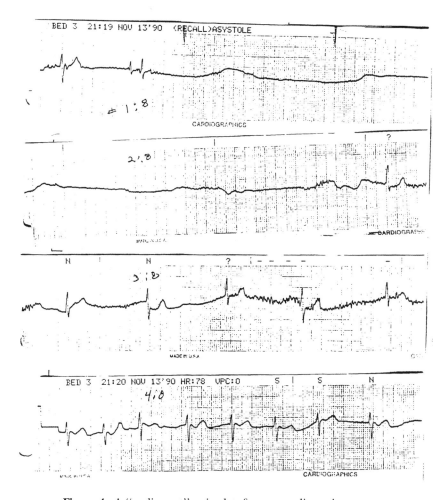

Figure 4. A "malignant" episode of neurocardiogenic syncope.

was eliminated in about half of the patients, while the remainder experienced fewer syncopal episodes of a lesser severity. Fitzpatrick then investigated tilt table testing performed with a temporary dual-chamber pacemaker in place.[126] He found that temporary DVI pacing with hysteresis could abort approximately 85% of the cases of neurocardiogenic syncope induced by 60° degree head-up tilt. Both Samoil et al[128] and McGuinn et al[127] also found that in a small number of patients, temporary dual-chamber pacing could prevent tilt-induced syncope or at least prolong the time from onset of symptoms to syncope.[127,128] These findings are in contrast to those of Sra et al,[32] who studied the effects of temporary pacing in 22 patients: 20 with sinus rhythm during AV sequential pacing and two with atrial fibrillation who had ventricular pacing alone. All 22 patients had an initial positive baseline tilt test after repeating the tilt with pacing (at a rate 20% higher than the supine resting heart rate): 1 patient remained asymptomatic, 1 had dizziness without hypotension, and 15 experienced presyncope rather than syncope. Only five patients had syncope during the following tilt. Afterward, all patients had repeat tilt table testing while on pharmacological therapy; metoprolol was effective in 10 of 22 patients, theophylline in 3 of 12 patients, and disopyramide in 6 of 9 patients. From this, they concluded that pacing was of little benefit, although it can also be concluded that pacing offered a clear benefit for some patients.

Finally, Petersen et al[129] present data on the long-term effects of permanent pacing in patients with severe recurrent syncope and reproducible tilt-induced neurocardiogenic syncope (with a pronounced bradycardic component). Dual-chamber permanent pacemakers were implanted in 37 patients who were then followed for 50±24 months. Approximately 89% had a marked reduction in symptoms, while 27% had complete elimination of symptoms. There was a reduction in the overall frequency of syncopal episodes from 136 to 11 episodes per year. Interestingly, the clinical features that best predicted the usefulness of permanent pacing included a young age (56 years as compared to 76 years) and the absence of a prodrome before spontaneous syncopal episodes. It should be kept in mind however, that during neurocardiogenic syncope, the fall in blood pressure usually precedes the fall in heart rate. Thus, pacing determined by rate criteria alone often represents "too little too late." The development of sensor technology that allows for the direct or indirect measurement of blood pressure would permit for the onset of pacing at the earliest point in the syncopal episode. The optimum pacing algorithm for the prevention of neurocardiogenic syncope has not yet been established. At present, we use dual-chamber pacing combined with rate hysteresis. The device is triggered by the development of a low heart rate that then reacts by pacing at a rate fast enough to either prevent (or at least slow down) the increasing hypotension.

Pacing should not be considered as firstline therapy because many patients respond to medical treatment and because pacing alone is rarely effective. However in drug refractory patients who demonstrate a significant bradycardic component to their syncope, cardiac pacing may significantly prolong the time from onset of symptoms to loss of consciousness and occasionally prevent syncope altogether.[130] In patients who experience little or no warning prior to syncope (drop attacks), cardiac pacing may cause a more gradual fall in blood pressure that can be perceived by the patient as a prodrome, thereby allowing him or her to take appropriate evasive actions (such as lying down).

At our institution, we will usually perform tilt table testing with a temporary pacemaker in place on patients in whom permanent pacemaker placement is being considered. Benefit from temporary pacing should be demonstrated prior to committing the patient to permanent pacing. In the vast majority of cases, permanent pacing must be combined with pharmacotherapy to be truly effective for elimination of symptoms.

The assessment of the efficacy of therapy may be made by noting a reduction or absence in the patient's clinical episodes or by repeat tilt table testing. Based on the reproducibility studies alluded to earlier, Grubb et al,[91] Gamache et al,[131] and Sra et al[132] report that the absence of syncope during repeat upright tilt table testing after the initiation of therapy (in patients with an initial positive response) appears to predict the absence of clinical recurrences over the long term.

This concept, however, has been questioned by Brignole et al,[133] who report on a group of 30 patients with similar responses to therapy in both treated and untreated patients. Their study group, however, was small and the frequency of syncopal episodes prior to study was not specified. In addition, most of the previously mentioned therapies were not used. A study by Fitzpatrick et al[134] revealed that regardless of treatment, the frequency of syncope in patients studied fell in the first year after the study. It is unclear why this occurred, but it may be that there is a beneficial psychological response to finally receiving a diagnosis after suffering from recurrent idiopathic syncopal episodes. This amount of variability in rates of recurrence makes evaluation of any therapeutic modality difficult. This is highlighted by Fitzpatrick et al,[135] who report a randomized double-blind trial with atenolol, transdermal scopolamine, and clonidine in patients with syncope and positive tilt studies. While clonidine and scopolamine appeared more efficacious than placebo, the effect was not statistically significant.

The wide range of treatment options just outlined, often tends to leave one confused over how to initiate any rational treatment plan. Indeed, at present, treatment seems somewhat more an art than a science. This having been said, we offer these suggestions (based on our experiences) for treatment of patients with recurrent syncope. First one must consider any concomitant illness or conditions that are present in the patient to be sure that potential therapy will be compatible. Next, look at the patient's age and tilt-response pattern. For children or adolescents with either a classic vasovagal or dysautonomic pattern, we begin therapy with fludrocortisone and continue it for at least 2 to 3 weeks. If no response is seen, we will usually add a second agent to it. Although β-blockers are useful in patients with either a classic vasovagal or POTS response, they are frequently ineffective (or counterproductive) in those patients with a dysautonomic pattern. Presently, for many patients we use the serotonin reuptake inhibitors (usually nefazadone) as a secondline agent. In severely refractory patients we will add a third agent, usually a vasoconstrictor such as methylphenidate or midodrine (these agents are particularly useful in dysautonomic patients and those with POTS patterns). It has been our experience that the use of two to three different agents (that work through different mechanisms) at lower dosages is often more effective and better tolerated than huge dosages of a single agent. Also keep in mind that the human body is a dynamic entity that changes over time. Thus, therapies that were initially effective may become less so over the course of years, especially if concomitant medical disorders develop.

Prognosis

Data on the long-term outcomes of patients are quite limited, however some general trends have been observed. One of the most important is that adolescents who develop recurrent syncope will usually "grow out of it" by the time they are in their twenties. Thus, the philosophy of treatment should be to get them through the "bad years" and then discontinue therapy. For this reason we are extremely reluctant to consider permanent pacing in this group, and we use it only when the life of the patient is considered to be in jeopardy. Our usual practice in adolescents is to treat for 1 to 2 years, and if the patient has remained completely symptom free during that time, to discontinue therapy. Roughly 80% of adolescents will not require further therapy, while the remaining 20% will experience recurrent symptoms and need to be placed back on treatment. The majority of these will be able to discontinue therapy after an additional 1 to 2 years. Older patients with recurrent neurocardiogenic syncope are a different matter. For this group, it may be necessary to continue therapy indefinitely, as we have observed a high recurrence rate when treatments are stopped.

Concurrent conditions seem to either reactivate a prior tendency toward syncope or exacerbate a previously unrecognized predisposition toward it. Principal among these conditions are pregnancy and the postpartum period.[136] During pregnancy there is a major increase in circulating blood volume to approximately 50% higher than the nonpregnant level. Concomitant with this increase in circulating blood volume is a decrease in systemic vascular resistance, resulting in a fall in blood pressure (principally diastolic) and a widening of the pulse pressure.[137] In some women the fall in blood pressure is severe, leading to recurrent syncope. For these individuals we often advise the use of elastic support hose and bed rest. We attempt to avoid pharmacotherapy during pregnancy, but when this is impossible, either fludrocortisone or disopyramide appear to be safe.

During the postpartum period, there is usually a rapid return to the nonpregnant state. While the fall in circulating blood volume appears to occur quite promptly, the aforementioned alterations in peripheral blood flow may persist to 6 or more weeks postpartum.[138] The combination of reduced volume and a continued low systemic vascular resistance would seem to create the ideal setting for hypotension and, possibly, syncope. Grubb et al[136] report on 12 women who developed episodic hypotension resulting in syncope in the immediate postpartum period. All 12 had their hypotension and symptoms reproduced during tilt table testing, all during the baseline tilt, and all with a dysautonomic pattern. Given enough time, the majority of these patients slowly return to normal. This "postpartum syncope" is important to recognize because maternal syncope can have a disastrous effect on the infant as well as the mother.

Other conditions that seem to reactivate a prior tendency to neurocardiogenic syncope are severe viral infections and treatment with chemotherapeutic agents (in particular cis-platinum and vincristine). We have also noted the return of syncope following trauma or severe emotional stress, and following exposure to extreme heat.

Summary

The disorder now known as neurocardiogenic syncope is a complex one with a wide clinical spectrum of presentations. Indeed, it often seems more like a group of related disorders rather than a single clinical entity. Currently understood as an exaggerated form of an otherwise normal response, the mechanism seems to involve sudden mechanoreceptor activation following a rapid increase in peripheral vascular pooling. Tilt table testing has emerged as an invaluable tool for reproducing episodes of neurocardiogenic syncope, allowing not only for the confirmation of the diagnosis, but also for more detailed investigations into the pathophysiology of the condition. Furthermore, detailed studies will be necessary to better understand this common, fascinating, and yet enigmatic condition and to elaborate optimal diagnostic and therapeutic modalities.

References

1. Kapoor W, Karpf M, Wieand S, et al. A prospective evaluation and follow-up of patients with syncope. *N Engl J Med* 1983;309:197–204.

2. Calkins H, Byrne M, El-Atassi R, et al. The economic burden of unrecognized vasodepressor syncope. *Am J Med* 1993;95:473–479.

3. Eagle KA, Black HR, Cook EF, Goldman L. Evaluation of prognostic classification for patients with syncope. *Am J Med* 1985;79:455–460.

4. Linzer M, Pontinen M, Gold GT. Impairment of physical and psychosocial function in recurrent syncope. *J Clin Epidemiol* 1991;44:1037–1043.

5. Decter BM, Goldner B, Cohen TJ. Vasovagal syncope as a cause of motor vehicle accidents. *Am Heart J* 1994;127:1619–1621.

6. Kenny RA, Ingram A, Bayless J, Sutton R. Head up tilt: A useful test for investigating unexplained syncope. *Lancet* 1989;1:1352–1355.

7. Kosinski D, Grubb BP, Temesy-Armos P. Pathophysiological aspects of neurocardiogenic syncope. *Pacing Clin Electrophysiol* 1995;18:716–721.

8. Hunter J. *Works of John Hunter, Vol. 3.* London: J.F. Palmer; 1837.

9. Foster M. *Textbook of Physiology.* London: Macmillan and Company; 1888;297, 345.

10. Lewis T. A lecture on vasovagal syncope and the carotid sinus mechanism: With comments on Gower's and Nothnagel's syndrome. *Br Med J* 1932;1:873–876.

11. Allen SC, Taylor CL, Hall VE. A study of orthostatic insufficiency by the tilt board method. *Am J Physiol* 1945;143:11–20

12. Wieling W, Lieshout J. Maintenance of postural normotension in humans. In: Low P (ed): *Clinical Autonomic Disorders.* Boston: Little, Brown, and Company; 1993;69–73.

13. Mehdriad AA, Janosik D, Fredman C. Mechanisms of tilt table-induced hypotension and bradycardia in patients with neurally mediated syncope. (Abstr) *J Am Coll Cardiol* 1993;17:216A.

14. El-Bedawi KM, Hainsworth R. Combined head up tilt and lower body suction: A test of orthostatic tolerance. *Clin Auton Res* 1994;4:41–47.

15. Hainsworth R, El-Bedawi KM. Orthostatic tolerance in patients with unexplained syncope. *Clin Autonom Res* 1994;4:239–244.

16. Tseng CJ, Tung CS. Brainstem and cardiovascular regulation. In: Robertson D, Biaggioni I. (eds): *Disorders of the Autonomic Nervous System.* London: Harwood Academic Publishers; 1995;9–24.

17. Benarroch E. The central autonomic network: Functional organization, dysfunction, and perspective. *Mayo Clin Proc* 1993;68:988–1001.

18. Smith ML, Carlson MD, Thames MD. Reflex control of the heart and circulation: Implications for cardiovascular aelectrophysiology. *J Cardiovasc Electrophysiol* 1991;2:441–449.

19. Fitzpatrick A, Williams T, Ahmed R, et al. Echocardiographic and endocrine changes during vasovagal syncope induced by prolonged head up tilt. *Eur J Cardiac Pacing Electrophysiol* 1992;2:121–128.

20. Morita H, Vatner SF. Effects of haemorrhage on renal nerve activity in conscious dogs. *Circ Res* 1985;57:788–793.

21. Lightfoot JT, Rowe SA, Fortney SM. Occurrence of presyncope in subjects without ventricular innervation. *Clin Sci* 1993;85:695–700.

22. Fitzpatrick AP, Banner N, Cheng A et al. Vasovagal syncope may occur after orthotopic heart transplantation. *J Am Coll Cardiol* 1993;21:1132–1137.

23. Waxman MB, Cameron DA, Wald RW. Role of ventricular afferents in vasovagal reactions. *J Am Coll Cardiol* 1993;21:1138–1141.

24. Rudas L, Pflugfelder PW, Kostuk WJ. Vasodepressor syncope in a cardiac transplant recipient: A case of vagal re-innervation? *Can J Cardiol* 1992;8:403–405.

25. Scherrer U, Vissing S, Morgan BJ, et al. Vasovagal syncope after infusion of a vasodilator in a heart transplant patient. *N Engl J Med* 1990;322:602–604.

26. Lofring V. Cardiovascular adjustments induced from the rostral cingulate gyrus: With specific reference to sympatho-inhibiting mechanisms. *Acta Physiol Scand* 1961;51(suppl 184):5–82.
27. Constantin L, Martins JB, Fincham RW, et al. Bradycardia and syncope as manifestations of partial epilepsy. *J Am Coll cardiol* 1990;15:900–915.
28. Dickinson CJ. Fainting precipitated by collapse firing of venous baroreceptors. *Lancet* 1993;342:970–972.
29. Landgren S. On the excitation mechanism of carotid baroreceptors. *Acta Physiol Scand* 1952;26:1–34.
30. Banner NR, Williams M, Patel N, et al. Altered cardiovascular and neurohumeral response to head up tilt after heart-lung transplantation. *Circulation* 1990;82:863–871.
31. Rea R, Thames M. Neural control mechanisms and vasovagal syncope. *J Cardiovascular Electrophysiology* 1993;4:587–595.
32. Sra J, Jazayeri M, Avitall B, et al. Comparison of cardiac pacing with drug therapy in the treatment of neurocardiogenic syncope with bradycardia or asystole. *N Engl J Med* 1993;328:1085–1090.
33. Öberg B, Thoren P. Increased activity in left ventricular receptors during hemorrhage or occlusion of caval veins in the cat: A possible cause of the vasovagal reaction. *Acta Physiol Scand* 1972;85:164–173.
34. Wallin BG, Sundläff G. Sympathetic outflow to the muscles during vasovagal syncope. *J Auton Nerv Syst* 1982;6:284–291.
35. Sra J, Jazayeri M, Murthy V, et al. Sequential catecholamine changes during upright tilt: Possible hormonal mechanisms responsible for pathogenesis of neurocardiogenic syncope. *J Am Coll Cardiol* 1991;17:216A.
36. Lewis W, Smith M, Carlson M. Peripheral sympathoinhibition precedes hypotension and bradycardia during neurally mediated vasovagal syncope. *Pacing Clin Electrophysiol* 1994;17:747.
37. Waxman MB, Asta JA, Cameron DA. Vasodepressor reaction induced by inferior vena cava occlusion and isoproterenol in the rat. *Circulation* 1994;89:2401–2411.
38. Chosy JJ, Graham DT. Catecholamines in vasovagal fainting. *J Psychosom Res* 1965;9:189–194.
39. Mouta H, Nishida Y, Motochigawa H, et al. Opiate receptor-mediated decrease in renal nerve activity during hypotensive hemorrhage in conscious rats. *Circ Res* 1988;63:165–172.
40. Evans RG, Ludbrook J, Potonick SJ. Intracisternal naloxone and cardiac nerve blockade prevent vasodilation during simulated haemorrhage in awake rabbits. *J Physiol (Lond)* 1989; 409:1–14.
41. Ferguson DW. Naloxone potentiates cardiopulmonary baroreflex sympathetic control in normal humans. *Circ Res* 1992;70:172–183.
42. Perna GP, Ficola U, Salvatori P et al. Increase of plasma β-endorphins in vasodepressor syncope. *Am J Cardiol* 1990;65:929–930.
43. Wallbridge DR, MacIntyre HE, Gray CE, et al. Increase in plasma β-endorphins precedes vasodepressor syncope. *Br Heart J* 1994;71:446–448.
44. Foldager N, Bonde-Petersen F. Human cardiovascular reactions to simulated hypovolemia, modified by the opiate antagonist naloxone. *Eur J Appl Physiol* 1988;57:507–513.
45. Smith ML, Carlson MD, Sheehan HM, et al. Naloxone does not prevent vasovagal syncope during simulated orthostasis in humans. *Physiologist* 1991; 34:238–239.
46. Grubb BP, Kosinski D. Serotonin and syncope: An emerging connection? *Eur J Cardiac Pacing Electrophysiol* 1996:5;306–314.

47. Kuhn D, Wolfe W, Loyenburg W. Review of the central serotonergic neuronal system in blood pressure regulation. *Hypertension* 1980;2:243–255.
48. Baum T, Shropshire AT. Inhibition of efferent sympathetic nerve activity by 5-hydroxytryptophan in centrally administered 5-hydroxytryphamine. *Neuropharmacology* 1975;14:227–233.
49. Tadepelli A, Mills E, Schanberg S. Central depression of carotid baroreceptor pressor response, arterial pressure, and heart rate by 5-hydroxytryptophan: Influence of the supramolecular areas of the brain. *Journal of Pharmacology and Experimental Therapeutics* 1977;202:310–319.
50. Abboud FM. Neurocardiogenic syncope. *N Engl J Med* 1993;328:1117–1119.
51. Bauer K, Dietersdorfer F, Kaik G. Assessment of β-adrenergic receptor blockade after isamoltane, a 5HT₁ recedptor active compound in healthy volunteers. *Clin Pharmacol Ther* 1993;53(6):675–683.
52. Elam RF, Bergman F, Feverstein G. The use of antiserotonergic agents for the treatment of acute hemorrhagic shock in cats. *Eur J Pharmacol* 1985;107:275–278.
53. Hasser E, Schadt J, Grove K. Serotonergic and opioid interactions during acute hemorrhagic hypotension in the conscious rabbit. (Abstr) *FASEB J* 1989; 3:A1014.
54. Morgan DA, Thoren P, Wilczynski E, et al. Serotonergic mechanisms mediate renal sympatho-inhibition during severe hemorrhage in rats. *Am J Physiol* 1988;255:H496–H502.
55. Theodorakis G, Markianos M, Sourlas N, et al. Central serotonergic and adrenergic activity in patients with vasovagal syncope (Abst). *Circulation* 1995; 92:414.
56. Matzen S, Secher NH, Knigge U, et al. Effect of serotonin receptor blockade on endocrine and cardiovascular responses to upright tilt in humans. *Acta Physiol Scand* 1993;149:163–176.
57. Samoil D, Grubb BP. Neurally mediated syncope and serotonin reuptake inhibitors. *Clin Auton Res* 1995;5:251–255.
58. Sakuma J, Togashi H, Yoshioka M, et al. N-methyl-L-arginine, an inhibitor of L-arginine-derived nitric oxide synthesis, stimulates renal sympathetic nerve activity in vivo: A role for nitric oxide in the central regulation of autonomic tone. *Circ Res* 1992;70:607–611.
59. Grubb BP, Gerard G, Roush K, et al. Cerebral vasoconstriction during head upright tilt-induced vasovagal syncope: A paradoxic and unexpected response. *Circulation* 1991;84:1157–1164.
60. Janasik D, Gomez C, Njemanze P, et al. Abnormalities in cerebral blood flow autoregulation during tilt-induced syncope. (Abstr) *Pacing Clin Electrophysiol* 1992;15:542.
61. Gomez CR, Janosik DL, Lewis ML. Transcranial Doppler in the evaluation of global cerebral ischemia: Syncope and cardiac arrest. In: Babikian VL, Wechsler LR. (eds): *Transcranial Doppler Ultrasonography*. St. Louis: Mosby Year Book, Inc.; 1993;141–149.
62. Njemanze P. Cerebral circulation dysfunction and hemodynamic abnormalities in syncope during upright tilt test. *Can J Cardiol* 1993;9:238–242.
63. Kaminer S, Truemper E, Fisher A. Recurrent syncope in children. Intracranial hemodynamics. (Abstr) *Pacing Clin Electrophysiol* 1993;1:532.
64. Fredman CS, Bierman KM, Patel V, et al. Transcranial Doppler ultrasonography during head upright tilt table testing. *Ann Int Med* 1995;123:848–849.
65. Folkow B, Neil E. *Circulation*. New York: Oxford University Press; 1971.
66. Linzer M, Felder A, Hackel A, et al. Psychiatric Syncope. *Psychosomatics* 1990;31:181–188.

67. Wayne HH. Syncope: Physiologic considerations and an analysis of the clinical characteristics in 510 patients. *Am J Med* 1961;30:418–438.
68. Luft NC, Nowell WK. Manifestations of brief instantaneous anoxia in men. *J Appl Physiol* 1956;8:444–454.
69. Duvoisin RC. Convulsive syncope induced by the Weber maneuver. *Arch Neurol* 1962;7:219–226.
70. Grubb BP, Gerard G, Roush K, et al. Differentiation of convulsive syncope and epilepsy with head up tilt table testing. *Ann Int Med* 1991;115:871–876.
71. Grubb BP, Rubin AM, Wolfe D, et al. Head upright tilt table testing: A useful tool in the evaluation and management of recurrent vertigo of unknown origin associated with syncope or near syncope. *Otolaryngol Head Neck Surg* 1992; 107:570–575.
72. Grubb BP, Samoil D, Temesy-Armos P, et al. Episodic periods of neurally mediated hypotension and bradycardia mimicking transient ischemic attacks in the elderly. *Cardiol Elderly* 1993;1(3):221–226.
73. Sutton R. Vasovagal syndrome: Could it be malignant? *Eur J Cardiac Pacing Electrophysiol* 1992;2:89.
74. Grubb BP, Temesy-Armos P, Moore J, et al. Head upright tilt table testing in the evaluation and management of the malignant vasovagal syndrome. *Am J Cardiol* 1992;69:904–908.
75. Gatzoulis KA, Mamarelis I, Apostolopoulos T, et al. Polymorphic ventricular tachycardia induced during tilt table testing in a patient with syncope and probable dysfunction of the sinus node. *Pacing Clin Electrophysiol* 1995;18:1075–1079.
76. Kosinski DJ, Grubb BP, Elliott L, Dubois B. Treatment of malignant neurocardiogenic syncope with dual chamber cardiac pacing and fluoxetine hydrochloride. *Pacing Clin Electrophysiol* 1995;18:1455–1457.
77. Engle GL. Psychologic stress, vasodepressor (vasovagal) syncope and sudden death. *Ann Int Med* 1978;89:403–412.
78. Linzer M, Varia I, Pontinen M, et al. Medically unexplained syncope: Relationship to psychiatric illness. *Am J Med* 1992;92:185–255.
79. Bou-Holaigh I, Rowe P, Kan J, Calkins H. The relationship between neurally mediated hypotension and the chronic fatigue syndrome. *JAMA* 1995;274:961–967.
80. Stevens H, Fazekas J. Experimentally induced hypotension. *Arch Neurol Psych* 1955;73:416–424.
81. Milstein S, Reyes W, Benditt D. Upright body tilt for evaluation of patients with recurrent syncope. *Pacing Clin Electrophisiol* 1989;12:117–124.
82. Fitzpatrick AP, Theodorakis G, Vardas P, Sutton R. Methodology of head up tilt table testing in patients with unexplained syncope. *J Am Coll Cardiol* 1991;17:125–130.
83. Shvartz E. Reliability of quantifiable tilt table data. *Aerospace Med* 1968;39:1094–1096.
84. Shvartz E, Meyerstein N. Tilt tolerance of young men and women. *Aerospace Med* 1970;41:253–255.
85. Vogt FB. Tilt table and volume changes with short term deconditioning experiments. *Aerospace Med* 1967;38:564–568.
86. Sutton R, Peterson M. The clinical spectrum of neurocardiogenic syncope. *J Cardiovasc Electrophysiol* 1995;6:569–576.
87. Strasberg B, Rechavia E, Sagie A, et al. Usefulness of head up tilt table test in evaluating patients with syncope of unknown origin. *Am Heart J* 1989;118:923–927.

88. Raviele A, Gasparini G, DePede F, et al. Usefulness of head up tilt table test in evaluating syncope of unknown origin and negative electrophysiologic study. *Am J Cardiol* 1990;65:1322–1327.

89. Abi-Samra F, Maloney J, Fouad FM, Castbe L. Usefulness of head up tilt table testing and hemodynamic investigations in the workup of syncope of unknown origin. *Pacing Clin Electrophisiol* 1987;10:406–410.

90. Almquist A, Goldenburg I, Milstein S, et al. Provocation of bradycardia and hypotension by isoproterenol and upright posture in patients with unexplained syncope. *N Engl J Med* 1989;320:346–351.

91. Grubb BP, Temesy-Armos P, Hahn H, Elliott L. Utility of upright tilt table testing in the evaluation and management of syncope of unknown origin. *Am J Med* 1991;90:6–10.

92. Pongiglione G, Fish FA, Strasberger JF, Benson DW. Heart rate and blood pressure response to upright tilt in young patients with unexplained syncope. *J Am Coll Cardiol* 1990;16:165–170.

93. Sheldon R, Killam S. Methodology of isoproterenol tilt table testing in patients with syncope. *J Am Coll Cardiol* 1992;19:773–779.

94. Kapoor WN, Brant N. Evaluation of syncope by upright tilt testing with isoproterenol. *Ann Intern Med* 1992;116:358–363.

95. Morillo CA, Klein G, Zandri S, Yee R. Diagnostic accuracy of a low dose isoproterenol head up tilt protocol. *Am Heart J* 1995;129:901–906.

96. Natale A, Akhtar M, Jazayeri M, et al. Provocation of hypotension during head up tilt testing in subjects with no history of syncope or presyncope. *Circulation* 1995;92:54–58.

97. Grubb BP, Kosinski D, Temesy-Armos P, Brewster P. Responses of normal subjects during head upright tilt table testing with and without low dose isoproterenol infusion. *Pacing Clin Electrophisiol* (in press).

98. Hackel A, Linzer M, Anderson N, Williams R. Cardiovascular and catecholamine responses to head-up tilt in the diagnosis of recurrent unexplained syncope in elderly patients. *J Am Geriatr Soc* 1991;39:663–669.

99. Grubb BP, Wolfe D, Gerard G, et al. Syncope and seizures of psychogenic origin: Identification with upright tilt table testing. *Clin Cardiol* 1992;15:839–842.

100. Grubb BP, Kosinski D, Boehm K, Kip K. The postural orthostatic tachycardia syndrome: A neurocardiogenic variant identified during head up tilt table testing. *Pacing Clin Electrophisiol* (in press).

101. Streeten DH. Abnormal orthostatic changes in blood pressure and heart rate in subjects with intact sympathetic nervous function: Evidence for excessive venous pooling. *J Lab Clin Med* 1988;111:326–335.

102. Sutton R, Peterson M, Brignole M, et al. Proposed classification for tilt-induced vasovagal syncope. *Eur J Cardiac Pacing Electrophysiol* 1992;2:180–183.

103. Blanc JJ, Mansourati J, Maheu B, et al. Reproducibility of a positive passive upright tilt test at a seven day interval in patients with syncope. *Am J Cardiol* 1993;72:469–471.

104. Fish FA, Strasburger JF, Benson W. Reproducibility of a sympomatic response to upright tilt in young patients with unexplained syncope. *Am J Cardiol* 1992;70:605–609.

105. Chen XC, Chen MY, Remole S, et al. Reproducibility of head up tilt table testing for eliciting susceptibility to neurally mediated syncope in patients without structural heart disease. *Am J Cardiol* 1992;69:755–760.

106. Grubb BP, Wolfe D, Temesy-Armos P, et al. Reproducibility of head upright tilt table test results in patients with syncope. *Pacing Clin Electrophisiol* 1992;15:1477–1481.

107. Benditt D, Ferguson D, Grubb BP, et al. Tilt table testing for assessing syncope: An American College of Cardiology Consensus document. *J Am Coll Cardiol* 1996;28:263–275.

108. Cox MM, Perlman B, Mayor MR, et al. Acute and long-term β-adrenergic blockade for patients with neurocardiogenic syncope. *J Am Coll Cardiol* 1995;26:1293–1298.

109. Mahanonda N, Bhuripanyo K, Kangkagate C, et al. Randomized placebo-controlled trial of oral atenolol in patients with unexplained syncope and positive upright tilt table test results. *Am Heart J* 1995;130:1250–1253.

110. Hjorth S, Sharp T. In vivo microdialysis evidence for central serotonin 1A and 1B autoreceptor of the β-receptor antagonist penbutolol. *J Pharmacol Exp Therap* 1993;265:707–712.

111. Hjorth S. Penbutolol as a blocker of central 5HT1A receptor-mediated responses. *Eur J Pharmacol* 1992;222:121–127.

112. Davgovian M, Jarardilla R, Frumin H. Prolonged aystole during head upright tilt table testing after β-blockage. *Pacing Clin Electrophisiol* 1992;15:14–16.

113. Milstein S, Buetikofer J, Durmigan A, et al. Usefulness of disopyramide for prevention of upright tilt-induced hypotension bradycardia. *Am J Cardiol* 1990;65:1334–1344.

114. Moullis CA, Leitch JW, Yee R, Klein GJ. A placebo-controlled trial of disopyramide for neurally mediated syncope induced by head up tilt. *J Am Coll Cardiol* 1993;22:1843–1848.

115. Bannister R. Multiple system atrophy and pure autonomic failure. In: Low P (ed): *Clinical Autonomic Disorders*. Boston: Little Brown Co.; 1993;517–525.

116. Nelson S, Stanley M, Love C, Schaal S. Autonomic and hemodynamic effects of oral theophylline in patients with vasodepressor syncope. *Arch Int Med* 1991;51:2425–2429.

117. Strieper M, Campbell R. Efficacy of α-adrenergic agonist therapy for the prevention of pediatric neurocardiogenic syncope. *J Am Coll Cardiol* 1993:22:594–597.

118. Susmano A, Volgman A, Buckingham T. Beneficial effects of dextroamphetamine in the treatment of vasodepressor syncope. *Pacing Clin Electrophisiol* 1993;16:1235–1238.

119. Grubb BP, Kosinski D, Kip K. Utility of methylphendiate in the therapy of refractory neurocardiogenic syncope. *Pacing Clin Electrophisiol* 1996;19:836–840.

120. Grubb BP, Wolfe D, Samoil D, et al. Usefulness of fluoxetine hydrochloride for prevention of resistant upright tilt-induced syncope. *Pacing Clin Electrophisiol* 1993;16:458–464.

121. Grubb BP, Samoil D, Kosinski D, et al. The use of sertraline hydrochloride in the treatment of refractory neurocardiogenic syncope in children and adolescents. *J Am Coll Cardiol* 1994;24:490–494.

122. Williamson BD, Strickberger A, Ching Men K, et al. A randomized trial of sertraline vs. atenolol and disopyramide in the treatment of neurocardiogenic syncope. (Abstr) *Pacing Clin Electrophisiol* 1994;17:747.

123. McGrady A, Bernal G. Relaxation-based treatment of stress-induced syncope. *J Behav Ther Exp Psychiatry* 1986;17:23–27.

124. Fitzpatrick AP, Travill CM, Yardas PE, et al. Recurrent symptoms after ventricular pacing in unexplained syncope. *Pacing Clin Electrophisiol* 1990;13:619–624.

125. Fitzpatrick A, Sutton R. Tilting toward a diagnosis in recurrent unexplained syncope. *Lancet* 1989;1:658–660.

126. Fitzpatrick A, Theodorakis G, Ahmed R. Dual chamber pacing aborts vasovagal syncope induced by head up 60° tilt. *Pacing Clin Electrophisiol* 1991;14:13–19.

127. McGuinn P, Moore S, Edel T, et al. Temporary dual chamber pacing during tilt table testing for vasovagal syncope: Predictor of therapeutic success. (Abstr) *Pacing Clin Electrophisiol* 1991;14:734.
128. Samoil D, Grubb BP, Brewster P, et al. Comparison of single and dual chamber pacing techniques in the prevention of upright tilt-induced vasovagal syncope. *Eur J Cardiac Pacing Electrophysiol* 1993;3:36–41.
129. Petersen ME, Chamberlain-Weber R, Fitzpatrick A, et al. Permanent pacing for prevention of recurrent vasovagal syncope. *Ann Int Med* 1995;122:204–209.
130. Benditt D, Petersen ME, Lurie K, et al. Cardiac pacing for prevention of recurrent vasovagal syncope. *Ann Int Med* 1995;122:204–209.
131. Gamachie C, Janosik D, Redd R, et al. Long-term outcome of head up tilt guided therapy in patients with neurally mediated syncope. (Abstr) *Pacing Clin Electrophisiol* 1991;14:663.
132. Sra JS, Anderson AJ, Sheikh SH, et al. Unexplained syncope evaluated by electrophysiologic studies and head up tilt testing. *Ann Int Med* 1991;114:1013–1019.
133. Brignole M, Menozzi C, Gianfranchi, et al. A controlled trial of acute and long-term medical therapy in tilt-induced neurally mediated syncope. *Am J Cardiol* 1992;70:339–342.
134. Fitzpatrick A, Theodorakis G, Travill C, Sutton R. Incidence of the malignant vasovagal syndrome in patients with recurrent syncope. *Eur Heart J* 1992; 12:389–394.
135. Fitzpatrick A, Ahmed R, Williams S, et al. A randomized trial of medical therapy in "malignant vasovagal syndrome" or "neurally mediated bradycardia/hypotension syndrome." *Eur J Cardiac Pacing Electrophysiol* 1991;1:99–102.
136. Grubb BP, Kosinski D. Samoil D, et al. Postpartum syncope. *Pacing Clin Electrophisiol* 1995;18:1028–1031.
137. Metcalfe J, Ueland K. Maternal cardiovascular adjustments to pregnancy. *Prog Cardiovasc Dis* 1974;16:363–374.
138. Elkayam U, Gleicher N. Cardiovascular physiology of pregnancy. In: U Elkayam, N Gleicher (eds): *Cardiac Problems in Pregnancy*. New York: Alan R Liss, Inc.; 1982;5–26.
139. Low P, McLeod J. The autonomic neuropathies. In: Low P (ed): *Clinical Autonomic Disorders*. Boston: Little Brown Co., Inc.; 1993;395–421.

Dysautonomic (Orthostatic) Syncope

Blair P. Grubb, MD

Introduction

One of the truly defining moments in the long process of human evolution was the adoption of upright posture. Although it greatly enhanced mobility, upright posture placed a new burden on a blood pressure control system that had evolved principally to meet the needs of an animal in the dorsal position. Thus, humans demonstrate an enhanced susceptibility to the effects of gravity on circulation. Indeed, the very organ that defines our humanity—the brain—is in the most precarious of locations in regard to vascular perfusion. The greatest challenge imposed on the body by upright posture is the downward shift of blood to a level below the heart. Via the sympathetic efferent pathways, the autonomic nervous system is the principal source of both short- and medium-term responses to these positional changes.[1] Although other mechanisms such as the renin-angiotensin-aldosterone system also contribute, their responses are seen over a much longer period. Thus, disturbances in autonomic function resulting in sympathetic failure can result in orthostatic (or positional) hypotension, which may be of a degree sufficient to lead to cerebral hypoperfusion and ultimately to loss of consciousness (syncope).

This chapter focuses on autonomic dysfunction as a cause of orthostatic hypotension leading to syncope. In it we review the physiological and biochemical abnormalities associated with these disorders, as well as the signs and symptoms commonly associated with them. We also provide an outline of both neurogenic and non-neurogenic causes of orthostatic hy-

From Grubb BP, Olshansky B (eds.). *Syncope: Mechanisms and Management.* Armonk, NY: Futura Publishing Co., Inc.; © 1998.

potension, a suggested plan of evaluation, and potential treatment options that are available.

Maintenance of Postural Normotension

In the normal human subject, approximately 25% to 30% of the circulating blood volume is in the thorax.[2] Assumption of the upright posture results in the gravity-mediated displacement of about 300 mL to 800 mL of blood (or 6 to 8 mL/kg) to the abdomen and lower extremities.[3] This represents a volume drop of 26% to 30%, with up to 50% of this fall occurring within seconds of standing. This rapid fall in central blood volume results in a drop in venous return to the heart. Since the heart cannot pump out what it does not receive, there is a reduction in stroke volume of about 40% due to the decrease in cardiac filling pressure.[3] This brings about a decrease in intravascular pressure above, and an increase in intravascular pressure below, what is referred to as the venous hydrostatic indifference point (HIP). The HIP represents the site in the vascular tree where pressure is independent of posture.[4] In humans, the venous HIP is at roughly the diaphragmatic level, while the arterial HIP is around the level of the left ventricle. Since the level of the venous HIP is to a large extent dependent on venous compliance, it can be affected by muscular activity.[5] During standing, leg muscle contractions combined with the venous valve system actively drive blood back to the heart, moving the HIP upward toward the right atrium. Respiratory activity also contributes to an increase in venous return. During deep inspiration there is a reduction in thoracic pressure favoring inward flow, while at the same time the intraabdominal pressure increases, reducing retrograde flow because of compression of the iliac and femoral veins.[6]

In addition to the aforementioned changes, upright posture also results in a large increase in the transmural capillary pressure in the dependent regions of the body, resulting in a net increase in fluid filtration into the tissue spaces. Equilibration of this transcapillary fluid shift occurs after about 30 minutes upright, during which there can be a net fall in plasma volume of up to 10%.[7]

In order for standing to occur successfully, a series of cardiovascular regulating mechanisms are brought into play, all aimed at preserving a constant level of arterial pressure and cerebral perfusion despite the effects of gravity. In normal subjects, orthostatic stabilization is achieved in 1 minute or less.[1] Interestingly, recent investigations have disclosed differences between the initial circulatory responses elicited by standing (active change) and those brought on by head-up tilt (passive change).[8] Wieling and van Lieshout[4,9] have divided the orthostatic response into three phases: 1) initial response (the first 30 seconds), 2) the early "steady state" circulatory adjustment (after 1 to 2 minutes upright), and 3) prolonged orthostasis (at least 5 minutes upright). As mentioned, these responses seem to differ somewhat according to whether the orthostatic stress is passive (tilt) or active (standing).

Immediately following head-up tilt, cardiac stroke volume remains normal for about six beats despite a fall in venous return (largely due to the blood in the pulmonary circulation). Next there is a gradual decline in both cardiac filling and arterial pressure.[10] These changes activate two groups of pressure receptors: high-pressure sites in the carotid sinus and the aortic arch, and low-pressure sites in the cardiac and pulmonary areas.[11] In regard to the latter, mechanoreceptors subserved by unmyelinated vagal afferents are present in all four cardiac chambers. These mechanoreceptors produce a tonic inhibitory effect on the cardiovascular centers of the medulla (in particular the nucleus tractus solitarii).[2] The reduction in venous return and filling pressure that results from the assumption of upright posture unloads these receptors, decreasing their firing rates thereby eliciting a reflex increase in sympathetic outflow with a resultant increase in vascular constriction in both the systemic resistance vessels and the splanchnic capacitance vessels.[1] A second local axon reflex, called the venoarteriolar axon reflex, also constricts arterial flow to muscle, skin, and adipose tissue.[12] This reflex can account for up to half of the increase in limb vascular resistance seen during standing.

Head-up tilt also seems to activate high-pressure receptors located in the carotid sinus. The initial increase in heart rate seen during tilt appears to be modulated by a fall in carotid arterial pressure.[4] The gradual increase in diastolic pressure seen during tilt appears more closely related to an increase in peripheral vascular resistance.

The initial circulatory response to standing is somewhat different.[10] The more active process of standing causes contraction of muscles in the legs and abdomen, resulting in the compression of both the capacitance and resistance vessels and an increase in peripheral vascular resistance. This actually results in a mild transient elevation in right atrial pressure and cardiac output that causes activation of low-pressure cardiac receptors. This increase in neural traffic to the brain stem causes a sudden decrease in peripheral vascular resistance that may drop by as much as 40%.[3] This in turn can allow for a fall in mean arterial blood pressure of up to 20 mm Hg that will last for up to 6 to 8 seconds. This drop is then addressed by the aforementioned mechanisms.

The early steady state period during upright posture is characterized by a steady increase in diastolic pressure of about 10%, with little or no change in systolic blood pressure. There is also an increase in heart rate of approximately 10 beats per minute. Compared with supine position, there is 30% less blood in the thorax, the cardiac output is 30% less, and the heart rate goes up by 10-15 beats per minute.[8]

Prolonged upright posture also brings neurohumoral mechanisms into play. The exact extent to which these mechanisms are activated depends, to a large extent, on the volume status of the patient. The greater the degree of volume depletion, the greater the degree of activation by the renin-angiotensin-aldosterone, as well as that of vasopressin.[13] However, the principal mechanism by which prolonged upright posture is compensated for lies in the arterial baroreceptor (especially carotid sinus) influence on peripheral vascular resistance.[4] Failure of any component in these complex responses can lead to a failure of normal compensation to postural change, which can lead to hypotension and resultant syncope.

Causes of Orthostatic Hypotension (Table 1)

The neurogenic causes of profound orthostatic hypotension can be subdivided into primary causes and secondary causes. Primary causes are for the most part idiopathic in nature, while secondary causes are associated with a known biochemical or structural anomaly, or are seen as part of a particular disease or syndrome.

Primary Causes

Chronic

Clinical dysautonomic syndromes may be either acute or chronic in nature. The chronic idiopathic form of this disorder was first described by Bradbury and Eggleston in 1925 and was termed "idiopathic orthostatic hypotension" because of its apparent lack of association with other gross neurological features.[14] The term "idiopathic orthostatic hypotension," however, is felt to ill represent the fact there is usually a general state of autonomic failure present with disturbances in bladder, sudomotor, and sexual function. Most investigators now prefer the term "pure autonomic failure" to describe this syndrome.[15] There is some evidence suggesting that autonomic failure in isolation may be due to degeneration of the peripheral postganglionic autonomic neurons (although definitive pathological confirmation of this has not yet been made).[16]

Primary chronic autonomic failure that is associated with other idiopathic neurological defects was first described by Shy and Drager[17] in 1960. More recently, the term "multiple system atrophy" (MSA) has been used to describe this devastating disorder.[18] There is little that can match the eloquence of the original report:

> *The full syndrome consists of the following features; orthostatic hypotension, urinary and rectal incontinence, loss of sweating, iris atrophy, external ocular palsies, rigidity, tremor, loss of associated movements, impotence, the findings of*

_____ **Table 1** _____

A Classification of Autonomic Disorders

Primary Autonomic Failure
  Pure Autonomic Failure
  Multiple System Atrophy
    Parkinsonian
    Cerebellar/Pyramidal
    Mixed
  Acute and Subacute Dysautonomias
Secondary Autonomic Failure
  Central Origin
    Age-related
    Multiple Sclerosis
    Cerebral Tumors (in particular those of the posterior fossa or third ventricle)
    Syringobulbia
  Peripheral Origin
    Afferent
      Gillian-Barré Syndrome
      Tabes Dorsalis
      Holmes-Adie Syndrome
    Efferent
      Diabetes Mellitus
      Amyloidosis
      Dopamine-β-Hydroxylase Deficiency
      Nerve Growth Factor Deficiency
    Afferent/Efferent
      Familial Dysautonomia
    Spinal Origin
      Transverse Myelitus
      Spinal Transverse Myelitus
      Spinal Tumors
      Syringomyelia
    Miscellaneous
      Renal Failure
      Neoplasia
      Autoimmune And Collagen Diseases
      Human Immunodeficiency Virus Infection

Adapted from Mathias.[27]

> *an atonic bladder, and loss of rectal sphincter tone, fasciculations, wasting of*
> *distal muscles, evidence of a neuropathic lesion in the electro-myogram that sug-*
> *gests involvement of the anterior horn cells, and the finding of a neuropathic*
> *lesion in the muscle biopsy. The date of onset is usually in the 5th to 7th decade*
> *of life.*[17]

Recent investigators have divided this form of autonomic failure into three major clinical subtypes.[18,19] The first subgroup consists of patients who have parkinsonian features (also referred to as the striatonigral degeneration group), those with cerebellar and/or pyramidal features (also referred to as the cerebellar or olivopontocerebellar atrophy/degeneration form), and finally, those patients who seem to exhibit features of both forms. It may be quite difficult to distinguish the parkinsonian form from classic idiopathic Parkinson's disease. Recent studies have found that somewhere between 7% and 22% of patients thought to have Parkinson's disease while alive were, at autopsy, found to exhibit neuropathological features consistent with multiple system atrophy.[18]

Acute

Acute panautonomic neuropathy, causing orthostatic hypotension and syncope is uncommon, but often dramatic in its presentation. The principal features that characterize acute panautonomic neuropathy (also called pandysautonomia) are elaborated by Low and McLeod[20] and consist of 1) acute or subacute onset, 2) widespread and severe sympathetic and parasympathetic failure, and 3) relative or total sparing of somatic nerve fibers. In almost every case, this acute onset of sympathetic and parasympathetic failure occurs in relatively young people who were previously quite healthy.[21] Malfunction of the sympathetic nervous system results in severe orthostatic hypotension of such a degree that patients are unable to sit upright in bed without losing consciousness. There is often a loss of sweating. Failure of the parasympathetic system results in dry mouth and eyes and a disruption in both bladder and bowel function. The latter is manifested by abdominal pain, bloating, nausea, vomiting, and severe constipation that may occasionally alternate with profuse diarrhea.[22] One of the most prominent features of the disorder is that patients often have a fixed heart rate of approximately 40 to 55 beats per minute with complete chronotropic incompetence. Many patients will also have fixed dilated pupils. Occasionally acute autonomic failure is accompanied by acute and inexorable neuropathic pain that may be truly agonizing to the patient.[23]

The rapidness of the onset of symptoms is often quite dramatic, and many of our patients have been able to relate the exact moment the illness began. Many patients complain of an antecedent febrile illness (presumed to be a viral infection), suggesting that the illness may be immune mediated.[20]

On physical examination these patients display profound orthostatic hypotension, a fixed heart rate, and fixed dilated pupils.[20,24] Patients often have urinary retention and dry, flaky skin. Gross motor strength and sensory perception are usually normal, although occasionally patients have abnormal pain and temperature perception.

There has been little systematic evaluation of the course and long-term prognosis of acute autonomic neuropathy. Although some patients make remarkable recoveries, for many the disease follows a chronic debilitating course that leaves significant residual deficits in its wake.

Secondary Causes

The secondary causes of autonomic failure or dysfunction include those disorders where the lesion has been identified or where there is a clear association with a known disease (for example diabetes mellitus or spinal cord transection). As noted in Table 1, there are a large variety of disorders that may be accompanied by autonomic dysfunction.

In older patients, a larger number of whom manifest orthostatic hypotension, a number of potential causes may coexist. Recent investigations have revealed that orthostatic hypotension may occur due to a single enzyme abnormality. An example of this is the condition known as isolated dopamine β-hydroxylase (DBH) deficiency.[25] Another cause can be nerve growth factor deficiency (which may actually cause DBH deficiency), or dopa decarboxylase deficiency and reduction in certain sensory neuropeptides.[26] Orthostatic hypotension may also be seen as a complication of neurological disorders that affect other neuronal systems (such as the thalamus), or with prior mediated disorders such as fatal familial dysautonomia. Orthostatic hypotension may also accompany conditions such as chronic renal failure, neoplastic disorders, and the acquired immune deficiency syndrome (AIDS).[27]

Pharmacological agents that affect the sympathetic nervous system may either cause or exacerbate orthostatic hypotension.[28] (Table 2) Drugs with central activity examples include reserpine, barbiturates, methyldopa, clonidine, and tricyclic antidepressants. Peripherally acting agents that may cause problems include prazosin, phenoxybenzamine, guanethidine, angiotensin-converting enzyme (ACE) inhibitors and β-blocking agents. Indeed, virtually any vasodilatory agent may exacerbate an otherwise mild tendency to orthostatic hypotension. On occasion, a patient may secretly use an agent to produce a factitious illness (Munchausen's syndrome) that simulates orthostatic hypotension. In addition, a patient may be covertly using illicit drugs (unbeknownst to family or friends) that result in orthostatic intolerance.

Clinical Features

The principal feature in virtually all of these various disorders is some form of impairment in cardiovascular regulation that manifests itself as orthostatic (or postural) hypotension. Orthostatic hypotension itself has been somewhat arbitrarily defined as a fall of >20 mm Hg systolic blood pressure within 3 minutes of standing.[15] However, it should be kept in mind that a smaller drop in pressure that is associated with symptoms may be

_____ Table 2 _____

Drugs That Cause Orthostatic Hypotension

Diuretics	β-Blockers
ACE Inhibitors	Calcium Channel Blockers
α-Blockers	Phenothiazines
Tricyclic Antidepressants	Bromocriptine
Ethanol	Opiates

equally important. In addition, some patients may exhibit a slow but steady decline in blood pressure over a somewhat longer period of time (10 to 15 minutes) that may be associated with symptoms. Whether a particular drop in blood pressure will produce symptoms is not determined solely by the absolute blood pressure, but is also dependent on the rate of change during the fall and the ability of cerebral autoregulation to maintain perfusion in the face of systemic hypotension.[27] It is also important to remember that postural hypotension is only one manifestation of disordered cardiovascular control. Patients suffering from autonomic failure may respond in an exaggerated fashion to any physiological or pharmacological stimulus that is capable of raising or lowering blood pressure.[19]

The syncopal spells that accompany orthostatic hypotension may sometimes appear as "drop attacks" that occur with little or no prodrome.[29] More commonly however, there is a gradual loss of consciousness over half a minute or so while the patient is standing or walking. Some patients report experiencing a neckache, proceeding syncope, that radiates to the shoulders and occipital region of the skull.[18] Other commonly reported prodromata include blurred vision and a sensation of dizziness, after which the patient may stumble or fall to his or her knees, then experience loss of consciousness. The visual disturbances seen also include tunnel vision, scotomata, and hallucinations. As opposed to classic vasovagal syncope, there is no associated diaphoresis and the episodes are not accompanied by bradycardia.[19] Episodes tend to be more common in the early morning hours and following meals, particularly if accompanied by alcohol consumption. Hot weather and exertion may also worsen episodes, presumably because each of these conditions leads to a redistribution of blood flow to peripheral or mesenteric areas. The primary autonomic failure syndromes tend to be slowly progressive over a number of years before the patient becomes significantly incapacitated. Although orthostatic hypotension may represent the most disabling aspect of autonomic failure, abnormalities of cardiovascular control may also be manifested by a fixed heart rate and supine hypertension. Both extremes in blood pressure may contribute to the functional disability in patients with orthostatic hypotension, and make therapy difficult.

Many patients with primary autonomic failure may develop impairment of body temperature regulation due to either hypohidrosis or anhidrosis, which predisposes them to hyperpyrexia and collapse during periods of hot weather.[18] Male patients will quite frequently experience impotence early in the course of these disorders, followed later by ejaculatory failure. In some patients multiple gastrointestinal complaints may be present. Constipation is a common finding, and it may alternate with diarrhea. Rectal incontinence may occur, as may dysphagia, although these usually do not occur until the later stages of the disease. A surprisingly common complaint is that of nocturnal polyuria.[27] This is presumed to occur because of the redistribution of blood from the peripheral areas to central areas during recumbency. Patients with severe nocturnal polyuria may lose as much as one liter of fluid in a single night, which may account for the greater frequency of postural symptoms in the early morning hours. Even in the presence of normal coronary arteries, classic angina pectoris may develop during periods of profound hypotension. Patients with advanced multiple system atrophy may experience a central form of sleep apnea associated with loud snoring and involuntary inspiratory gasps.

In patients with MSA, parkinsonian features may be quite prominent and can lead to a misdiagnosis of Parkinson's disease.[18] In these patients the most common features are rigidity and bradykinesia. As opposed to true Parkinson's disease, which often begins unilaterally, the involvement in MSA is usually bilateral at onset. Dysarthria and micrographia are common features. In contrast to Parkinson's disease, a resting tremor is uncommon in MSA. Dementia is no more common among patients with MSA than it is among the general population.

Investigation of Autonomic Disorders

As with any clinical disorder, the investigation begins with a detailed history and physical examination. Laboratory evaluation is then undertaken in a directed manner and the information obtained from all of these endeavors is merged together to make a diagnosis and arrive at a reasonable plan of management.

The first aim of the clinical evaluation is to determine whether or autonomic dysfunction is present, and if it is, in what distribution it occurs. At the same time one should endeavor to recognize any specific patterns that can be related to known syndromes (some of which may require special investigations), and in particular to recognize potentially treatable problems. Finally, it is most important to determine the effects on the patient of the autonomic dysfunction.

Outlining of all the various patterns of autonomic dysfunction that may be present is beyond the scope of this chapter. The interested reader is directed to several excellent texts of autonomic disorders, which include several pertinent (and illustrative) examples.[30-33] Autonomic dysfunction due to amyloid polyneuropathy is diffuse in nature, with a selective loss of pain and temperature sensation, orthostatic hypotension, and weight loss.[34] Amyloid infiltration can be demonstrated in the subcutaneous fat, rectal tissue, and nerves.[35] In patients with diabetic neuropathy, not only is there obvious hyperglycemia, there are also signs and symptoms of diffuse autonomic failure involving the cardiovagal, postganglionic sympathetic, sudomotor, and adrenergic systems. It is particularly important to identify any drugs the patient may be taking that could result in orthostatic hypotension (such as antihypertensive agents).[28] In young people with severe autonomic dysfunction it is important to consider the possibility of street drugs (such as cocaine, amphetamines, crack, or phencyclidine) as well as alcohol as contributing factors. Other potentially treatable problems are autonomic dysfunction associated with thallium or arsenic neuropathy.[27]

In the patient's history, the physician should endeavor to identify any cyclic or fluctuating nature to his or her symptoms. Orthostatic hypotension may exhibit spontaneous variations throughout the course of the day, and may vary in respect to medication, meals, and with the menstrual cycle in women. Knowledge of these variations can be quite useful in planning a therapeutic program.

The anatomic location of the preganglionic autonomic nervous system makes it relatively inaccessible to direct physiological assessment. Therefore, tests used to evaluate the adequacy of autonomic function are not direct assessments, rather, they measure end organ responses to various physiological and pharmacological challenges. In addition, it is possible to determine the levels of both autonomic neurotransmitters and neuromodulators in the plasma, urine, and cerebrospinal fluid. Quantification of autonomic receptor density and affinity can also be performed.

The first and simplest test is to test blood pressure in the supine, sitting, and standing positions. The fall in blood pressure that is regarded as significant is somewhat variable between laboratories, but is generally felt to be 20-30 mm Hg systolic and 10-15 mm Hg diastolic.[15] Care should be taken to measure blood pressure when standing with the arm extended horizontally to prevent the hydrostatic effects of a fluid column in the dependent arm (which could potentially result in a falsely elevated reading). Since, as previously alluded to, the nature of the orthostatic response to active standing differs from that of passive tilting, we often perform tilt table testing on these subjects. Tilting also provides a stable setting for the measurement of other determinants of autonomic function, and it seems to provide an adequate degree of reproducibility.[36] Presently, we perform head-upright tilt table testing while the patient is fasting. A standard tilt table with a foot board made for weight bearing is used and a standard sphygmomanometer is used for blood pressure measurements. Patients are also connected to a standard cardiographic monitor for continuous evaluation of heart rate and rhythm. The tilt table is then inclined at an angle 70° from horizontal for a period of 45 minutes, with blood pressures measured every 3 minutes until hypotension begins. At this time, measurements are made every 30 seconds. We now also routinely measure cerebral blood flow during tilt by means of transcranial Doppler ultrasonography.[37,38] In addition to measuring blood pressure, heart rate responses are also determined at rest and in response to standing and head-up tilt, to deep respiration, and to Valsalva maneuver. Resting heart rate is principally determined by vagal tone, which normally declines upon standing, resulting in an increase in heart rate of between 10 and 30 beats per minute.[39] The normal maximum heart rate response to standing occurs after 15 beats, then slows to a stable rate by the 30th beat.[3] This response depends on a normal parasympathetic innervation of the heart.

Other tests include assessment of thermoregulatory sweating by raising the body temperature using an external heat source. The sweat response is then measured by the degree of color change of an indicator substance (which is spread over the body) such as iodine with starch, quinizarin, or alizarin red.[40] Cutaneous bioelectric recordings that measure the degree of skin conductance, skin resistance, or the sympathetic skin potential are also used as another method of ascertaining sudomotor function.[41]

The serum levels of norepinephrine and the way they change between the supine and head-up tilt positions can also be used to determine the nature of suspected autonomic failure.[42,43] In patients suffering from deficits in the postganglionic sympathetic vasomotor fibers, the supine plasma norepinephrine levels can be abnormally low, whereas in patients with multiple system atrophy, supine plasma levels are usually normal.[27] With both disorders, however, the expected increase in plasma norepinephrine levels during tilt may either be blunted or absent, indicating a sympathetic outflow dysfunction. Plasma vasopressin levels may also be measured in order to determine the function of the afferent limb of the baroreflex. Failure of vasopressin to increase during hypotension in a patient documented to have a normal response to an infusion of hypertonic saline can be due to lesions affecting the baroreceptor afferents in the vagus nerve or their central connections to the paraventricular hypothalamic nuclei.[24]

The response of the body to pharmacological challenges with a number of different agents has also been used. These agents include epinephrine, norepinephrine, isoproterenol, clonidine, and atropine.[29] Each is used to determine the sensitivity of different groups of receptors as well as the functional status of the cardiac vagus and sympathetic nerve terminals. The interested reader is directed to several excellent references on these tests.[43]

Therapeutic Measures (Table 3)

Foremost in the treatment of orthostatic hypotension is the identification and treatment of potentially reversible causes. For example,

_____ **Table 3** _____

Treatment Options

Therapy	Method or Dose	Common Problems
Head-up tilt of bed	45° head-up tilt of bed, (often will need footboard)	Hypotension, sliding off bed, leg cramps
Elastic support hose	Require at least 30–40 mm Hg ankle counterpressure, work best if waist high	Uncomfortable, hot, difficult to get on
Diet	Fluid intake of 2–2.5 liters/day Na^+ intake of 150–250 mEq/day	Supine hypertension peripheral edema
Exercise	Aerobic exercise (mild) may aid venous return. Water exercise particularly helpful	May lower blood pressure if done too vigorously
Fludrocortisone	Begin at 0.1–0.2 mg/day may work up to doses not exceeding 1.0 mg/day	Hypokalemia, hypomagnesemia peripheral edema, weight gain, congestive heart failure
Methylphenidate	5–10 mg PO TID given with meals, give last dose before 6 pm	Agitation, tremor, insomina, supine hypertension
Midodrine	2.5–10 mg every 2–4 hours. May use up to 40 mg/day	Nausea, supine hypertension
Clonidine	0.1–0.3 mg PO BID or patches placed 1/week	Dry mouth, bradycardia hypotension, bradycardia
Yohimbine	8 mg PO BID to TID	Diarrhea, anxiety nervousness
Ephedrine sulfate	12.5–25 PO TID	Tachycardia, tremor, supine hypertension
Fluoxetine	10–20 mg PO Q day (requires 4–6 weeks of therapy)	Nausea, anorexia, diarrhea

continues

_____ Table 3   Continued _____

Treatment Options

Therapy	Method or Dose	Common Problems
Erythopoiten	4,000 IU sq twice a week	Requires injections, burning at site, increase hematocribe CVA
Pindolol	2.5–5.0 mg PO BID to TID	Hypotension, congestive heart failure, bradycardia
Desmopressin	An analog of vasopressin used as a nasal spray	Hyponnatremia

PO = _per os_ (by mouth); TID = three times a day; BID = twice daily; sq = subcutaneous; CVA = cerebrovascular accident.

problems such as volume depletion, blood loss, and drug-induced hypotension all represent treatable causes. When the cause of the hypotension is not reversible, treatments aimed at improving symptoms are initiated.

Primary in the therapy of these disorders is the education of the patient and family as to the nature of the disorder. Any potential precipitating factors, such as extreme heat, should be avoided. Neurogenic orthostatic hypotension is often greatly worsened when the patient becomes dehydrated or sodium depleted (or both), thus, patients should be encouraged to maintain an adequate intake of salt and water. Since large meals may cause a great amount of splanchnic shunting and aggravate symptoms, patients are advised to eat smaller and more frequent meals with a reduced carbohydrate content. Alcohol, a vasodilator, can markedly aggravate symptoms and should be avoided.

Patients should understand that these disorders are chronic in nature, and that for the most part treatments tend to be palliative, rather than curative in nature. It has been our experience that many patients will go through a period of depression, sometimes accompanied by a period of denial and occasional anger, after being given this information. However most patients, with time, learn to accept their illness and continue on despite it. Some patients and their families may require psychological counseling to help them cope with their condition.

Sleeping with the head of the bed elevated upright is often helpful.[44] It seems to moderate the sudden pooling of blood that can occur on arising in the morning, and it may lessen the degree of nocturnal diuresis. In addition to reducing the degree of supine hypertension, remaining at mildly elevated levels seems to condition the cerebrovasculature to low pressures. If a hospital bed is used, a 45° head-up angle is used; alternatively the head of the bed can be elevated to approximately 6 to 12 inches. Some patients may need a footboard to keep them from sliding off the edge of the bed. Upon waking, patients should sit on the edge of the bed for several minutes before standing, and then do so slowly.[45]

For a number of years, physicians have prescribed custom fitted elastic support hose to create a counterpressure gradient in the lower extremities in order to reduce the degree of venous pooling. The garments are constructed such that maximum pressure is exerted at the ankles with less pressure at the top. Usually, at least 30 to 40 mm Hg ankle counterpressure must be used in order to be effective. Although they are helpful, they may be difficult to put on and quite uncomfortable in hot climates.

A number of pharmacological measures have been used in the treatment of orthostatic hypotension. One of the mainstays of therapy for orthostatic hypotension is 9-α-fludrocortisone. First reported by Hickler et al[46] in 1959, it is a mineral corticoid that acts on the distal renal tubule to promote the reabsorption of sodium in exchange for a loss of potassium and hydrogen ions. This retention of sodium promotes a retention of water and thereby affects an increase in total blood volume. As previously noted, patients with autonomic failure tend to have a reduced blood volume, and are quite sensitive to changes in their fluid balance. However, this increase in blood volume seems to be transient and after a month or so, it cannot be detected even though at this point, tissue stores of fluid are often increased. In addition, fludrocortisone appears to increase the sensitivity of blood vessels to the effects of norepinephrine, thereby increasing the peripheral vascular resistance.[18] Some recent evidence suggests that fludrocortisone may even increase the number of α-receptors in the vasculature.[47,48] The starting dosage is 0.1 mg once or twice a day and can be slowly titrated up to 1.0 mg PO (by mouth) twice a day (although it is unclear if dosages in excess of 0.4 mg/day provide much additional benefit). Patients should be encouraged to increase their salt and fluid intake. The patient should be monitored for hypokalemia and hypomagnesemia while on therapy. Many patients may have a transient period of peripheral edema lasting approximately 1 week. In patients with reduced cardiac function, care must be taken not to precipitate congestive heart failure from increase in fluid volume. Care must also be taken not to cause excessive supine hypertension. Most patients for whom fludrocortisone is effective will have supine blood pressures in the range of 190/90 to 180/100 mm Hg. However, persistent supine pressures above 200/120 mm Hg should be avoided, and if they occur, a change in dosage is required. Fludrocortisone may worsen preexisting migraines or acne, and occasional patients complain of hair loss.

Another longstanding form of therapy is the sympathetic "stimulators." These agents augment the actions of the patient's own sympathetic nervous system to increase vascular tone. An example of such an agent is yohimbine, an α_2-receptor antagonist.[49] Central α_2 stimulation inhibits the sympathetic activity, thus, by blocking this, yohimbine augments sympathetic outflow. The drug causes a small, but nonetheless significant, rise in serum norepinephrine and it increases blood pressure. Dosages are in the range of 8 mg PO twice daily (BID) or three times a day (TID), with the major side effects being anxiety, nervousness, and diarrhea.

A number of sympathomimetic drugs have been used for the treatment of orthostatic hypotension.[50] These agents act via either direct or indirect stimulation of α-adrenergic receptors, which promote both arteriolar and venous vasoconstriction. It should be kept in mind that many patients with orthostatic hypotension are extremely sensitive to the effects of these agents, and extreme supine hypertension may result from their use. The earliest agents used included ephedrine, phenylephrine, and vasopressin. Biaggioni et al[51] report that phenylpropanolamine can be effective. The amphetamine-like agent, methylphenidate, may sometimes be quite useful for controlling postural hypotension, but central nervous system (CNS) stimulation and potential for dependence limit its utility.[50] A somewhat more attractive agent with similar degrees of α-adrenergic activity is midodrine. This drug causes vasoconstriction in both the arteriolar and venous capacitance vessels without producing stimulation in the CNS or cardiac systems.[52] Studies have demonstrated that it is a safe and effective therapy for orthostatic disorders.[53]

While it sounds somewhat paradoxical, the α_2-adrenergic agonist, clonidine, may be quite useful when the hypotension occurs secondary to a profound efferent postganglionic sympathetic lesion.[54] Postjunctional vascular α_2-receptors are widespread (particularly in veins), and appear to be hypersensitive in autonomic failure.[55] Even though the drug's central activity inhibits sympathetic outflow (resulting in hypotension), patients with severe autonomic failure often have little or no remaining sympathetic activity and the peripheral effects are allowed to predominate.

Some investigators advocate the use of β-blockers, particularly when the postural hypotension is associated with supine hypertension.[48] β-blockers have been shown to elevate peripheral resistance, an effect most likely due to blockage of the β_2 (vasodilatory) receptors. Their negative inotropic and chronotropic actions, however, often limit their use. Pindolol, a drug with intrinsic sympathomimetic activity, is advocated by some as a potential alternative.

Recently, two novel therapeutic approaches have emerged: erythropoietin and the serotonin reuptake inhibitors.[4] Erythropoietin has been found to cause a remarkable improvement in orthostatic tolerance when administered to patients with autonomic failure.[56,57] The mechanism of action is unclear, but it appears to be independent of the drug's ability to raise red blood cell count.[58] Its major drawbacks are its expense and the fact that it needs to be injected. Despite these drawbacks it can be remarkably effective for some people.

A large body of research has demonstrated that central serotonergic activity plays a major role in central regulation of blood pressure.[59] Recent evidence suggests that the serotonin reuptake inhibitors (or SSRIs) may be an effective therapy in the prevention of the sudden hypotension seen during episodes of neurocardiogenic syncope.[60] At the same time, it has been realized that some of the SSRIs (venlafaxine in particular) may produce hypertension in patients. Grubb et al report some success in treating patients who have orthostatic hypotension with the agent fluoxetine hydrochloride[61] as well as with venlafaxine hydrochloride.[62] The mechanism by which this effect may occur is unknown.

Patients with autonomic failure are often noted to have a resting bradycardia as well as a marked chronotropic incompetence. Moss et al[62] and Weissman et al[63] report that continuous tachypacing can be effective for treatment of otherwise refractory cases of orthostatic hypotension. However, continuous tachypacing virtually eliminates any degree of heart rate variability, and it may exacerbate supine hypertension (not to mention the stress that pacing at high rates may place on the heart). Grubb et al[65] report on the use of an adaptive-rate pacing system controlled by right ventricular preejection interval in a patient with refractory orthostatic hypotension. The pacemaker adequately sensed the fall in blood pressure while sitting or standing, and increased the pacing rate accordingly, thereby preventing syncope. While supine, the pacing rate fell to a preprogrammed 60 pulses per minute, thus avoiding any exacerbation of the patient's concomitant hypertension. Further improvements in pacemaker sensors that would allow for the direct or indirect measurement of blood pressure would allow these devices to alter their rate according to need, and potentially make pacing a more attractive option in the management of orthostatic hypotension.[66]

It is important to remember that the aforementioned therapies are principally aimed at controlling orthostatic hypotension, and that the patient with autonomic failure will often have multiple other complaints that these treatments will not address. It should also be kept in mind that autonomic disorders are often progressive in nature, thus any treatment plan may have to be significantly modified over time.

Conclusions

Autonomic dysfunction is a common and frequently unrecognized cause of syncope. There is a huge spectrum in the etiology and severity of disorders, which may all manifest themselves by orthostatic intolerance. As the overall age of the western societies increases, autonomic dysfunction will likely become an increasingly important cause of syncope.

References

1. Joyner MJ, Shepherd JT. Autonomic control of the circulation. In: Low P. (ed): *Clinical Autonomic Disorders*. Boston: Little Brown Co.; 1993;55–67.
2. Shepherd JT, Shepherd RFJ. Control of the blood pressure and circulation in man. In: Bannister R, Mathias C. (eds): *Autonomic Failure: A Textbook of Clinical Disorders of the Autonomic Nervous System*. Oxford: Oxford Medical Publishers; 1992;78–93.
3. Smith JJ. *Circulatory Response to the Upright Posture*. Ann Arbor: CRC Press; 1990;187.
4. Wieling W, van Lieshout JJ. Maintenance of postural normotension in humans. In: Low P. (ed): *Clinical Autonomic Disorders*. Boston: Little Brown Co.: 1993;69–75.
5. Blomquist CG, Stone HL. Cardiovascular adjustments to gravitational stress. In: Shepherd JJ, Abboud FM (eds): *Handbook of Physiology, Section 2: The Cardiovascular System*. Bethesda: The American Physiological Society; 1983;1025–1063.
6. Rowell LB. *Human Circulation Regulation During Physical Stress*. Oxford: Oxford University Press; 1986.
7. Thompson WO, Thompson PK, Dailey ME. The effect of posture upon the composition and volume of the blood in man. *J Clin Invest* 1988;5:573–609.
8. Streeten DHP. *Orthostatic Disorders of the Circulation: Mechanisms, Manifestations and Treatment*. New York: Plenum Publishing; 1957.
9. Wieling W, TenHarkel A, van Lieshout JJ. Classification of orthostatic disorders based on the short-term circulatory response upon standing. *Clin Sci* 1991; 99:241–248.
10. Wieling W, van Lieshout JJ. Circulatory adaptation upon standing. In:Yoshikawa M. (ed): *New Trends in Autonomic Nervous System Research, Excerpt 2 Medica*. Amsterdam: 1991;200–204.
11. Angell-James JE, Daily MB. Comparison of the reflex vasomotor responses to separate and combined stimulation of the carotid sinus and aortic arch baroreceptors by pulsatile and nonpulsatile pressures in the dog. *J Physiol (Lond)* 1970;209:257–293.
12. Henriksen O, Sejrsen P. Local reflex in microcirculation in human skeletal muscle. *Acta Physiol Scand* 1977;99:19–26.
13. Sancho J. The role of the renin-angiotensin-aldosterone system in cardiovascular homeostasis in normal human subjects. *Circulation* 1976;53:400–405.
14. Bradbury S, Eggleston C. Postural hypotension: A report of three cases. *Am Heart J* 1925;1:73–86.
15. Mathias CJ. The classification and nomenclature of autonomic disorders: Ending chaos, resolving conflict and hopefully achieving clarity. *Clin Auton Res* 1995;5:307–310.
16. Freeman R. Pure Autonomic Failure. In: Robertson D, Biaggioni I (eds): *Disorders of the Autonomic Nervous System*. London: Harwood Academic Publishers; 1995;61–82.
17. Shy GM, Drager GA. A neurological syndrome associated with orthostatic hypotension. *Arch Neurol* 1960;3:511–527.
18. Bannister R. Multiple system trophy and pure autonomic failure. In Low P (ed): *Clinical Autonomic Disorders*. Boston: Little Brown Co.; 1993;517–526.

19. Polinsky RJ. Shy-Drager syndrome and multiple system atrophy. In: Robertson D, Biaggioni I (eds): *Disorders of the Autonomic Nervous System.* London: Harwood Academic Publishers; 1995;107–141.
20. Low P, McLeod J. The autonomic neuropathies. In Low P (ed): *Clinical Autonomic Disorders.* Boston: Little Brown Co.; 1993;395–421.
21. Suarez GA, Fealey RD, Camilleri M, Low P. Idiopathic autonomic neuropathy: Clinical, neurophysiological, and followup studies on 27 patients. *Neurology* 1994;44:1675–1682.
22. Appenzeller O, Kornfeld M. Acute Pandysautonomia. *Arch Neurol* 1973;29:334–339.
23. Thomashefsky AJ, Horowitz SJ, Feingold MH. Acute autonomic neuropathy. *Neurology* 1972;22:251–255.
24. Appenzeller O. Peripheral autonomic neuropaties. In: Robertson D, Biaggioni I (eds): *Disorders of the Autonomic Nervous System.* London: Harwood Academic Publishers;1995;141–145.
25. Robertson D, Perry SE, Hollister AS, et al. Dobamine-hydroxylase deficiency: A genetic disorder of cardiovascular regulation. *Hypertension* 1991;18:1–8.
26. Robertson D. Genetic disorders of the autonomic nervous system. In: Robertson D, Biaggioni I (eds): *Disorders of the Autonomic Nervous System.* London: Harwood Academic Publishers; 1995;197–215.
27. Mathias CJ. Orthostatic hypotension: Causes, mechanisms and influencing factors. *Neurology* 1995;45(suppl):6–11.
28. Wynne HA, Schofield S. Drug-induced orthostatic hypotension. In Kenny R (ed): *Syncope in the Older Patient.* London: Chapman and Hall Ltd.; 1996:137–154.
29. Mathias CJ, Bannister R. Clinical features and investigation of the primary autonomic failure syndromes. In: Bannister R, Mathias C (eds): Autonomic Failure: A Textbook of Clinical Disorders of the Autonomic Nervous System. Oxford: Oxford Medical Publishers; 1992;531–547.
30. Low P (ed). *Clinical Autonomic Disorders.* Boston: Little Brown Co.; 1993.
31. Robertson D, Biaggioni I (eds): *Disorders of the Autonomic Nervous System.* London: Harwood Academic Publishers; 1995.
32. Bannister R, Mathias C. *Autonomic Failure: A Textbook of Clinical Disorders of the Autonomic Nervous System.* Oxford: Oxford Medical Publications; 1992.
33. Robertson D, Polinsky R. *A Primer on the Autonomic Nervous System.* San Diego: Academic Press, Inc.; 1996.
34. Kelly JJ. The natural history of peripheral neuropathy in primary systemic amyloidosis. *Ann Neurol* 1979;6:1–7.
35. Kyle RA, Greipp PR. Amyloidosis; clinical and laboratory features in 229 cases. *Mayo Clinic Proc* 1983;58:665–683.
36. Grubb BP, Kosinski D. Current trends in the etiology, diagnosis, and management of neurocardiogenic syncope. *Curr Opin Cardiol* 1996;11:32–41.
37. Grubb BP, Gerard G, Roush K, et al. Cerebral vasoconstriction during head upright tilt-induced vasovagal syncope. *Circulation* 1991;84:1157–1164.
38. Brooks DJ, Redmond S, Mathias CJ, et al. The effect of orthostatic hypotension on cerebral blood flow and middle cerebral artery velocity in autonomic failure, with observations on the effect of ephedrine. *J Neurol Neurosurg Psychiatry* 1989;50:962–966.
39. Bannister R, Sever P, Gross M. Cardiovascular reflexes and biochemical responses in progressive autonomic failure. *Brain* 1977;100:327–344.
40. Sato K. One step iodine starch method for direct visualization of sweating. *Am J Med Sci* 1988;259:528–531.

41. Low PA. Quantitative sudomotor axon reflex test in normal and neuropathic subjects. *Ann Neurol* 1983;14:573–580.
42. Lipsitz L. Abnormalities in blood pressure regulation. In: Kenny R (ed): *Syncope in the Older Patient.* London: Chapman and Hall Ltd.; 1996;33–46.
43. Mathias C, Bannister CJ. Investigation of autonomic disorders. In: Bannister R, Mathias C (eds): *Autonomic Failure: A Textbook of Clinical Disorders of the Autonomic Nervous System.* Oxford: Oxford Medical Publishers.; 1992;255–290.
44. MacLean AR, Allen EY. Orthostatic hypotension and orthostatic tachycardia: Treatment with the "head up" bed. *JAMA* 1940;115:2162.
45. Wieling W, van Lieshout JJ, van Leeuwen AM. Physical manoeuvres that reduce postural hypotension in autonomic failure. *Clin Autonomic Res* 1993;3:57–66.
46. Hickler RB, Thompson GR, Fox LM, Hamlin JT. Successful treatment of orthostatic hypotension with 9-α-fluorohydrocortisone. *N Engl J Med* 1959;261:788–791.
47. Davies B. The pressor actions of noradrenaline, angiotensin II, and saralasin in chronic autonomic failure treated with fludrocortisone. *Br J Clin Pharmacol* 1979;8:253–260.
48. Robertson D, Davis TL. Recent advances in the treatment of orthostatic hypotension. *Neurology* 1995;45 (suppl 5)526–532.
49. Goldberg MR, Hollister AS, Robertson D. Influence of yohimbine on blood pressure, autonomic reflexes, and plasma catecholamines in humans. *Hypertension* 1983;5:772–778.
50. Onrot J. Pharmacological treatment of orthostatic hypotension. In: Robertson D, Biaggioni I (eds): *Disorders of the Autonomic Nervous System.* London: Harwood Academic Publishers; 1995;419–435.
51. Biaggioni I, Onrot J, Parrish CK, Robertson D. The potent pressor effect of phenylpropanolamine in patients with autonomic impairment. *JAMA* 1987; 258:236–239.
52. McTavish D, Goa KL. Midodrine: A review of its pharmacological properties and therapeutic use in orthostatic hypotension and secondary hypotensive disorders. *Drugs* 1989;38:757–777.
53. Jankovic J, Gilden JL, Hiner BC, et al. Neurogenic orthostatic hypotension: A double blind placebo-controlled study with midodrine. *Am J Med* 1993;95:38–48.
54. Robertson D, Goldberg MR, Hollister AS, et al. Clonidine raises blood pressure in idiopathic orthostatic hypotension. *Amer J Med* 1983;74:193–199.
55. Onrot J, Goldberg MR, Biaggioni I, et al. Post junctional vascular smooth muscle α_2- adrenoreceptors in human autonomic failure. *Clin Invest Med* 1987;10:26–31.
56. Hoeldtke RD, Streeten DH. Treatment of orthostatic hypotension with erythropoietin. *N Engl J Med* 1993;329:611–615.
57. Biaggioni S, Robertson D, Krantz S, et al. The anemia of primary autonomic failure and its reversal with recombinant erythropoietin. *Ann Int Med* 1994; 121:181–186.
58. Kuhn D, Wolfe W, Loyenburg W. Review of the role of the central serotonergic neuronal system in blood pressure regulation. *Hypertension* 1980;2:243–255.
59. Grubb BP, Lachant N, Kosinski D. Erythropoietin as a therapy for severe refractory orthostatic hypotension. *Clin Auton Res* 1994;4:212.
60. Grubb BP, Kosinski D. Serotonin and Syncope: An emerging connection? *Eur J Cardiac Pacing Electrophysiol* 1996;5:306–314.
61. Grubb BP, Samoil D, Kosinski D, et al. Fluoxetine hydrochloride for the treatment of severe refractory orthostatic hypotension. *Am J Med* 1994;97:366–368.

62. Moss AJ, Glasser W, Topol E. Atrial tachypacing in the treatment of a patient with primary orthostatic hypotension. *N Engl J Med* 1980;302:1456–1457.
63. Weissman P, Chin M, Moss A. Cardiac tachypacing for severe refractory idiopathic orthostatic hypotension. *Ann Int Med* 1992;116:650–651.
64. Grubb BP, Wolfe DA, Samoil D et al. Adaptive rate pacing controlled by right ventricular pre-ejection interval for severe refractory orthostatic hypotension. *PACE* 1993;16:801–805.
65. Grubb BP. New concepts in sensor technology for rate adaptive pacing. In: Barold S, Mugica J (eds): *New Perspectives in Cardiac Pacing III.* Armonk: Futura Publishing, 1997.

Bradyarrhythmias as a Cause of Syncope

David G. Benditt, MD and
Richard Sutton, DScMed

Introduction

It has been long recognized that excessively slow heart rates may cause syncope. Prior to the invention of electrocardiographic recordings, careful physical examination yielded the necessary clues. In this regard, description of dissociated "a" and "cv" waves during examination of the neck veins, such as that reported by Stokes[1] in the mid 1800s, provided the earliest documentation of atrioventricular (AV) block as a possible cause of syncope. In 1913, in reviewing his considerable clinical experience, Sir James Mackenzie[2] wrote, "*I have made observations and tracings of several patients during syncopal attacks, and have found a variety of conditions...The most common has been a slowing of the heart rate, with great weakness of the pulse, so that only a slight tracing was obtained by the sphygmograph.*"

Despite the relative ease with which bradyarrhythmias can now be recorded in even free-living individuals, it is crucial to recognize that the relationship between syncope and documented bradycardia may not be clear-cut. For instance, in some such patients the presence of underlying heart disease may result in susceptibility to any of a number of other symptomatic arrhythmias (eg, ventricular tachycardia or atrial fibrillation with very rapid ventricular response), which may be the real culprits. In other patients, even severe symptomatic bradycardia may be of neural reflex origin, and concomitant vasodilation may play an important role in eliciting

From Grubb BP, Olshansky B (eds.). *Syncope: Mechanisms and Management*. Armonk, NY: Futura Publishing Co., Inc.; © 1998.

symptomatic hypotension. In the latter instance, treatment of bradycardia alone (eg, cardiac pacing) may not completely resolve the problem.

Classification of Bradyarrhythmic Causes of Syncope

Symptomatic bradyarrhythmias imply a disturbance of sinus node function, of AV conduction, or of both. Causes of these abnormalities may be broadly classified as: 1) Intrinsic disturbances usually associated with congenital or acquired structural cardiac disease, 2) Extrinsic disturbances initiated by or exacerbated by drug effects, or 3) Neurally mediated reflex functional disturbances. In the latter case, apart from the bradycardia, important peripheral vascular phenomena are usually additional critical elements.

Bradyarrhythmias Associated with Intrinsic Sinus Node or AV Conduction Disease

Disturbances of sinus node function and atrioventricular conduction may be of either congenital or acquired origin.[3] In this regard, acquired sinus node dysfunction is thought to be a relatively frequent cause of transient neurological symptoms (Table 1), and currently accounts for more than half of the permanent pacemakers implanted in most Western countries. Similarly, acquired AV conduction system disease is ubiquitous, especially in an aging society. However, given the propensity for acquired AV conduction system disease to be associated with ventricular dysfunction, the importance of ventricular tachyarrhythmias as a cause of syncope in these patients should not be overlooked.

Drug-Induced Bradycardia

Drug-induced disturbances of sinus node function are well described.[3,4] Sympatholytic antihypertensive agents have been especially incriminated. However, as most of these agents (eg, guanethidine, α-methyl dopa) are of diminishing clinical importance, the β-adrenergic blockers, calcium channel blockers, cardiac glycosides, and "membrane-active" antiarrhythmic drugs have become of proportionally greater concern. In regard to drug-induced disturbances of AV conduction, antiarrhythmic agents offer the greatest potential for harm. The risk is, of course, greatest in the setting of a preexisting conduction disturbance (eg, underlying bundle branch block).

Neurally Mediated Reflex Disturbances

The neurally mediated reflex syncopal syndromes (Table 2), and especially the so-called vasovagal or "common faint" are the most common

_____ Table 1 _____

Causes of Sinus Node Dysfunction

Intrinsic Sinus Node Dysfunction

- Idiopathic degenerative disease (probably most common)
- Ischemic
    -chronic coronary artery disease occasionally involving sinus node artery
    -during acute myocardial infarction [particularly inferior wall (see "extrinsic")]
- Infiltrative disorders: amyloidosis, hemochromatosis, tumors
- Inflammatory or postinflammatory: pericarditis, myocarditis
- Musculoskeletal disorders: Duchenne's or myotonic dystrophy, Friedreich's ataxia
- Collagen-vascular disease: Lupus erythematosus, scleroderma
- Postoperative: Mustard's procedure, atrial septal defect repair

Extrinsic Sinus Node Dysfunction

- Drug effects (see Table 7)
- Electrolyte disturbances: particularly hyperkalemia
- Endocrine conditions: hypothyroidism, or less commonly, hyperthyroidism
- Myocardial infarction, acute inferior wall (neural reflex effects)
- Neurally mediated bradycardia-hypotension syndromes
    -carotid sinus syndrome
    -vasovagal syncope
    -postmicturition syncope
    -cough, sneeze syncope
    -others
- Miscellaneous
    -intracranial hypertension
    -obstructive jaundice

_____ Table 2 _____

Neurally Mediated Syncopal Syndromes

Emotional syncope (common or "vasovagal" faint, "malignant" vasovagal faint)
Carotid sinus syncope
Gastrointestinal stimulation
  swallow syncope, defecation syncope
Micturition syncope
Cough syncope
Sneeze syncope
Glossopharyngeal neuralgia
Airway stimulation
Raised intrathoracic pressure
  brass wind instrument-playing, weight-lifting

causes of syncope.[5-15] It is currently believed that the various conditions comprising the neurally mediated syncopal syndromes exhibit many common pathophysiological elements, with the principal clinically relevant differences among them being the "trigger factors" (eg, pain, carotid sinus stimulation, cough, micturition, etc.).

The afferent neural signals that initiate neurally mediated syncopal events may originate from the central nervous system (CNS) directly (as in the case of syncope associated with fear or anxiety) or from any variety of peripheral "receptors" that respond to mechanical or chemical stimuli, pain, or possibly even temperature change (eg, carotid sinus syncope, postmicturition syncope, etc). The subsequent electrophysiological and hemodynamic picture may be quite variable. Certain patients exhibit a predominantly "cardioinhibitory" picture, with an extended period of bradycardia (or asystole) as the proximate cause of the faint. Most, however, present a mixed vasodepressor and cardioinhibitory response.[14-19] Only on rare occasions does a pure vasodepressor syndrome occur. A detailed classification of these responses, as observed during tilt table testing, was recently summarized by a multicenter European working group (VASIS, Vasovagal International Study).[18]

Syncope Due to Bradyarrhythmias in the Setting of Intrinsic Sinus Node or AV Conduction System Disease

Sinus Node Dysfunction

Sinus node dysfunction (also termed "sick sinus syndrome" or "sinoatrial disease") encompasses an array of sinus node and/or atrial arrhythmias that result in persistent or intermittent periods of inappropriate slow or fast heart beating (Figures 1–4).[3] Clinical manifestations of sinus node dysfunction vary from seemingly asymptomatic electrocardiographic findings to a wide range of complaints including syncope, dizziness, shortness of breath, palpitations, fatigue, lethargy, and dementia. For the patient experiencing syncopal symptoms, the cause may be a transient severe bradyarrhythmia or tachyarrhythmia, or both. On occasion, and particularly when the patient is being treated with antiarrhythmic drugs, atrial bradycardia may be associated with the development of symptomatic ventricular tachyarrhythmias (Figure 5). Most often though, it is believed that the arrhythmias associated with syncope in sinus node dysfunction patients are those that produce relatively long periods (in the range of 10 to 15 seconds) of severe bradycardia with consequent inadequate cerebral blood flow (ie, sinus pauses and sinoatrial block).

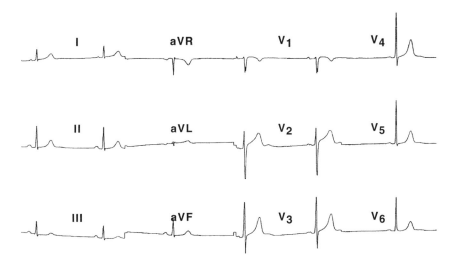

Figure 1. 12-lead ECG illustrating sinus bradycardia in a 72-year-old patient with recurrent lightheadedness on exertion. This patient exhibited marked sinus bradycardia at rest and symptomatic chronotropic incompetence during exertion.

Brady- or tachyarrhythmias may also be the cause of presyncopal symptoms. For example, atrial fibrillation with a slow ventricular response or chronotropic incompetence (inadequate heart rate responsiveness during physical exertion or emotional stress) may play a role. However, dizziness and lightheadedness are relatively common complaints in many patients (especially in the elderly, who comprise a large proportion of the sinus node dysfunction population), and their causes are often difficult to pinpoint. Although arrhythmic etiologies are perhaps among the easier possibilities to evaluate, it is often difficult to establish an unequivocal relationship between symptoms and arrhythmia.

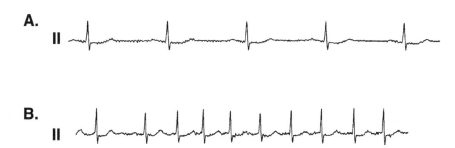

Figure 2. Rhythm strips from a patient who exhibited intermittent atrial tachyarrhythmias as the principal manifestation of sinus node dysfunction. Panel A: Sinus rhythm. Panel B: Paroxysmal primary atrial tachycardia.

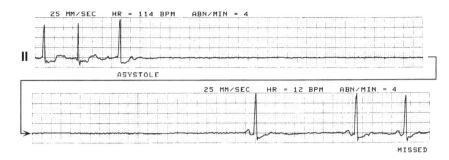

Figure 3. Asystolic pause recorded during in-hospital monitoring of a 68-year-old patient with recurrent syncope.

Etiology of Intrinsic Sinus Node Dysfunction

Although congenital or familial disorders of sinus node function occur, most clinically important disturbances of sinus node dysfunction are acquired due to the aging process or concomitant disease (Table 1). Specifically, degenerative and/or fibrotic changes within the sinoatrial node region may accompany aging or result from disease states such as hypertension, cardiomyopathy, atherosclerotic cardiovascular disease, inflammation (eg, pericardial disease, myocarditis, collagen vascular diseases), or surgical trauma (particularly well known to occur after the Mustard procedure for transposition of the great arteries, and with closure of atrial septal defects, especially of the sinus venous type). The role of ischemic heart disease is difficult to ascertain. The significance of finding a close association between sinus node dysfunction and coronary artery disease is uncertain because both conditions are inherently more common in older individuals, especially in Western countries. Overall, it is believed that ischemia caused by sinus node artery disease appears to account for the disturbance in only about one third of adult patients with sinus node disease.[3] In some additional patients, however, the consequences of previous myocardial infarction may be relevant, especially if myocardial damage was extensive and complicated by congestive heart failure or hypotension. Ex-

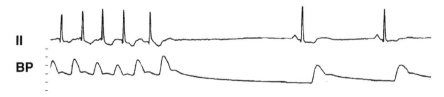

Figure 4. Prolonged pause following termination of atrial tachycardia in a patient with recurrent dizziness. Symptoms were primarily associated with the tachyarrhythmias.

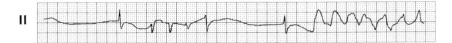

II

Figure 5. Recording from an 80-year-old patient with recent onset of recurrent syncope. The individual had been taking a type IA antiarrhythmic agent for control of paroxysmal atrial fibrillation. ECG monitor reveals junctional bradycardia, marked QT interval prolongation, and polymorphous ventricular tachycardia (torsades de pointes). Syncopal symptoms in this case were due to the bradycardia-dependent tachycardia. The bradycardia could be attributed to the adverse antiarrhythmic drug action on native cardiac pacemaker function in a patient in whom sinus node dysfunction presented initially as paroxysmal atrial fibrillation.

trinsic factors such as cardioactive drugs or autonomic influences are considered separately, later.

Orthotopic cardiac transplantation has provided an important new group of patients with an apparently high propensity for exhibiting disturbance of sinus node function in the early postoperative period. Fortunately, however, despite the combination of surgical trauma, ischemic time, rejection, and drug effects, only a small proportion of transplant patients (approximately 2% in the University of Minnesota experience) develop sufficiently severe bradycardia to require implantation of cardiac pacemakers, and in the majority of these cases the indication is chronotropic incompetence. Syncope due to sinus node dysfunction appears to be rare in this setting.

Syncope in Sinus Node Dysfunction

The frequency with which bradyarrhythmias due to intrinsic disturbances of sinus node function cause symptoms in free-living individuals is unknown. However, among those selected symptomatic sinus node dysfunction patients who were referred to centers that have taken an interest in reporting their clinical experience, syncope and dizziness were relatively common presenting features [range, 40% to 92%; (Table 3)]. In part, this apparently high frequency may be due both to the fact that these symptoms are more readily recognized by patients and physicians than some of the other symptoms associated with sinus node dysfunction, and to the fact that they are often considered among the most worrisome of all symptoms. Thus, among 56 patients with either severe bradyarrhythmias or bradycardia-tachycardia syndrome described by Rubenstein et al,[20] 25 (45%) presented with syncope and an additional 15 (27%) reported various presyncopal symptoms. In the vast majority of these cases (80%), bradyarrhythmias were considered to be the principal responsible rhythm disturbance. Similarly, among 22 patients with sinus node dysfunction and syncope, Sutton and Perrins[21] report resolution of symptoms with preven-

_____ **Table 3** _____

Syncope in Sinus Node Dysfunction

Ref	All Pts (Ages)	Synope/Dizziness	Brady-Induced*
Easley & Goldstein (1971)	13 (63–82 yrs)	12 (92%)	13 (100%)▯
Rubenstein et al (1972)	56 (26–92 yrs)	40 (71%)	32/40 (80%)
Wan et al (1972)	15 (20–85 yrs)	6 (40%)	5/6 (83%)
Kulbertus et al (1973)	13 (57–95 yrs)	12 (92%)	12 (100%)
Obel et al (1974)	34 (25–82 yrs)	26 (78%)	NA
Hartel & Talvansaari (1975)	90 (22–86 yrs)	49 (54%)	32/49 (65%)
Strauss et al (1975)	20 (32–87 yrs)	12 (60%)	NA
Sauerwein et al (1976)	30 (53–81 yrs)	22 (73%)	22/22 (100%)
Scheinman et al 1978‡	28 (24–80 yrs)	23 (82%)	23 (100%)
Sutton & Perrins (1979)#	37 (36–89 yrs)	22 (59%)	NA

* = Differentiation of syncope etiology (brady vs. tachy) was not always clear; best estimate provided here; ▯ = syncope due to brady alone in 6 pts, and due to post-tachy bradyarrhythmia in 7 pts; # = only syncope patients included from this study; ‡ = pts were selected based on the presence of sinus pauses or sinoatrial exit block; Pts = patients.

tion of bradycardia by cardiac pacing in 16 (73%) cases. Of the patients with residual symptoms, treatment failure due to pacing system dysfunction occurred in one case, while symptomatic tachyarrhythmias were ultimately uncovered in several others.

The electrocardiographic manifestations of sinus node dysfunction may include both bradyarrhythmias (most importantly, sinus bradycardia, sinus pauses, sinoatrial exit block, inexcitable atrium, and chronotropic incompetence) and tachyarrhythmias (principally paroxysmal or persistent atrial fibrillation or atrial flutter). Although bradyarrhythmias are more often associated with syncope in published reports of patients classified as having sinus node dysfunction, every effort should be made to keep an open mind in the assessment of such patients and to identify the specific arrhythmia(s) responsible. Of concern is the fact that sinus node dysfunction patients tend to be in an age group in which other cardiac disease is also present. Therefore susceptibility to ventricular tachyarrhythmias or AV conduction disturbances must be considered.

Sinus bradycardia, even if relatively severe, is rarely a cause of syncope. However, presyncopal symptoms, especially during periods of physical exertion, may be expected. While such symptoms are probably primarily the result of inadequate cerebral nutrient flow due to bradycardia, the presence of junctional rhythm with retrograde atrial capture or isorhythmic AV dissociation may be an exacerbating factor (Figure 6). In the latter circumstance, the basis for symptomatology may be both due to diminished cardiac output (ie, loss of atrial contribution) and neurohumoral factors (including release of atrial peptides). In essence, the mechanism is comparable to that associated with "pacemaker syndrome."[22,23]

Sinus pauses or sinus arrest imply failure of normal pacemaker discharge with consequent lack of an expected atrial activation of sinus node origin. The duration necessary for qualification as a sinus pause or sinus arrest remains difficult to define, and in a given individual depends in part on the magnitude of underlying sinus arrhythmia (ie, the degree with which that individual's sinus rate varies on a regular basis). As a rule, however, asymptomatic sinus pauses of up to 3 seconds in duration are relatively common and without clear-cut adverse prognostic implications.[24–26] On the other hand, pauses in excess of 3 seconds are rare during ambulatory monitoring (were detected in 2.4% and 0.8% of patients in two reports).[27,28] Although the apparent clinical significance of pauses greater than 3 seconds' duration may vary, they warrant careful assessment to detect symptomatic correlations. Thus, in patients presenting with syncope or dizziness, the identification of pauses greater than 3 seconds suggests (but does not prove) a basis for the symptoms. The same general rules may be applied to sinoatrial exit block.

Coexistence of periods of bradyarrhythmias and atrial tachycardias (usually atrial fibrillation, but possibly atrial flutter or other primary atrial tachycardias) is a common manifestation of sinus node dysfunction, often termed bradycardia-tachycardia syndrome.[3,29,30] Symptoms may result from either an excessively rapid heart beat or bradycardia, or both. One of the most frequent causes of syncope and dizziness in sinus node dysfunction patients is

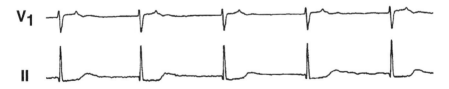

Figure 6. ECG recording depicting junctional rhythm with retrograde atrial activation (P waves superimposed on the T waves) in a patient with "fluttering in the chest, weakness, and lightheadedness." In cases such as this, atrial contraction against a closed AV valve can be expected to cause a clinical picture comparable to that associated with "pacemaker syndrome." In essence, symptoms are believed to be multifactorial in origin, including regurgitation of blood into systemic and pulmonary veins, diminished contribution of atrial systole to cardiac output, and neurohumoral effects presumably triggered by atrial wall stretch.

a prolonged pause following termination of a tachycardia episode (Figure 4). Such pauses may be aggravated by antiarrhythmic drug therapy that was initiated to suppress tachycardia susceptibility. Finally, it is important to bear in mind that bradyarrhythmias may increase susceptibility to tachycardia, and that the tachyarrhythmia may be responsible for symptoms. A common example is the tendency for atrial fibrillation to occur in the setting of excessive atrial bradycardia. However, symptomatic ventricular ectopy (Figure 7) and ventricular tachyarrhythmias (especially torsade de pointes) may also become a problem in bradycardic patients, especially if the patient is being treated with antiarrhythmic drugs (Figure 5).

Persistent atrial fibrillation, particularly in association with a very slow ventricular response (unrelated to drugs), is considered part of the spectrum of sinus node dysfunction. Unless the ventricular rate is exceedingly slow, syncope or dizziness is unlikely. Nevertheless, intermittently very long R-R intervals may occur, thereby causing bradycardia-related symptoms. Concomitant AV conduction system disease may be part of the problem for individuals with such slow ventricular rates,. However, although diffuse conduction system disease may occur as part of the sinus node dysfunction picture, the predilection for development of clinically worrisome AV block has probably been overemphasized (see below). In fact, many sinus node dysfunction patients manifest surprisingly rapid ventricular responses during atrial tachycardias.

Concomitant disturbances of AV conduction in patients with sinus node dysfunction is a well-recognized and important, although poorly understood, phenomenon. Its importance becomes most apparent when subsidiary pacemaker sites (junctional or ventricular) fail to provide expected "back-up" in the setting of an inadequate sinus rate. Additionally, a propensity to AV conduction failure has substantial implications with respect to the choice of cardiac pacing mode for symptomatic patients. Sutton and Kenny[31] provide a succinct assessment of this issue. In their review of published reports encompassing 1808 patients, 300 (16.6 %) manifested con-

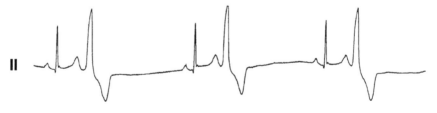

Figure 7. Rhythm strip obtained during a symptomatic period in an elderly man who presented with near syncope associated with modest exertion. In this case, chronotropic incompetence further complicated by ventricular bigeminy resulted in an inappropriately low "effective" heart rate. Atrial rate-adaptive pacing in conjunction with antiarrhythmic drug therapy proved beneficial.

duction system disease at the time sinus node dysfunction was diagnosed. However, severe degrees of AV block that might be expected to cause syncope (eg, high-grade AV block) were uncommon (5% to 10% of cases). In studies in which follow-up was available, only 117 of 1395 patients (8.4%) evolved conduction system disturbances over a mean follow-up time of 34.2 months (ie, approximately 2.7 percent/year) and for the most part these new conduction disturbances were of relatively minor forms (eg, first-degree AV block, Wenckebach block at slower heart rates than before).

The acuteness with which new AV conduction system disturbances develop is a crucial factor in determining the likelihood for the development of syncope. This aspect cannot be assessed from the Sutton and Kenny report.[31] However, findings such as those reported by Rosenqvist and coworkers,[32] Stangl and coworkers,[33] and Sutton and Bourgeois[34] suggest that the rate of progression is typically slow and should be detectable by careful periodic clinical and electrocardiographic follow-up. For example, in the Rosenqvist report,[32] only 1 of 30 patients experienced high-grade AV block (ie, <1% incidence of progression/year) during a 5-year follow-up, and that patient had marked HV interval prolongation on entry into the study. Similarly, in the experience reported by Stangl et al,[33] only 6 of 110 patients observed over a period of 52±28 months exhibited conduction disease progression, and in most cases the progression was minor (third-degree AV block, none; Mobitz II second-degree AV block, 1; first-degree AV block, 5).

It appears that susceptibility to subsequent conduction system involvement or aggravation of existing conduction system disease in patients with sinus node dysfunction is largely unrelated to the nature of the presenting electrocardiographic abnormalities.[35] Among 17 patients with bradycardia followed for 36 months, high-grade AV block developed in 1 (about 2 percent/year) compared with 3 instances among 22 patients with bradycardia-tachycardia syndrome followed for 53 months (about 3.1 percent/year). On the other hand, iatrogenic influences may be important. van Mechelen and colleagues[36] note that during serial electrophysiological evaluation of 24 sinus node dysfunction (SND) patients followed over a 3-year period, deterioration of AV conduction system performance (as assessed by serial estimation of the atrial paced rate at which type I second-degree AV block was observed) appeared to correlate more closely with the use of antiarrhythmic drugs than with conduction system degeneration itself. Santini et al[37] make a similar observation. Thus, careful control of patient exposure to antiarrhythmic drugs may be among the most important factors for diminishing risk of developing clinically significant conduction system disease in patients with sinus node dysfunction.

Sinus node dysfunction patients, largely due to their age and tendency to harbor coexisting diseases (especially cardiovascular disorders), are also susceptible to "loss of consciousness spells," which may not be due to a primary arrhythmia. Thromboembolic complications, myocardial ischemia, or new-onset seizure disturbances are important considerations. The first of these considerations, thromboembolism, is primarily responsible for the excess morbidity and mortality associated with sinus node disease.[3,31,38,39] As a rule, medical history, physical examination, and relatively straightforward testing distinguish these conditions from syncope of arrhythmic origin.

Many aspects of sinus node dysfunction remain poorly understood. Among the more curious of these is the relationship between sinus node disease and apparent dysfunction of subsidiary pacemaker sites, which leads to risk of prolonged symptomatic asystole. Whether a common disease process is responsible for both remains to be clarified. Autonomic disturbances are potentially contributory. In this regard, Brignole et al[40] propose that sinus node dysfunction incorporates (and perhaps in some patients may be considered a variant of) the autonomic dysfunction associated with carotid sinus syndrome and vasovagal syncope. Conceivably, in such circumstances, neural influences may explain the diffuse nature of native pacemaker dysfunction.

Treatment

Appropriate treatment for the patient with sinus node dysfunction and syncope necessitates consideration of the underlying electrophysiological and arrhythmic disturbance, the effects of drugs on sinus node function, current indications for and available modes of cardiac pacing, and the role of anticoagulation.[3] In addition, the currently evolving role of transcatheter or surgical ablation for arrhythmia control also warrants examination. At present, only a relatively small proportion of sinus node dysfunction patients undergo ablation, and in the majority of these cases His bundle ablation is used to facilitate control of ventricular rate.[41] Transcatheter ablation for control of atrial flutter is best reserved for a select subset of patients in whom atrial flutter is the solitary primary atrial tachycardia. Similarly, surgical methods for direct treatment of atrial fibrillation are currently confined to a selected small number of patients, and are undertaken at relatively few centers[42,43] In addition, transcatheter techniques for altering atrial electrophysiological milieu and reducing susceptibility to atrial fibrillation are as yet in early stages of evolution.[44] The ultimate role surgery and catheter ablation may play in this setting remains to be seen.

In general, cardiac pacemaker therapy has proved to be highly effective in patients with sinus node dysfunction when bradyarrhythmia has been demonstrated to account for symptoms (Table 4). For the most part, modern pacing practice is moving away from use of single-chamber ventricular pacing (VVI, VVIR modes) in sinus node dysfunction patients unless persistent atrial fibrillation precludes atrial pacing. Pacing techniques that endeavor to maintain a normal atrioventricular relationship not only offer

_____ Table 4 _____

Indications for Pacing in Sinus Node Dysfunction

Class I: Indicated
Documented bradycardia-related symptoms

Class II: Possibly Indicated
Symptomatic sinus node dysfunction in which a relationship between symptoms
  and bradycardia has been sought, but not established

Class III: Not Indicated
Asymptomatic sinus node dysfunction

_____

better hemodynamic responses, but also eliminate symptoms commonly
associated with "pacemaker syndrome," and tend to diminish the likelihood of later development of atrial fibrillation and its consequent risk of
thromboembolism.[31-33,37,45,46] Finally, since a diagnosis of sinus node dysfunction is inherently associated with an inappropriate chronotropic
response, the use of rate-adaptive pacing (ie, implantable devices incor-
porating one or more physiological sensors) is usually warranted for purposes of optimizing exertional tolerance.

Although, theophylline is reported to be helpful in a few cases (predominantly autonomically mediated bradyarrhythmias), drug therapy is
now, as a rule, only rarely used to treat bradyarrhythmias in patients with
sinus node dysfunction. On the other hand, by virtue of their age and
associated disease processes, sinus node dysfunction patients are often ex-
posed to a wide range of drugs that may exacerbate or unmask underlying
susceptibility to bradycardia. This problem is considered in more detail
later in this chapter (see section entitled _Extrinsic Disturbances of Sinus Node
Function and AV Conduction_).

As noted earlier, thromboembolic complications (probably primarily
associated with atrial fibrillation) are an important contributing factor to
excess mortality and morbidity in sinus node dysfunction patients. While
these complications do not cause true syncope, they do cause neurological
disturbances that may be interpreted as dizziness or syncope. Consequently,
stroke risk reduction by anticoagulation is an important element in the
treatment of individuals with sinus node dysfunction, particularly in those
with paroxysmal or persistent atrial fibrillation. The reader is referred to a
recent review of the major anticoagulation trials.[47] In this regard, there is
solid evidence supporting the use of warfarin therapy, and while the merits
of full-dose (325 mg) aspirin therapy remain to be resolved, warfarin is
clearly superior to "mini-dose" aspirin (75 mg). In brief, long-term oral
anticoagulant therapy should be considered for all patients older than 65
years, and for younger patients with the following risk factors: a previous

transient ischemic attack (TIA) or stroke, hypertension, heart failure, diabetes, clinical coronary artery disease, mitral stenosis, prosthetic heart valve, or thyrotoxicosis.

Finally, innovative pacing and/or atrial defibrillation techniques may become a part of the treatment strategy in sinus node dysfunction patients. Multiple-site atrial pacing is currently being evaluated as a technique to prevent atrial fibrillation by reducing intra-atrial conduction delays.[48] Additionally, the development of low-energy implantable atrial defibrillators has reached the early clinical trial stage.[49,50] These devices used in conjunction with drugs or pacemakers offer an opportunity to reverse atrial tachyarrhythmia breakthroughs promptly, thereby reducing the need for aggressive antiarrhythmic drug therapy. It seems unlikely that they will prove helpful in syncope prophylaxis, especially if hypotension occurs as a transient event associated with tachyarrhythmia onset.

AV Conduction Disturbances

Disturbances of AV conduction range from slowing of AV conduction (first-degree AV block), to intermittent failure of impulse transmission (second-degree AV block), to complete conduction failure (third-degree AV block). In terms of clinical importance in the syncope patient, both the type of block and the site at which block occurs must be considered. While it is true that certain patterns of block are more frequently associated with abnormalities in a particular element of the conduction system (eg, first-degree AV block is most often due to AV nodal delay), substantial variability may occur and often multiple sites of delay contribute and can be identified during cardiac electrophysiological study.[51–53] A complete discussion of these issues is beyond the scope of this chapter. However, by way of example, in both first- and second-degree (type 1) AV block, the AV node (prolonged AH interval) is almost always responsible when there is no evidence of underlying cardiac disease and when the QRS morphology is normal. In the presence of a narrow QRS complex, first-degree AV block has been reported to be due to AV nodal delay in more than 85% of patients, and due to delay within the His bundle in only 13%.[51] On the other hand, in the setting of a wide QRS complex, first-degree AV block was AV nodal in origin in only 22% of cases, infranodal in 45%, and as a result of delay in more than one site in approximately 33% of cases. Similarly, in patients with a narrow QRS complex, type I second-degree AV block was AV nodal in origin in approximately 70% of cases, whereas in the presence of a wide QRS complex, infranodal conduction delay may account for 60% to 70% of cases.

Etiology

Table 5 summarizes the principal recognized causes of AV block. Progressive idiopathic fibrosis of the cardiac conduction system is the most

_____ Table 5 _____

Causes of AV Block

Atherosclerotic disease
  Acute myocardial infarction
  Healed myocardial infarction
Calcific infiltration
  Calcific valvular heart disease
Cardiomyopathy
Collagen-vascular diseases
  Ankylosing spondylitis, dermatomyositis, rheumatoid arthritis, scleroderma,
    systemic lupus erythematosis
Congenital AV block
  Associated with congenital heart disease (ostium primum ASD, transposition of
    the great vessels)
  Associated with maternal systemic lupus erythematosis
Drug effects
  β-adrenergic blockers, cardiac glycosides, "membrane-active" antiarrhythmic
    agents
Idiopathic fibrosis (Lev's disease)
Infiltrative diseases
  Amyloidosis, hemochromatosis, sarcoidosis
Inflammatory diseases
  Endocarditis
  Myocarditis
    Bacterial (diphtheria, Lyme disease, rheumatic fever, tuberculosis)
    Viral (measles, mumps)
    Parasitic (Chagas' disease)
Neurally mediated AV block
  Carotid sinus syndrome, other neurally mediated syncopal syndromes
    (eg, vasovagal syncope)
Trauma
  Catheter trauma/ablation, radiation, cardiac surgery
Tumors
  Mesothelioma, rhabdomyoma

AV = atrioventricular; ASD = atrial septal defect.

common cause of acquired conduction system disease.[54,55] In general, this process can be considered an aging-related process of sclerosis of the cardiac skeleton, and it is particularly likely in patients without evidence of significant underlying structural heart disease. Acute myocardial infarction is associated with the various forms of AV block, and is another common cause of acquired complete AV block. Chronic ischemic heart disease is also commonly associated with various degrees of AV block, although it is often impossible to be certain of a causal relationship.

Studies that examine the association of acute myocardial infarction and the development of AV block largely predate the thrombolytic era, and are consequently suspect in the context of current treatment and natural history.[56–59] Nevertheless, the older reports suggest that in individuals with inferior wall myocardial infarction, complete AV block occurs in 10% to 15%.[56] Many of these cases occur early following onset of symptoms, and over 60% of those who will develop AV block manifest it within the first 24 hours. Fortunately, complete AV block in this setting is usually transient, often evolves from less severe degrees of block (first-degree, type I second-degree), is most often at the level of the AV node, and can often be reversed or ameliorated with atropine. The mechanisms eliciting this form of AV block are multiple, including nodal ischemia, adenosine release, and enhanced parasympathetic tone. Approximately 5% of patients with anterior myocardial infarctions develop complete heart block.[57,59] Among these latter patients, the site of block tends to be within the specialized cardiac conduction system and is associated with a poor prognosis due to the magnitude of associated ventricular damage. As a rule, patients who develop transient or fixed AV block during acute myocardial infarction tend to be older and to have sustained a more severe myocardial infarction as evidenced by higher enzyme levels, left ventricular failure, right ventricular infarction, or evidence of bundle branch block preceding the development of complete heart block.

Other causes of infranodal AV block include certain complications of valvular heart disease, especially aortic stenosis. In many of these cases, extension of calcification or fibrosis into the nearby conducting system is at fault. The specialized cardiac conduction system may also be damaged by infiltrative cardiomyopathies such as amyloidosis, hemochromatosis, and sarcoid, as well as by certain noninfectious inflammatory conditions including ankylosing spondylitis, lupus erythematosus, and scleroderma.[60–63] On the other hand, while abnormalities of cardiac conduction are relatively common in many patients with congestive or hypertrophic cardiomyopathy, the development of clinically significant AV block is unpredictable.

Cardiac surgery is an important cause of acquired AV block.[64] AV block most frequently complicates aortic valve replacement, but is seldom associated with coronary artery bypass grafting in the absence of an exceedingly prolonged procedure, lengthy ischemic time, or myocardial infarction. Repair of certain forms of congenital heart disease, especially those physically close to the conducting system (eg, ostium primum atrial septal defects, ventricular septal defects), is frequently complicated by AV block.

Syncope Associated with AV Conduction Disease

As a rule, it is the acquired disturbances of AV conduction that are most often associated with syncopal symptoms. The risk of syncope or life-threatening bradycardia being associated with the various forms of AV block is dependent on the underlying disease process. Thus, even in the case of high-grade AV block, the long-term outcome may be excellent in terms of survival when the disturbance is due to neurally mediated hypervagotonia (eg, carotid sinus syndrome, vasovagal syncope). Conversely, high-grade AV block occurring during the course of an anterior myocardial infarction is associated with a high propensity for syncope and sudden death (the latter is largely due to the magnitude of myocardial damage and consequent risk of ventricular arrhythmia).

First-Degree AV Block

As a rule, first-degree AV block is generally nonprogressive and an essentially benign finding. Among almost 4000 pilots followed for 27 years, this finding was noted in 148 individuals (approximately 3.5%).[65] Outcomes in the first-degree AV block group did not differ from those observed in the normal population. An exception to the benign nature of first-degree AV block are those cases in which the condition occurs in conjunction with bifascicular block; infranodal conduction disease may contribute directly to the apparent conduction delay.[51,52,66] These latter individuals are susceptible to development of progressively higher degrees of AV block with associated symptoms. There is also a rare familial form of conduction system disease (autosomal dominant) in which first-degree AV block is known to progress to more severe conduction system disturbances.

As a solitary finding, first-degree AV block is almost never the cause of syncope. When syncope does occur in this setting, there is usually no direct causal relationship. However, the presence of first-degree AV block, especially in the absence of structural heart disease, may suggest hypervagotonia and thereby raise suspicion of neurally mediated syncope (discussed later in this chapter). Rarely, presyncopal symptoms (but only exceptionally, true syncope) may occur if the PR interval is sufficiently prolonged such that during exercise, successive P waves are so far in front of the QRS complex that they are superimposed on preceding T waves. In this case, the mechanism of symptomatic hypotension is comparable to that in "pacemaker syndrome,"[22,23] and may be due to a combination of several factors, including loss of atrial contribution to cardiac output, neurohumoral influences triggered by excessive stretch on the atrial walls, and retrograde ejection of blood into the systemic and pulmonary veins.

Second-Degree AV Block

Type I second-degree AV block is generally considered a relatively innocent conduction disturbance when the QRS complex is narrow and there is no evidence of associated infranodal conduction system involvement (Figure 8). In this setting, bradycardia is rarely of sufficient severity to account for syncope. However, some doubt remains regarding the

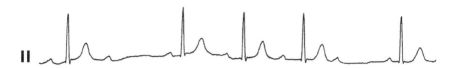

Figure 8. Mobitz type I AV block (4:3) in a patient with recurrent dizziness. Note the progressive PR interval prolongation prior to the blocked P wave. The ECG findings proved to be incidental and were unrelated to the cause of symptoms.

supposedly benign nature of Mobitz I block in older individuals. Shaw et al[67] followed 214 patients with chronic second-degree block prospectively. The 5-year survival was similar in those with Mobitz type I (mean age 69 years; 57% survival), Mobitz type II (mean age 74 years; 61% survival), and patients with 2:1 and 3:1 block (mean age 75 years; 53% survival). The authors concluded that Mobitz I and Mobitz II AV block were associated with similar risks in this older population, that the presence of bundle branch block did not affect their conclusion, and that pacing improved prognosis.

When type I second-degree block occurs in healthy physically fit individuals, the cause is most often increased vagal tone, and in the absence of certain drug toxicities (eg, cardiac glycosides), there is no clinical concern. Similarly, in the setting of acute inferior wall myocardial infarction, this form of AV block tends to resolve without the need for permanent pacing. On the other hand, analogous to the case for first-degree AV block, when second-degree type I block occurs in the setting of evident infranodal conduction system disease (eg, wide QRS), the delay is often within the intraventricular specialized conduction system (ie, documented by intracardiac recordings), and risk of progression to complete block is substantial.

In contrast to the type I form, it is widely agreed that type II second-degree AV block carries a worrisome prognosis (Figure 9). Type II block is most often seen in conjunction with bundle branch block and is indicative of severe disease of the infranodal specialized cardiac conduction system. In this case, there is a predilection for Stokes-Adams attacks and the development of higher grades of AV block. Cardiac pacing is indicated.

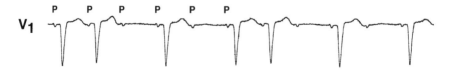

Figure 9. Mobitz type II AV block in a patient who also exhibited intermittent high-grade AV block and syncope. Note that the PR interval is unchanging and that there is intermittent absence of a QRS complex.

2:1 AV Block

As noted above, 2:1 AV block may be the result of AV nodal or infra-nodal disease. In such instances, the site(s) of block may be suspected by the presence of other observations occurring in temporal proximity to the 2:1 event (eg, periods of second-degree type I block may suggest an AV nodal site), but only intracardiac recordings can provide positive proof. The natural history of 2:1 AV block and its association with syncopal symptoms may be expected to parallel, for comparable sites of disease, the clinical pictures described above for second-degree AV block.

Third-Degree AV Block

Third-degree AV block may be high grade [in which multiple P waves are blocked (Figure 10)] or complete. In both cases there is failure of conduction of multiple atrial impulses to the ventricles. The cardiac rhythm, therefore, depends on subsidiary pacemakers located within either the proximal portions of the specialized cardiac conduction system (ie, His bundle), which may result in relatively narrow QRS complexes, or within its much more distal ramifications, resulting in wide QRS complexes.

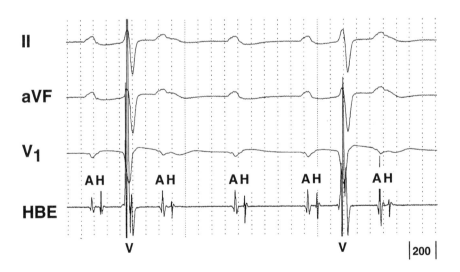

Figure 10. ECG recordings (leads II, aVF, and Vl) and intracardiac recording from the vicinity of the His bundle (HBE) revealing infra-His block. Dissociation of the ventricular escape rhythm from the His potential was demonstrable during a prolonged recording period, thereby supporting a diagnosis of complete AV block. Pacemaker therapy was instituted.

Syncope is a common symptom in patients with high-grade and complete AV block, and has been variously reported to occur in 38% to 61% of such cases.[68,69] In acute anterior myocardial infarction with associated AV block, the prognosis is ultimately related to the magnitude of ventricular damage. By contrast, complete AV block after inferior wall myocardial infarction rarely persists, and its occurrence is often preceded by a progression through stages, beginning with PR interval prolongation and/or type I second-degree AV block. The site of block in this setting is usually within the AV node, and its transient occurrence has no adverse long-term prognostic implications.[70]

In general, the risk for syncope or dizziness is greatest at onset of block, prior to establishment of a subsidiary rhythm. Thereafter, the ventricular rhythm often regularizes, and averages 35 to 40 bpm in acquired third-degree AV block. In fixed complete AV block, syncope may occur as a result of the unreliability of subsidiary pacemakers, or due to inability of the circulation to provide sufficient cerebral blood flow during periods of exercise or stress. In both cases, the close association with severe underlying heart disease also raises concern regarding tachyarrhythmia-induced syncope (including increased proarrhythmia risk in patients who are taking antiarrhythmic drugs).

For the most part, congenital complete AV block is considered to have a more benign outcome (ie, is less often accompanied by syncope or life-threatening consequences) than does the acquired form. In patients with congenital AV block, the site of block is typically at the level of the AV node (ie, His bundle potentials are recorded before each ventricular electrogram), the QRS complexes are narrow, and the block usually is associated with a relatively rapid subsidiary rhythm and one that tends to increase in rate with exercise. Consequently, affected individuals exhibit sufficient heart rate excursion to remain physically active in their younger years. Ultimately, however, exertional intolerance often becomes an issue by middle age, at which time cardiac pacing may be necessary.

The prognosis for patients with congenital complete heart block is determined primarily by the presence of any associated congenital heart disease (eg, corrected transposition of the great vessels, atrial septal defect, etc.), and in the absence of concomitant abnormalities, children with this disease tend to grow normally. Recently, however, concern has been raised regarding the supposedly benign natural history of congenital AV block,[71,72,73] and further evaluation of this issue is needed. In the meantime, syncope and dizziness (along with exertional intolerance) are accepted indications for pacing in these patients. For instance, among 14 adult patients in one series[72] who had been followed for 25 years, cardiac pacemakers were deemed necessary in 7 cases. The indications for pacing were syncope in 5 patients and dizziness in 2.

Bundle Branch and Fascicular Blocks

Syncope in patients with various forms of bundle branch block and fascicular blocks depends on the risk of developing high-grade or complete AV block, as well as on the risk of occurrence of ventricular tachyarrhythmias. In the Framingham study,[74,75] an 18-year follow-up of approximately 5200 individuals initially believed free of cardiovascular disease, revealed a 2.4% incidence of new bundle branch block (0.13% annually). Right bundle branch block (RBBB) was most common (70 of 125 patients), and was not associated with acute events, but was associated with hypertension and was accompanied by greater incidence of coronary artery disease (2.5 times greater), congestive heart failure (4 times greater) and cardiovascular mortality (3 times greater) than that observed in age-matched controls. In contrast, in almost one half of patients developing left bundle branch block (LBBB), an acute event was identified. The subsequent 10-year follow-up of these patients was accompanied by a mortality five times that of age-matched controls.

In patients with chronic infranodal conduction system disease manifest by bifascicular block, progression to second- or third-degree AV block is usually slow. However, susceptibility increases the longer the HV interval and appears to be particularly great when the HV interval exceeds 100 msec.[76–78] Evidence of susceptibility to potentially significant infranodal conduction system disease may be uncovered by demonstration of HV prolongation or infranodal block during incremental atrial pacing studies,[79] or after parenteral antiarrhythmic drug administration (eg, procainamide, ajmaline).

Indications for undertaking electrophysiological study in patients with AV conduction system disease have been outlined by a task force of the American College of Cardiology and the American Heart Association (Table 6).[80] The classes of indications are analogous to those used for cardiac pacing: Class I, general agreement that electrophysiological study provides useful patient management information; Class II, less certainty regarding the utility of the information, but electrophysiological study still often used; Class III, general agreement that electrophysiological study does not provide useful information.

Treatment

Apart from the use of atropine in certain forms of transient AV block (eg, associated with inferior wall myocardial infarction, during the course of invasive cardiovascular procedures), cardiac pacing has replaced pharmacological therapy in the treatment of patients with symptomatic AV block. Syncope, when clearly documented to be associated with bradycardia or when bradycardia is strongly suspected in the setting of AV block, is a well-defined indication for pacing.[81,82]

_____ Table 6 _____

Guidelines for Undertaking Electrophysiological Study for Acquired AV Block or Chronic Intraventricular Conduction Delay

Class I: Indicated
1. Syncope or near syncope in patients with suspected, but not electrocardiographically documented, infranodal block.
2. Patients with a pacemaker for treatment of AV block, but in whom symptoms persist and tachyarrhythmias are suspected as the cause.
3. In the setting of bundle branch block, when tachyarrhythmias are a suspected cause of symptoms.

Class II: Possibly Indicated
1. AV block or chronic bundle branch block when it is thought that determining site of block is of value for treatment or prognostic purposes.
2. Suspected concealed junctional extrasystoles as cause of AV block.

Class III: Not Indicated
1. Symptomatic AV block or intraventricular conduction delay already correlated with electrocardiographic findings.
2. Neurally mediated (vagally mediated) AV block (usually recognized by concomitant sinus slowing)
3. Asymptomatic patients with intraventricular conduction delays.

AV = atrioventricular.

Extrinsic Disturbances of Sinus Node Function and AV Conduction

Extrinsic Disturbances of Sinus Function

Numerous extrinsic factors may affect sinus node function without inducing structural disturbances. Of these, autonomic nervous system influences, cardioactive drugs, and less importantly, metabolic disturbances, are the most common.[3,4,83-88] Drug-induced disorders are dealt with in this section, while neurally mediated causes are considered separately, below. Cardioactive drugs may initiate or aggravate sinus bradyarrhythmias, or induce chronotropic incompetence (Table 7). Cardiac glycosides may aggravate sinus node dysfunction, but this group of agents only rarely causes clinical problems.[4,89-91] The drugs most often known to cause or aggravate bradyarrhythmic aspects of sinus node dysfunction include the now infrequently used (in "developed" countries) sympatholytic antihypertensive agents (eg, α-methyldopa, guanethidine), as well as widely used agents such as β-adrenoceptor blockers, calcium channel blockers, membrane-active antiarrhythmics (especially amiodarone, sotalol, flecainide, and propafen-

_____ Table 7 _____

Drugs Affecting Sinus Node Function

Antiarrhythmic drugs:
- *amiodarone:* may be associated with de novo evidence of sinus node dysfunction
- *flecainide, propafenone, sotalol:* may be expected to exacerbate sinus node dysfunction
- *quinidine, dispoyramide, procainamide:* less often worsens sinus node function possibly due to vagolytic properties
- *bretylium, lidocaine, mexiletine:* rarely a problem.

Antihypertensives (sympatholytic):
- α-methyldopa, reserpine, clonidine

β-adrenergic blocking drugs:
- without intrinsic sympathomimetic action (ISA): propranolol, nadolol, etc.
- with ISA, less severe affects: pindolol, acebutolol, etc.

Calcium channel blockers:
- verapamil and diltiazem more prominently than nifedipine

Cardiac Glycosides (rarely a clinical problem)

Miscellaneous:
- carbamazepine
- cimetidine
- lithium
- phenytoin

_____

one), and the antiepileptic drug, carbamazepine (Tegretol®).[3,4] Less commonly, lithium carbonate, cimetidine, amitriptyline, and the phenothiazines may be responsible.[3,4] On the other side of the coin, certain antiarrhythmic drugs may result in difficult to recognize proarrhythmic effects in the atrium (ie, an unexpected increase in the frequency of atrial tachyarrhythmias), as well as ventricular proarrhythmia.

Extrinsic Disturbances of AV Conduction

The AV nodal region is heavily innervated, and in the normal resting state sympathetic and parasympathetic influences tend to be approximately balanced (in contrast to the sinus node, where parasympathetic influences usually dominate). However, in some situations (eg, well-trained athletes, cardiac glycoside excess, transient hypervagotonia associated with conditions such as carotid sinus syndrome, cough syncope, vasovagal syncope, etc.), parasympathetic control may become predominant;[92–96] first-degree, second-degree type I, or even paroxysmal high degree of AV block may then occur. In paroxysmal AV block, bradycardia may be severe enough to account for syncope. More often though, syncope in the setting of demonstrable hypervagotonia is the result of neurally mediated reflex activity in which bradycardia is associated with peripheral vascular dilatation (see section of this chapter entitled *Syncope of Neurally Mediated Reflex Origin*). Consequently, recurrent syncope in association with extrinsic disturbances of AV conduction may be multifactorial in origin.

Drug effects are a common cause of AV nodal conduction disturbances,[97] and may be the most important factor in the deterioration of AV conduction in patients with sinus node dysfunction.[3,36] A variety of cardioactive drugs affect the AV node in this way, either due to direct pharmacological actions (eg, adenosine, many conventional antiarrhythmic drugs), or indirectly, as a result of their actions on the autonomic nervous system (eg, β-adrenergic blocking drugs), or both. Cardiac glycosides are perhaps the most widely recognized drugs to have such an effect, and are well known for inducing first-degree or Mobitz type I second-degree AV block by enhancing the effects of vagal tone at the AV node. β-blockers, by diminishing sympathetic effects on the AV node, are equally important in this regard. Calcium channel blockers and other antiarrhythmic drugs (eg, quinidine or sotalol) may act directly, as well as through effects on the autonomic nervous system, to alter conduction in the AV node. At usual doses, however, antiarrhythmic drugs are rarely associated with de novo development of complete AV block at the AV nodal level. On the other hand, especially in patients with wide QRS morphology indicative of intrinsic infranodal conduction system disease, symptomatic AV block may occur within the intraventricular specialized conduction system tissues. Once again, however, syncope in this setting cannot be assumed to be bradycardic in origin because drug-induced tachycardias (ie, proarrhythmic effects of antiarrhythmic drugs) are also more common in this situation.

Syncope of Neurally Mediated Reflex Origin

Neurocardiogenic syncope includes vasovagal syncope, carotid sinus syndrome, and other unusual forms of neurally mediated syncope such as cough, deglutition, and micturition syncope. All of these conditions involve both an element of vasodepression as well as the more easily recognized bradycardia (which in some cases may be prolonged asystole) (Figure 11). The advent of tilt table testing for the clinical investigation of syncope[98] greatly increased the capability to confirm the diagnosis of these conditions in symptomatic patients. Optimum treatment, however, remains less well defined.

Clinical Presentation

Vasovagal syncope is essentially the "simple" or "common" faint. In young people, this type of faint tends to be easy to diagnose because a clear history of preceding dizziness together with other typical phenomena is obtained (see review by Sutton and Petersen[99]). The patient often reports

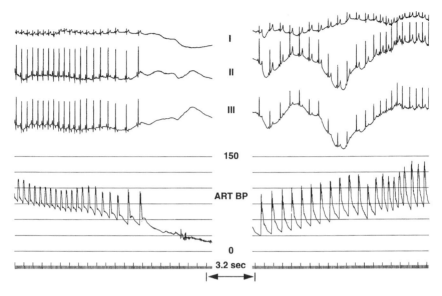

Figure 11. ECG recordings and arterial pressure tracing revealing onset of hypotension and bradycardia during head-up tilt table testing in a patient with recurrent unexplained syncope and a structurally normal heart. The findings reproduced the patient's symptoms, thereby supporting a diagnosis of neurally mediated (vasovagal) syncope.

feelings of lack of air, a change in breathing pattern, detachment from surroundings, sweating, loss of hearing, and nausea prior to total loss of consciousness. Witnesses commonly report that the patient exhibited marked pallor. During the recovery phase, there is rapid resumption of orientation, but weakness, nausea, and headache may last from minutes to hours. In older subjects, the premonitory symptoms may be very brief, and therefore entirely unrecognized, or completely lacking. In such patients, syncope occurs without warning and may result in falls and physical injury. This presentation may be difficult to distinguish, by history alone, from syncope complicating conduction disturbances of the heart. This variant of the vasovagal faint has been termed "malignant vasovagal syndrome."[100]

Vasovagal syncope may be triggered by any of a variety of situational factors. Some of the latter include unpleasant sights (eg, sight of blood), pain, extreme emotion, prolonged standing, stuffy rooms, boredom, and previous consumption of alcohol. Typical venues for fainting are churches, hospitals, the sports field (usually in association with injury), parties, queues, airplanes, and restaurants. When prodromal symptoms are lacking, of a suspicious venue may be helpful in determining the correct diagnosis.

Carotid sinus syndrome usually presents with syncope without warning, but with a slower recovery than is expected in Stokes-Adams attacks. Although rare, this diagnosis can be supported by a history suggesting that head movements trigger dizziness or syncope. As a rule, the condition almost exclusively afflicts older people with a substantially higher incidence among males. These features are in contrast to those of vasovagal syncope, which affects the sexes equally and occurs at all ages. Abrupt bradycardia tends to be a more prominent feature in carotid sinus syndrome than in vasovagal syncope. Prolonged attacks in both conditions usually involve a period of asystole and may be complicated by seizure-like activity and incontinence of urine.

Pathophysiological Mechanisms

The efferent reflex pathways (ie, central nervous system (CNS) to major organ systems and peripheral circulation) that cause hypotension and bradycardia in the various neurally mediated syncopes are relatively well understood. Essentially, enhanced efferent neural signals in the vagus nerve mediate bradycardia while almost simultaneous diminution of sympathetic neural activity is believed to be primarily responsible for causing dilatation of skeletal muscle arterioles[101,102] and splanchnic venules (ie, the vasodepression component).[103] On the other hand, the "trigger" factors, the afferent neural pathways (ie, from "trigger" sites to the CNS), and the processing in the vasomotor center are far less clear.

In general, the risk of triggering neurally mediated reflex syncope is accentuated by the loss of central venous volume. This may occur spontaneously as a result of dehydration, hemorrhage, or adoption of the erect posture. The latter has been associated with displacement of 500 to 1000 mL of blood from the central circulation to dependent regions (higher in patients with inadequate peripheral vascular compensation). Originally, in typical vasovagal syncope, cardiac baroreceptors (particularly those in the left ventricular wall) were implicated as principal sites of inappropriate triggering of the bradycardia-hypotension reflex.[94,104-106] However, given the documented occurrence of vasovagal syncope in orthotopic heart transplant recipients,[107] the focus of interest has shifted toward other residual central mechano- and chemoreceptors (eg, those baroreceptors that persist in the right atrial remnant in transplanted patients, receptors in the great vessels and pulmonary circulation). These various receptors may be triggered by very low filling pressures that are known to occur in developing vasovagal syncope.[108] The latter may simply reflect concomitant central volume diminution due to the factors noted above. Whether patients who are particularly susceptible to vasovagal syncope respond in an exaggerated manner to this "stress" is as yet uncertain. In carotid sinus syndrome, the afferent side of the reflex loop is somewhat more clear-cut. In this case, the mode of triggering is neurological, arising from stimulation of autonomic receptors in the cervical region,[109] potentially in conjunction with absence of parallel inputs from the sternocleidomastoid muscles.[110] This direct stimulation may account for the rapid onset often characteristic of carotid sinus syndrome. If there are central processing abnormalities, they are probably similar to those in vasovagal syncope. These abnormalities, if they exist, and shared efferent mechanisms may explain the observed clinical overlap between carotid sinus syndrome and vasovagal syncope.[111]

The principal afferent neural pathways from central mechano- and chemoreceptors to the medulla in classic vasovagal syncope are generally thought to be via vagal C-fibers.[94,104-106] In susceptible patients, activity triggered in these pathways initiates a poorly understood series of events within the medullary cardiovascular control areas that results in the efferent response noted above. For other nonvasovagal types of neurally mediated syncope (eg, carotid sinus syncope, postmicturition syncope, etc.) separate afferent neural pathways from the trigger site to the brain have been identified, although central chemo- and mechanoreceptors may also contribute secondarily in these settings.[112]

The factors that impart ''susceptibility'' to neurally mediated syncope in humans remain to be elucidated. It seems that most humans are capable of experiencing vasovagal reactions from time-to-time, although a only a subset (and these often only for a brief period in their lives) seem to exhibit marked susceptibility to recurrent episodes. Potentially, susceptibility may arise from enhanced trigger site sensitivity, abnormal medullary response to an otherwise normal afferent signal, an excessive and/or inappropriately balanced efferent neural response, or an undesirable peripheral response (perhaps related to the concept of accentuated antagonism between sympathetic and parasympathetic pathways). Susceptibility may also be characterized by certain neurohumoral responses that have been recorded in fainters but not in control subjects. Thus, for example, marked elevation of circulating adrenaline, vasopressin, and β-endorphins[19,113,114] have been reported to precede vasovagal syncope. Whether these are causal, or a secondary phenomenon, is unknown. Finally, susceptibility to cerebral vasoconstriction may play a role in determining whether a faint occurs,[115] although further study of this phenomenon is needed to be certain that it is not a nonspecific response to systemic hypotension.

Incidence and Prognosis

The incidence of carotid sinus syndrome in the population has been calculated to be 35 to 40 new patients per million per year.[109,111] However, in clinical practice the condition is detected much less frequently. The reasons for this discrepancy include failure to perform carotid sinus massage and tilt table testing routinely in syncope patients and misclassification due to failure to record both blood pressure and heart rate response when carotid massage is undertaken (ie, in the absence of adequate arterial pressure measurements, predominant vasodepressor responses may be overlooked).

In general, carotid sinus syndrome is not considered a mortal condition; the 70-year-old patient at presentation has a 65% 5-year survival.[116] Nevertheless, given the usual effectiveness of appropriately selected pacing therapy, failure to recognize the diagnosis unduly exposes elderly patients (those most often afflicted) to risk of physical injury associated with recurrent syncope and dizzy spells.[117]

Vasovagal syncope is a condition that can occur in anybody given sufficiently adverse circumstances, and therefore, discussion of its incidence is not appropriate. One study has estimated that approximately 18% of presentations of two or more syncopal episodes that prompt referral for permanent pacing are vasovagal in origin.[118] Vasovagal syncope is also not thought to lead to a high fatality risk. However, since sudden asystole is known to be a cause of death,[119] the possibility of a rare association between vasovagal and sudden death has been considered.[120] Furthermore, the tendency for vasovagal syncope to occur in young physically fit individuals has raised concern regarding its possible contribution to sports-related syncope with the rare occurrence of physical injury or death as a result.[120,121]

Investigation

The most common form of carotid sinus syndrome (predominant cardioinhibitory form) is diagnosed when carotid sinus massage in the erect position for 5 to 10 seconds is associated with symptom reproduction due to the occurrence of asystole or paroxysmal AV block of at least 3 seconds in duration.[109,111] The vasodepressor component can be assessed separately by controlling the bradycardia with use of a temporary dual-chamber pacing system and beat-to-beat arterial pressure monitoring in the erect position. These tests are best performed on a tilt table using digital plethysmography to record beat-to-beat arterial pressure changes.[122]

Vasovagal syncope may be suspected based on the patient's clinical history, but as noted earlier, this is not always possible. Consequently, although protocols have been in a state of evolution in recent years, tilt-table testing techniques have proved very valuable.[14,18,19,94,98,112,118,123] As a rule, the first step is passive head-up tilt at 60° to 70°, during which the patient is supported by a footplate and gently applied body straps for a period not less than 30 minutes, and preferably 45 minutes.[123] Tilt angles <60° and >80° lead to loss of sensitivity and specificity.[118,125] Subsequently, if needed, tilt testing in conjunction with a drug challenge (eg, isoproterenol, edrophonium, nitroglycerin) may be undertaken either immediately or as a separate procedure.[94,126] The most frequently used drug is isoproterenol, usually given in escalating doses from 1 to 3 μ/min.[94] Nitroglycerin, intravenously or sublingually, has recently gained particular favor in Europe.[126]

Tilt testing has a false-positive rate of around 10%[94,125] and a repro-ducibility, in the short term, of 80% to 90%, and over longer than 1 year, approximately 60%.[118,127-130] Since there is no "gold standard" for diagnosis of neurally mediated syncope, the sensitivity of tilt testing cannot accurately be estimated. Thus, tilt table testing is an imperfect test. Nevertheless, its utility is clear inasmuch as it remains the only investigation that provides the opportunity to precipitate a typical attack under the eyes of the inves-tigator. Further, its specificity and reproducibility are comparable to many other widely accepted useful diagnostic procedures.

Treatment

The mainstay in treatment of typical vasovagal syncope is explanation and reassurance. This approach proves most effective when there is a pro-drome of sufficient duration to permit the patient to take suitable evasive action. Patients whose symptoms demand more than mere reassurance are those whose attacks have minimal or no prodrome (especially if they have had resulting injury), those who cannot be taught to abort attacks, and whose attacks are complicated by seizure-like activity or incontinence. Ad-ditionally, patients with "high risk" occupations or avocations in which syncope might lead to injury to themselves or to others (eg, pilots, com-mercial drivers, window washers, swimmers, etc.) present a concern.

There exists a vast literature on medication for patients with vasovagal syncope, but most of these are uncontrolled studies. The few small con-trolled studies that have been reported (atenolol, cafedrine, disopyramide, scopolamine and etilefrine) all have methodological problems. Nonethe-less, only one of these (the β-adrenergic blocker, atenolol) has shown a drug benefit over 1-month follow-up.[124,131-134] One report suggests that the magnitude of sinus tachycardia present before syncope offers a clue to the potential benefit of β-adrenergic blockade therapy. Other drugs that ap-pear to be useful in selected cases include serotonin-reuptake inhibitors and fludrocortisone. Again, controlled studies are unavailable.

Cardiac pacing has proved highly successful in carotid sinus syndrome when bradycardia has been documented.[117] Currently, pacing is acknowl-edged to be the treatment of choice in all but the most mild forms of carotid sinus syndrome. Debate only exists concerning the mode of pacing, simple VVI or DDD. In general, dual-chamber pacing is favored. A rate-drop response diagnostic and rapid pacing rate hysteresis are desirable (see below). The VVI or VVIR pacing modes should only be chosen if there is clear absence of both susceptibility to "ventricular pacing effect" (ie, a drop in systemic pressure as a result of ventricular pacing alone) and a substantial concomitant vasodepressor element.[117,135] Single-chamber atrial pacing (AAI or AAIR) is contraindicated in carotid sinus syndrome (and other forms of neurally mediated syncope) due to the propensity for these patients to exhibit paroxysmal high-grade AV block during the episodes . Incidentally, the presence of AV block may be masked by marked sinus bradycardia or asystole, but becomes immediately evident upon pacing the atrium.

In contrast to carotid sinus syndrome, experience with pacing in other forms of neurally mediated syncope has been much more limited.[136,137] In the case of vasovagal syncope, provided that it is reserved for severe cases with recurring dominant cardioinhibition, pacing may play a useful role. However, unlike in cases of AV block where almost total efficacy is expected, pacing in vasovagal syncope, has more limited capabilities. Given currently available pacing techniques, pacing can only be anticipated to prolong the prodrome sufficiently for evasive action to be taken. This may nevertheless prove beneficial in that it may permit the patient to avoid injury and perhaps complete loss of consciousness. If pacing is undertaken, atrial pacing is contraindicated due to the potential for paroxysmal AV block. Only a dual-chamber system is capable of maximizing cardiac output in the face of falling venous return while also avoiding provocation of retrograde (ventriculoatrial) conduction. Further, it is essential that the pacing system be capable of detecting imminent neurally mediated syncopal events (eg, by means of a rate drop diagnostic algorithm),[138] and it must provide a form of high-rate hysteresis in order to pace rapidly enough when necessary. Thus, significant abrupt bradycardia must develop before pacing is triggered, but when pacing is initiated, the rate must be relatively rapid in order to give maximum hemodynamic boost. The latter diagnostic element and "high rate" feature are not yet possessed by all dual-chamber devices.

Diagnostic Techniques

Given the overwhelming contribution of cardiac rhythm disturbances to the causes of syncope, fortuitous electrocardiographic documentation during a spontaneous symptomatic episode would be of obvious diagnostic value in the assessment of the basis of syncope. The additional documentation of ambulatory blood pressure would also be a great asset, especially in those patients where there is doubt regarding the actual occurrence of systemic hypotension.

The 12-lead electrocardiogram, which is only a brief sample of the cardiac rhythm, rarely provides specific findings in the syncope patient. Certain observations may, however, provide indirect clues leading to further investigation. For instance, the presence of ventricular preexcitation (eg, Wolff-Parkinson-White syndrome), QT interval prolongation, or evidence of acute cardiac injury (eg, evolving myocardial infarction) may suggest an explanation. Conversely, relatively common findings such as sinus bradycardia, right or left bundle branch block, or bifascicular conduction system disease, are, more often than not, nonspecific findings.

As a rule, if ambulatory electrocardiographic monitoring is successful in providing a symptom- arrhythmia correlation, the need for additional diagnostic testing may be substantially diminished (neurally mediated bradycardia with a concomitant vasodepressor element remains a consideration). However, outpatient monitoring necessitates exposing patients to recurrence of potentially serious arrhythmias. Furthermore, in most syncope patients symptoms are infrequent and transient, and the patient and/or family members must be willing and able to undergo the necessary training to effectively use long-term event recorders. In the end, ambulatory monitoring (with the possible exception of a newly developed implantable monitor)[139] often proves nondiagnostic.

Exercise testing is not typically very productive in the evaluation of the syncope patient, and is best reserved for patients with exercise-induced symptoms or for those in whom myocardial ischemia is suspected. In terms of bradyarrhythmias associated with syncope, certain exercise test observations may be pertinent in the management of individual cases. For example, exercise testing may identify severe degrees of chronotropic incompetence,[3] excessively rapid heart rate deceleration after exercise, tachycardia-related AV block, or the exercise-associated variant of neurally mediated syncope.[112,121] Similarly, echocardiography rarely provides a definitive basis for syncope, but may be highly suggestive in patients with hypertrophic obstructive cardiomyopathy (HOCM) or severe valvular aortic stenosis.

In general, invasive electrophysiological testing has proved useful for defining probable arrhythmic causes of syncope in selected clinical settings, specifically in those individuals with underlying structural heart disease. On the other hand, such testing has proved less successful among patients who have no apparent structural substrate for arrhythmia.[11,13,14,140,141] For example, in a recent review by Camm and Lau,[11] electrophysiological testing was deemed to have provided a diagnosis in 56% of all patients. However, the testing was clearly more successful in patients with (71%) than in patients without (36%) evident structural cardiac disease.

As with any test, care must be taken in interpreting the findings of invasive electrophysiological studies. For example, in one study in which bradyarrhythmias were known to be the cause of syncope (21 syncopal patients with known symptomatic atrioventricular block or sinus pauses),[142] electrophysiological testing only correctly identified 3 of 8 patients with documented sinus pauses (sensitivity 37.5%), and 2 of 13 patients with documented atrioventricular block (sensitivity 15.4%). On the other hand, other abnormalities not known to have occurred spontaneously in these individuals, were often induced during electrophysiological study. Potentially, tilt table testing may have proved helpful for these patients, and may have permitted placing the apparently false-positive electrophysiological findings in perspective.

Among all causes of syncope, the neurally mediated syncopal syndromes are the most frequent (especially the "common" or vasovagal faint). These conditions and their evaluation have been discussed in more detail previously. However, head-up tilt testing has become a particularly important diagnostic technique to identify susceptibility to the vasovagal faint.[143,144] Detailed discussion of tilt table testing protocols, test reproducibility, and estimated specificity and sensitivity is beyond the scope of this chapter.

The addition of tilt table testing to electrophysiological testing has substantially enhanced diagnostic capabilities in syncope patients. For example, Sra et al[140] report results of electrophysiological testing in conjunction with head-up tilt testing in 86 consecutive patients who were referred for evaluation of unexplained syncope. Electrophysiological testing was abnormal in 29 patients (34%), with the majority of these cases (21 patients) being inducible sustained monomorphic ventricular tachycardia. The remainder comprised inducible supraventricular tachycardias (5 patients), sinoatrial dysfunction (1 patient), and conduction system disease (2 patients). Among the remaining patients, head-up tilt testing proved positive in 34 cases (40%), while 23 patients (26%) remained undiagnosed. In general, patients exhibiting positive electrophysiological findings were older and more frequently male, and exhibited lower ventricular ejection fractions and higher frequency of evident heart disease than did patients with positive head-up tilt tests or patients in whom no diagnosis was determined. During follow-up, syncope recurrence occurred in approximately 13% of patients. Importantly, however, syncope recurrence in patients for whom treatment was directed by electrophysiological testing or tilt table testing seemed to be highly associated with discontinuation of recommended therapies.

A further evaluation of the combined use of electrophysiological testing and head-up tilt testing in the assessment of syncope is provided in the report by Fitzpatrick et al.[118] Among 322 syncope patients evaluated between 1984 and 1988, conventional electrophysiological testing provided a basis for syncope in 229 cases (71%), with 93 patients having a normal electrophysiological study. Among the patients with abnormal electrophysiological findings, AV conduction disease was diagnosed in 34%, sinus node dysfunction in 21%, carotid sinus syndrome in 10%, and an inducible sustained tachyarrhythmia in 6%. As noted above, in the 93 patients with normal conventional electrophysiological studies, tilt table testing was undertaken in 71 cases, and it reproduced syncope, consistent with a vasovagal mechanism, in 53 of the 71 cases (75%). A diagnosis of neurally mediated vasovagal syncope was made for 16% of the entire patient population, a percentage that largely reflects the selected nature of the study population and is therefore lower than would be expected in a broader range of syncope patients (eg, those presenting to emergency rooms or general medical clinics).

Summary

Bradyarrhythmias due to sinus node dysfunction, AV conduction disturbances, and neurally mediated reflex hypotension bradycardia (especially vasovagal syncope) are frequent causes of syncope. However, in symptomatic patients with sinus node and/or AV conduction disturbances, symptoms may be due to tachy- or bradyarrhythmias or both, and the etiology may be either intrinsic structural disease, extrinsic factors (especially drug effects), or a combination of the two. Consequently, the presence of sinus node abnormalities or AV conduction abnormalities is alone insufficient to use as a basis for the development of an effective treatment strategy, and additional careful evaluation is needed to define the precise role of such abnormalities in the occurrence of syncope in a given individual. Similar difficulties arise with respect to the neurally mediated syncopal syndromes. In these cases, the electrocardiographic manifestations encompass a spectrum of possibilities from severe sinus arrest and/or high-grade AV block to syncope in the absence of overt bradycardia (ie, predominantly, a vasodepressor effect). The first may be interpreted as suggesting the presence of underlying conduction system disease, whereas in the case of pure vasodepressor syncope the diagnosis may be missed entirely if electrocardiographic recordings are obtained in the absence of concomitant blood pressure recordings. Thus, even when electrocardiographic recordings documenting bradycardia during spontaneous symptoms are available, the ultimate basis for syncopal symptoms may still require further careful diagnostic assessment.

The principal diagnostic step in the syncope patient is the differentiation of those individuals with normal cardiovascular status and those with evident structural disease. In the former, assuming that the medical history or physical examination has not identified another system problem, tilt table testing should be undertaken. In the latter group, a functional assessment of the suspected structural disturbance (ie, hemodynamic, angiographic, and electrophysiological studies, as appropriate) and an evaluation of susceptibility to tachy- and bradyarrhythmias by conventional electrophysiological testing is appropriate at an early stage. Tilt table testing should follow if the diagnosis remains in doubt. In only a few instances should special neurological studies be selected as an initial step. In all cases, the ultimate objective is to obtain a sufficiently strong correlation between the syncopal symptoms and detected abnormalities to permit both an accurate assessment of prognosis and to initiate an appropriate treatment plan.

Acknowledgment: The authors would like to thank Wendy Markuson and Barry L.S. Detloff for assistance in preparation of the manuscript.

References

1. Stokes W. Observations on some cases of permanently slow pulse. *Dublin Quart J Med Sci* 1846;2;73–85.
2. Mackenzie J. *Diseases of the Heart.* London: Oxford Medical Press; 1913;48.
3. Benditt DG, Sakaguchi S, Goldstein MA, et al. Sinus node dysfunction: Pathophysiology, clinical features, evaluation and treatment. In: Zipes DP, Jalife J (eds): *Cardiac Electrophysiology: From Cell to Bedside, 2nd Edition.* Philadelphia: W.B. Saunders Co.; 1215–1246;1995.
4. Benditt DG, Benson DW Jr, Dunnigan A, et al. Drug therapy in sinus node dysfunction. In: E Rapaport E (ed): *Cardiology Update:1984.* New York: Elsevier; 1984;79–101.
5. Wayne HH. Syncope: Physiological considerations and an analysis of the clinical characteristics in 510 patients. *Am J Med* 1961;30:418–438.
6. Day SC, Cook EF, Funkenstein H, et al. Evaluation and outcome of emergency room patients with transient loss of consciousness. *Am J Med* 1982;72:15–23.
7. Silverstein MD, Singer DE, Mulley AG, et al. Patients with syncope admitted to medical intensive care units. *JAMA* 1982;248:1185–1189.
8. Gendelman HE, Linzer M, Gabelman M, et al. Syncope in a general hospital population. *N Y State J Med* 1983;83:116–165.
9. Martin GJ, Adams SL, Martin HG, et al. Prospective evaluation of syncope. *Ann Emerg Med* 1984;13:499–504.
10. Kudenchuk PJ, McAnulty JH. Syncope: Evaluation and treatment. *Mod Concept Cardiovasc Dis* 1985;54:25–29.
11. Camm AJ, Lau CP. Syncope of undetermined origin: Diagnosis and management. *Prog Cardiol* 1988;1:139–156.
12. Ross RT. *Syncope.* London: WB Saunders Co;1988.
13. Kapoor W. Evaluation and outcome of patients with syncope. *Medicine* 1990; 69:160–175.
14. Benditt DG, Remole S, Milstein S, et al. Syncope: Causes, clinical evaluation, and current therapy. *Ann Rev Med* 1992;43:283–300.
15. Benditt DG, Sakaguchi S, Shultz JI, et al. Syncope: Diagnostic considerations and the role of tilt table testing. *Cardiol Rev* 1993;1:146–156.
16. Chen M-Y, Goldenberg IF, Milstein S, et al. Cardiac electrophysiologic and hemodynamic correlates of neurally mediated syncope. *Am J Cardiol* 1989; 63:66–72.
17. Almquist A, Gornick CC, Benson DW Jr, et al. Carotid sinus hypersensitivity: Evaluation of the vasodepressor component. *Circulation* 1985;67:927–936.
18. Sunon R, Petersen M, Brignole M, et al. Proposed classification for tilt induced vasovagal syncope. *Eur J Cardiac Pacing Electrophysiol* 1992;2:180–183.
19. Fitzpatrick A, Williams T, Ahmed R, et al. Echocardiographic and endocrine changes during vasovagal syncope induced by prolonged head-up tilt. *Eur J Cardiac Pacing Electrophysiol* 1992;2:121–128.
20. Rubenstein JJ, Schulman CL, Yurchak PM, et al. Clinical spectrum of the sick sinus syndrome. *Circulation* 1972;46:5–13.
21. Sutton R, Perrins EJ. Neurological manifestations of the sick sinus syndrome. In: Busse EW (ed): *Cerebral Manifestations of Episodic Cardiac Dysrhythmias.* Amsterdam: Excerpta Medica; 1979;174–181.
22. Ausubel K, Funnan S. The pacemaker syndrome. *Ann Intern Med* 1985; 103:420–429.

23. Ellenbogen K, Wood MA, Stambler B. Pacemaker syndrome: Clinical, hemodynamic, and neurohumoral features. In: Barold SS, Mugica J (eds): *New Perspectives in Cardiac Pacing, Vol 3.* Mount Kisco, NY: Futura Publishing Co.; 1993;85–112.
24. Talan DA, Bauernfeind RA, Ashley WVV, et al. Twenty-four hour continuous ECG recordings in long-distance runners. *Chest* 1982;82:19–24.
25. Viitasalo MT, Kala R, Eisalo A. Ambulatory electrocardiographic recording in endurance athletes. *Br Heart J* 1982;47:213–220.
26. Hattori M, Toyama J, Ito A, et al. Comparative evaluation of depressed automaticity in sick sinus syndrome by Holter monitoring and overdrive suppression test. *Am Heart J* 1983;105:587–592.
27. Ector H, Rolies L, De Geest H. Dynamic electrocardiography and ventricular pauses of 3 seconds and more: Etiology and therapeutic implications. *Pacing Clin Electrophysiol* 1983;6:548–551.
28. Hilgard J, Ezri MD, Denes P. Significance of ventricular pauses of three seconds or more detected on twenty-four hour Holter recordings. *Am J Cardiol* 1985;55:1005–1008.
29. Ferrer MI. The sick sinus syndrome in atrial disease. *JAMA* 1968;206:645.
30. Kaplan BM, Langendorf R, Lev M, Pick A. Tachycardia-Bradycardia syndrome (So-called "sick sinus syndrome"). *Am J Cardiol* 1973;26:497–508.
31. Sutton R, Kenny R-A. The natural history of sick sinus syndrome. *Pacing Clin Electrophysiol* 1986;9:1110–1114.
32. Rosenqvist M, Brandt J, Schuller H. Atrial versus ventricular pacing in sinus node disease: A treatment comparison study. *Am Heart J* 1986;111:292–297.
33. Stangl K, Winzfeld A, Seitz K, et al. Atrial stimulation (AAI): Long-term followup of 110 patients. In: Belhassen B, Feldman S, Copperman Y (eds): *Cardiac Pacing and Electrophysiology. Proceedings of the VIIIth World Symposium on Cardiac Pacing and Electrophysiology.* Jerusalem: R & L Creative Communications; 1987;283–285.
34. Sutton R, Bourgeois I. *The Foundations of Cardiac Pacing, Pt 1.* Mount Kisco, NY: Futura Publishing Co., 1991;131.
35. Gijs Mast E, Van Hemel NM, Bakea L, et al. Is chronic atrial stimulation a reliable method for single chamber pacing in sick sinus syndrome? *Pacing Clin Electrophysiol* 1986;9:1127–1130.
36. van Mechelen R, Segers A, Hagemeijer F. Serial electrophysiologic studies after single chamber atrial pacemaker implantation in patients with symptomatic sinus node dysfunction. *Eur Heart J* 1984;5:628–636.
37. Santini M, Alexidou G, Ansalone G, et al. Relation of prognosis in sick sinus syndrome at age, conduction defects and modes of permanent cardiac pacing. *Am J Cardiol* 1990;565:729–735.
38. Skagen K, Hansen IF. The long-terrn prognosis for patients with sinoatrial block treated with pennanent pacemaker. *Acta Med Scand* 1975;199:13–15.
39. Sasaki S, Shimotori M, Akahane K, et al. Long-term follow-up of patients with sick sinus syndrome: A comparison of clinical aspects among unpaced, ventricular inhibited paced, and physiologically paced groups. *Pacing Clin Electrophysiol* 1988;11:1575–1583.
40. Brignole M, Menozzi C, Gianfranchi L, et al. Neurally mediated syncope detected by carotid sinus massage and head-up tilt test in sick sinus syndrome. *Am J Cardiol* 1991;68:1032–1036.
41. Scheinman MM, Evans-Bell T, the Executive Committee of the Percutaneous Cardiac Mapping and Ablation Registry. Catheter ablation of the atrioventricular junction: A report of the percutaneous mapping and ablation registry. *Circulation* 1984;70:1024–1029.

42. Cox JL. The surgical treatment of atrial fibrillation IV: Surgical technique. *J Thorac Cardiovasc Surg* 1991;101:5884–5892.
43. Cox JL, Boineau JP, Schuessler RB, et al. Modifications of the MAZE procedure for atrial flutter and atrial fibrillation: I - rationale and surgical results. *J Thorac Cardiovasc Surg* 1995;110: 473–484.
44. Haissaguerre M, Gencel L, Fischer B, et al. Successful catheter ablarion of atrial fibrillation. *J Cardiovasc Electrophysiol* 1994;5:1045–1052.
45. Rosenqvist M, Brandt J, Schuller H. Long-term pacing in sick sinus node disease: Effects of stimulation mode on cardiovascular morbidity and mortality. *Am Heart J* 1988;116:16–22.
46. Andersen HR, Thuesen L, Bagger JP, et al. Prospective randomised trial of atrial versus ventricular pacing in sick-sinus syndrome. *Lancet* 1994;344:1523–1528.
47. Laupacis A, Albers G, Dalen J, et al. Antithrombotic therapy in atrial fibrillation. *Chest* 1995;108:3525–3595.
48. Daubert C, Mabo P, Berder V, et al. Atrial tachyarrhythmias associated with high-degree interatrial conduction block: Prevention by permanent atrial resynchronisation. *Eur J Cardiac Pacing Electrophysiol* 1994;4:35–40.
49. Dunbar DN, Tobler HG, Fetter J, et al. Intracavitary electrode catheter cardioversion of atrial tachyarrhythmias in the dog. *J Am Coll Cardiol* 1986;7:1015–1027.
50. Murgatroyd FD, Johnson EE, Cooper RA, et al. Safety of low energy atrial defbrillation: World experience (Abstract). *Circulation* 1994;99(suppl I):14.
51. Puech P, Grolleau R, Guimond C. Incidence of different types of AV block and their localization by His bundle recordings. In: Wellens HJJ, Lie KI, Janse MJ (eds): *The Conduction System of the Heart*. Leiden, The Netherlands: Stenfert Kroese; 1976;467–484.
52. Rosen KM, Rahimtoola SH, Chuquimia R, et al. Electrophysiological significance of first degree atrioventricular block with intraventricular conduction disturbance. *Circulation* 1971;43: 491–502.
53. Nanila OS, Scherlag BJ, Javier RP, et al. Analysis of the AV conduction defect in complete heart block utilizing His bundle electrograms. *Circulation* 1970;41:437–448.
54. Lev M. The pathology of atrioventricular block. *Cardiovasc Clin* 1972;4:159–186.
55. Lev M, Bharati S. Atriovenuicular and intraventricular conduction system disease. *Arch Int Med* 1975;135:405–410.
56. Roanan M, Wagner GS, Wallace AG, Bradyarrhythmias in acute myocardial infarction. *Circulation* 1973:45:703–722.
57. Sutton R, Davies M. The conduction system in acute myocardial infarction complicated by heart block. *Circulation* 1968:38:987–992.
58. Rosen KM, Loeb HS, Chuquimia R, et al. Site of heart block in acute myocardial infarction. *Circulation* 1970:42:925–933.
59. Brown RW, Hunt D, Sloman IG. The natural history of atrioventricular conduction defects in acute myocardial infarction. *Am Heart J* 1969;78:460–466.
60. Vigorita VJ, Hutchins GM. Cardiac conduction system in hemochromatosis: Clinical and pathological features in six patients. *Am J Cardiol* 1979;44:418–423.
61. Bharati S, Lev M, Denes P, et al. Infiltrative cardiomyopathy with conduction disease and ventricular arrhythmia: Electrophysiologic and pathologic correlations. *Am J Cardiol* 1980;45:163–173.
62. Bharati S, de la Fuente DJ, Kallen RJ, et al. Conduction system in systemic lupus erythematosus with atrioventricular block. *Am J Cardiol* 1975;35:299–304.
63. Hassel D, Heinsimer J, Califf RM, et al. Complete heart block in Reiter's syndrome. *Am J Cardiol* 1984;53:967–968.
64. Smith R, Grossman W, Johnson L, et al. Arrhythmias following cardiac valve replacement. *Circulation* 1972;45:1018–1023.

65. Mathewson FA, Rabkin SW, Hsu PH. Atrioventricular heart block: 27 year follow-up experience. *Trans Assoc Life Ins Med Dir Amer* 1976;60:110–130.
66. McAnulty JH, Murphy E, Rahimtoola SH. A prospective evaluation of intra-Hisian conduction delay. *Circulation* 1979;59:1035–1039.
67. Shaw DB, Kekwick CA, Veale D, et al. Survival in second degree atrioventricular block. *Br Heart J* 1985;53:587–593.
68. Rowe JC, White PD. Complete heart block: A follow-up study. *Ann Intern Med* 1958;49:260–270.
69. Penton GB, Miller H, Levine SA. Some clinical features of complete heart block. *Circulation* 1956;13:801–824.
70. Berger PR, Roucco NA Jr, Ryan TI, et al. Incidence and prognostic implications of heart block complicating inferior myocardial infarction treated with thrombolytic therapy: Results from TIMI II. *J Am Coll Cardiol* 1992;20:533–540.
71. Michaelson M, Engle MA. Congenital complete heart block: An international study of the natural history. *Cardiovasc Clin* 1972;4:86–101.
72. Pordon CM, Moodie DJ. Adults with congenital complete heart block: 25-year follow-up. *Cleve Clin J Med* 1992;59:587–590.
73. Michaelsson M, Jonzon A, Riesenfeld T. Isolated congenital complete atrioventricular block in adult life. *Circulation* 1995;92:442–449.
74. Schneider JF, Thomas HE Jr, Kreger BE, et al. New acquired left bundle branch block: The Framingham Study. *Ann Intern Med* 1979;90:303–310.
75. Schneider JF, Thomas HE Jr, Kreger BE, et al. New acquired right bundle branch block: The Framingham Study. *Ann Intern Med* 1980;92:37-44.
76. Dhingra RC, Denes P, Wu D, et al. Syncope in patients with chronic bifascicular block. *Ann Intern Med* 1974;81:302–306.
77. Scheinman MM, Peters RW, Sauve MI, et al. Value of H-Q interval in patients with bundle branch block and the role of prophylactic permanent pacing. *Am J Cardiol* 1982;50:1316–1322.
78. Dhingra RC, Amat y Leon F, Pouget M, et al. Infranodal block: Diagnosis, clinical significance and management. *Med Clin North Am* 1976;60:175–192.
79. Dhingra RC, Wyndham CRC, Bauernfend RA, et al. Significance of bundle branch block distal to the His bundle induced by atrial pacing in patients with chronic bifascicular block. *Circulation* 1979;60:1455–1464.
80. Fisch C, DeSanctis RW, Dodge HT, et al. Guidelines for intracardiac electrophysiologic studies: A report of the American College of Cardiology/American Heart Association Task Force on Assessment of Diagnostic and Therapeutic Cardiovascular Procedures. *Circulation* 1989;80:1925–1939.
81. Dreifus LS, Fisch C, Griffin JC, et al. Guidelines for implantation of cardiac pacemakers and antiarrhythmia devices: A report of the American College of Cardiology/American Heart Association Task Force on Assessment of Diagnostic and Therapeutic Cardiovascular Procedures. *Circulation* 1991;84:455–467.
82. Rattes MF, Klein GJ, Shanna AD, et al. Efficacy of empirical cardiac pacing in syncope of unknown cause. *Can Med Assoc J* 1989;140:381–385.
83. Strauss HC, Prystowsky EN, Scheinman MM. Sino-atrial and atrial electrogenesis. *Prog Cardiovasc Dis* 1977;19:385–404.
84. Chung EK. Sick sinus syndrome: Current views. *Mod Concept Cardiovasc Dis* 1980;49:61–66.
85. Jordan JL, Yamaguchi I, Mandel WJ. Studies on the mechanism of sinus node dysfunction in the sick sinus syndrome. *Circulation* 1978;57:217–223.
86. Scheinman MM, Strauss HC, Evans GT, et al. Adverse effects of sympatholytic agents in patients with hypertension and sinus node dysfunction. *Am J Med* 1978;64:1013–1020.

87. Seipel L, Both A, Breithardt G, et al. Action of antiarrhythmic drugs on His bundle electrogram and sinus node function. *Acta Cardiol* 1974;18(suppl):251–267.
88. Linker NJ, Camm AJ. Drug effects on the sinus node. A clinical perspective. *Cardiovasc Drugs Ther* 1988;2:165–170.
89. Engel TR, Schaal SF. Digitalis in the sick sinus syndrome: The effect of digitalis on sinoatrial automaticity and atrioventricular conduction. *Circulation* 1973; 43:1201–1207.
90. Dhingra RC, Amat y Leon F, Wyndham C, et al. The electrophysiological effects of ouabain on sinus node and atrium in man. *J Clin Invest* 1975;56:555–562.
91. Strauss HC, Gilben M, Svenson RH, et al. Electrophysiologic effects of propranolol on sinus node function in patients with sinus node dysfunction. *Circulation* 1976;54:452–459.
92. Almquist A, Gornick C, Benson DW Jr, et al. Carotid sinus hypersensitivity: Evaluation of the vasodepressor component. *Circulation* 1985;71:927–936.
93. Lieshout JJV, Wieling W, Karemaker JM, et al. The vasovagal response. *Clin Sci* 1991;81:575–586.
94. Almquist A, Goldenberg IF, Milstein S, et al. Provocation of bradycardia and hypotension by isoproterenol and upright posture in patients with unexplained syncope. *New Engl J Med* 1989;320:346–351.
95. Smith ML, Carlson MD, Thames MD. Reflex control of the heart and circulation: Implications for cardiovascular electrophysiology. *J Cardiovasc Electrophysiol* 1991;2:441–449.
96. Chen M-Y, Goldenberg IF, Milstein S, et al. Cardiac electrophysiologic and hemodynamic correlates of neurally mediated syncope. *Am J Cardiol* 1989; 63:66–72.
97. Kocovic DZ, Friedman PL. Atriovenuicular nodal block. In: Podrid PJ, Kowey PR (eds): *Cardiac Arrhythmias. Mechanisms, Diagnosis, and Management.* Baltimore: Williams & Wilkins; 1995;1039–1050.
98. Kenny RA, Ingram A, Bayliss J, et al. Head-up tilt: A useful test for investigating unexplained syncope. *Lancet* 1986;2:1352–1354.
99. Sutton R, Petersen MEV. The clinical spectrum of neurocardiogenic syncope. *J Cardiovasc Electrophysiol* 1995;6:569–576.
100. Sutton R. Vasovagal syndrome: Could it be malignant? *Eur J Cardiac Pacing Electrophysiol* 1992;2:89.
101. Barcroft H, Edholm OG. On the vasodilatation in human skeletal muscle during posthaemorrhagic fainting. *J Physiol (Lond)* 1945;104:161–175.
102. Vallin BG, Sundlof G. Sympathetic outflow to muscles during vasovagal syncope. *J Auton Nerv Syst* 1982;6:287–291.
103. Bearn AG, Billing B, Edholm OG, Sherlock S. Hepatic blood flow and carbohydrate changes in man during fainting. *J Physiol (Lond)* 1951;115:442–445.
104. Sharpey-Schafer EP, Hayter CJ, Barlow ED. Mechanism of acute hypotension from fear and nausea. *Br Med J* 1958;2:878–880.
105. Thoren P. Role of cardiac C fibres in cardiovascular control. *Rev Physiol Biochem Pharmacol* 1979;86:1–94.
106. Oberg B, Thoren P. Increased activity in left ventricular receptors during hemorrhage or occlusion of caval veins in the cat: A possible cause of the vasovagal reaction. *Acta Physiol Scand* 1972;85:164–173.
107. Fitzpatrick AP, Banner N, Cheng A, et al. Vasovagal syncope may occur after orthotopic heart transplantation. *J Am Coll Cardiol* 1993;21:1132–1137.
108. Dickinson CJ. Fainting precipitated by collapse firing of venous baroreceptors. *Lancet* 1993;342:970–972.
109. Morley CA, Sutton R. Carotid sinus syncope. *Int J Cardiol* 1984;6:287–293.

110. Tea SH, Mansourati J, L'Heveder G, et al. New insights into the pathophysiology of carotid sinus syndrome. *Circulation* 1996;93:1411–1416.
111. Brignole M, Menozzi C, Gianfranchi L, et al. Neurally mediated syncope detected by carotid sinus massage and head-up tilt test in sick sinus syndrome. *Am J Cardiol* 1991;68:1032–1036.
112. Benditt DG, Goldstein MA, Adler S, et al. Neurally mediated syncopal syndromes: Pathophysiology and clinical evaluation. In: Mandel WJ (ed): *Cardiac Arrhythmias, 3rd Ed.* Philadelphia: JB Lippincott Co; 1995;879–906.
113. Sander-Jensen K, Secher NH, Astrup A, et al. Hypotension induced by passive head-up tilt: Endocrine and circulatory mechanisms. *Am J Physiol* 1986; 251:R743–R749.
114. Wallbridge DR, Maclntyre HE, Gray CE, et al. Increase in plasma β-endorphins precedes vasodepressor syncope. *Br Heart J* 1994;71:446–448.
115. Grubb BP, Gerard G, Roush K, et al. Cerebral vasoconstriction during head-upright tilt induced vasovagal syncope: A paradoxic and unexpected response. *Circulation* 1991;84:1157–1164.
116. Sutton R, Ahmed R, Ingram A. Twelve year experience of pacing in carotid sinus syndrome. (Abstract). *Pacing Clin Electrophysiol* 1989;12:1153.
117. Benditt DG, Remole S, Asso A, et al. Cardiac pacing for carotid sinus syndrome and vasovagal syncope. In: Barold SS, Mugica I (eds): *New Perspectives in Cardiac Pacing, 3.* Mount Kisco, NY: Futura Publishing Co.; 1993;15–28.
118. Fitzpatrick A, Theodorakis G, Vardas P, et al. Methodology of head-up tilt testing in patients with unexplained syncope. *J Am Coll Cardiol* 1991;17:125–130.
119. Pepine C, Morganroth J, McDonald J, et al. Sudden death during ambulatory electrocardiographic monitoring. *Am J Cardiol* 1991;68:785–788.
120. Milstein S, Buetikofer J, Lesser J, et al. Cardiac asystole: A manifestation of neurally mediated hypotension bradycardia. *J Am Coll Cadiol* 1989;14:1626–1632.
121. Sakaguchi S, Shultz J, Remole S, et al. Syncope associated with exercise: A manifestation of neurally mediated syncope. *Am J Cardiol* 1995;75:476–481.
122. Petersen MEV, Williams T, Sutton R. A comparison of non-invasive continuous finger blood pressure measurement [Finapres] with intra-arterial pressure during prolonged head-up tilt. *Eur Heart J* 1995;16:1647–1654.
123. Fitzpatrick A, Sutton R. Tilting towards a diagnosis in unexplained recurrent syncope. *Lancet* 1989;1:658–660.
124. Fitzpatrick AP, Ahmed R, Williams S, et al. A randomized trial of medical therapy in malignant vasovagal syndrome or neurally-mediated bradycardia/hypotension syndrome. *Eur J Cardiac Pacing Electrophysiol* 1991;1:991–202.
125. Natale A, Akhtar M, Jazayeri M, et al. Provocation of hypotension during head-up tilt testing in subjects with no history of syncope or presyncope. *Circulation* 1995;92:54–58.
126. Raviele A, Menozzi C, Brignole M, et al. Value of head-up tilt testing potentiated with sublingual nitroglycerin to assess the origin of unexplained syncope. *Am J Cardiol* 1995;76:267–272.
127. Chen XC, Chen MY, Remole S, et al. Reproducibility of head-up tilt-table testing for eliciting susceptibility to neurally-mediated syncope in patients without structural heart disease. *Am J Cardiol* 1992;69:755–760.
128. Grubb BP, Wolfe DA, Temesy-Armos PN, et al. Reproducibility of head upright tilt test results in patients with syncope. *Pacing Clin Electrophysiol* 1992; 15:1477–1481.
129. Sheldon R, Splawinski J, Killam S. Reproducibility of isoproterenol tilt-table tests in patients with syncope. *Am J Cardiol* 1992;69:1300–1305.

130. Petersen MEV, Price D, Williams T, et al. Short AV delay VDD pacing does not prevent vasovagal syncope in patients with cardioinhibitory vasovagal syndrome. *Pacing Clin Electrophysiol* 1994;17:882–891.
131. Brignole M, Menozzi C, Gianfranchi L, et al. A controlled trial of acute and long-term medical therapy in tilt-induced neurally mediated syncope. *Am J Cardiol* 1992;70:339–342.
132. Morillo CA, Leitch JU, Yee R, et al. A placebo-controlled trial of intravenous and oral disopyramide for prevention of neurally mediated syncope induced by head-up tilt. *J Am Coll Cardiol* 1993;22:1843–1848.
133. Moya A, Permanyer-Miralda G, Sagrista-Sauleda J, et al. Limitations of head-up tilt test for evaluating the efficacy of therapeutic interventions in patients with vasovagal syncope: Results of a controlled study of etilefrine versus placebo. *J Am Coll Cardiol* 1995;25:65–69.
134. Mahanonda N, Bhuripanyo K, Kangkagate C, et al. Randomized double-blind placebo-controlled trial of oral atenolol in patients with unexplained syncope and positive upright tilt table results. *Am Heart J* 1995;130:1250–1253.
135. Brignole M, Menozzi C, Lolli G, et al. Long term outcome paced and nonpaced patients with severe carotid sinus syndrome. *Am J Cardiol* 1992;69:1039–1043.
136. Benditt DG, Peterson M, Lurie K, et al. Cardiac pacing for prevention of recurrent vasovagal syncope. *Ann Intern Med* 1995;122:204–209.
137. Petersen MEV, Chamberlain-Webber R, Fitzpatrick AP, et al. Permanent pacing for cardioinhibitory malignant vasovagal syndrome. *Br Heart J* 1994;71:274–281.
138. Benditt DG, Sutton R, Gammage M, et al. Cardiac pacing in vasovagal syncope: Multi- center assessment of a rate-drop response algorithm (Abstract). *Pacing Clin Electrophysiol* 1996;19:592.
139. Krahn AD, Klein GJ, Norris C, et al. The etiology of syncope in patients with negative tilt table and electrophysiologic testing. *Circulation* 1995;92:1819–1824.
140. Sra JS, Anderson AJ, Sheikh SH, et al. Unexplained syncope evaluated by electrophysiologic studies and head-up tilt testing. *Ann Int Med* 1991;114:1013–1019.
141. DiMarco IB, Garan H, Hawthorne WJ, et al. Intracardiac electrophysiologic techniques in recurrent syncope of unknown cause. *Ann Int Med* 1981;95:542–548.
142. Fujimura O, Yee R, Klein GJ, et al. The diagnostic sensitivity of electrophysiologic testing in patients with syncope caused by bradycardia. *N Engl J Med* 1989;321:1703–1707.
143. Benditt DG, Ferguson DW, Grubb BP, et al. Tilt-table testing for assessing syncope and its treatment: An American College of Cardiology expert consensus document. *J Am Coll Cardiol* 1996;28:263–275.
144. Benditt DG, Lurie KG, Adler SW, et al. Rationale and methodology of head-up tilt table testing for evaluation of neurally mediated (cardioneurogenic) syncope. In: Zipes DP, Jalife J (eds): *Cardiac Electrophysiology. From Cell to Bedside* Philadelphia: WB Saunders Co.; 1995;1115–1128.

Chapter 6

Tachyarrhythmias as a Cause of Syncope

Mark N. Harvey, MD and Fred Morady, MD

Syncope is an important clinical problem, accounting for approximately 3% of emergency room visits and 1% of general hospital admissions.[1,2] The mechanism of tachycardia-induced syncope is most likely multifactorial.[3–6] The physiological causes of tachycardia-induced syncope may include the effects of tachycardia rate, alterations in hemodynamics, an altered autonomic state, and changes in atrial function. This chapter addresses the clinical features of tachycardia-induced syncope, the predominant physiological changes that occur during tachyarrhythmias, and the relationship between tachyarrhythmias and syncope.

Clinical Features of Syncope Due to Tachyarrhythmias

Ventricular Tachycardia

Ventricular tachycardia often results in syncope.[7] Other symptoms such as palpitations, dizziness, and presyncope may occur, although symptoms during ventricular tachycardia may be highly variable.[8] In one series, ventricular tachycardia was reported to be the etiology of unexplained syncope in 21% of patients evaluated.[9] In patients evaluated for sustained ventricular tachycardia, syncope was reported as the presenting symptom in

From Grubb BP, Olshansky B (eds.). *Syncope: Mechanisms and Management.* Armonk, NY: Futura Publishing Co., Inc.; © 1998.

15% of patients evaluated in one series, with near syncope in 15%, and lightheadedness in 35%.[8]

Decreased left ventricular function post myocardial infarction is a predisposing factor and can be an important clinical feature for sudden cardiac death due to ventricular tachycardia and ventricular fibrillation.[3] Thirty-five percent of patients with advanced congestive heart failure and syncope may have ventricular tachycardia as the cause of syncope.[10] Nonsustained ventricular tachycardia may also present an important clinical problem, with transient symptoms occurring during tachycardia. Nonsustained ventricular tachycardia has been reported during Holter monitoring in 29% of patients undergoing evaluation for syncope.[11,12] However, unless symptoms occur in association with the arrhythmia, it should not be assumed that nonsustained ventricular tachycardia is the cause of syncope.

A history of syncope may correlate with the occurrence of syncope during induction of ventricular tachycardia at the time of an electrophysiological test. In one study of patients with ventricular tachycardia presenting with syncope, 80% developed syncope when ventricular tachycardia was induced by programmed stimulation; a clinical history of syncope was found to be a significant predictor for the occurrence of syncope during induced ventricular tachycardia.[13] These observations have been confirmed in other studies of patients with ventricular tachycardia.[4]

Supraventricular Tachycardia

In patients evaluated for unexplained syncope, supraventricular tachycardia is infrequently found to be the etiology, accounting for approximately 2% of such patients.[14] In contrast, syncope may be a symptom of supraventricular tachycardia and may be an important clinical feature.[15–17] The type and rate of supraventricular tachycardia induced by programmed stimulation during an electrophysiological test correlates well with the features of the clinically occurring supraventricular tachycardia.[18] However, there is no correlation between syncope during clinical supraventricular tachycardia and syncope associated with supraventricular tachycardia induced during electrophysiological evaluation.[15,16]

The historical features of syncope due to supraventricular tachycardia may be less useful in distinguishing patients with syncope due to supraventricular tachycardia from those with other etiologies of syncope, because syncope during supraventricular tachycardia is often related to an abnormal vasomotor response to the hemodynamic stress of supraventricular tachycardia.[19–23] Additionally, the posture of the patient during supraventricular tachycardia may augment the vasomotor response and may contribute to the development of syncope. The symptoms that occur as the result of this abnormal vasomotor response may mimic vasodepressor syncope, making it difficult to distinguish patients with syncope due to supraventricular tachycardia from patients with vasodepressor syncope.

There are other clinical situations in which syncope may occur due to tachyarrhythmias. In patients with syncope and ventricular preexcitation syndromes, ventricular tachycardia may infrequently be found as the etiology of syncope.[24] In addition, atrial fibrillation in the setting of Wolff-Parkinson-White syndrome may result in syncope from rapid ventricular rates or in induction of ventricular fibrillation by rapid ventricular rates, as may supraventricular tachycardia by use of a rapidly conducting accessory pathway.[24]

Effect of Tachycardia Rate

Ventricular Tachycardia

The ventricular tachycardia rate is an important determinant of syncope due to ventricular tachycardia. Significantly more patients with sustained ventricular tachycardia present with syncope or near syncope when the tachycardia rate is ≥200 bpm.[8] In the electrophysiological evaluation of patients presenting with syncope caused by ventricular tachycardia, significantly faster rates of induced ventricular tachycardia are observed when compared to the tachycardia rates of patients without syncope.[13] One study found that spontaneous episodes of ventricular tachycardia associated with rates >220 bpm were associated with syncope, whereas ventricular tachycardia rates from 130 to 220 bpm often were hemodynamically stable, without syncope.[13] In this same study, ventricular tachycardia rates were evaluated as a predictor for syncope. It was found that a ventricular tachycardia rate >230 bpm was predictive of syncope during ventricular tachycardia compared to rates <200 bpm, which were predictive of ventricular tachycardia occurring without syncope. The concomitant use of antiarrhythmic medications is important, as their presence may slow the rate of ventricular tachycardia, resulting in the subsequent prevention of syncope.[13]

Supraventricular Tachycardia

The influence of the tachycardia rate in patients with syncope associated with supraventricular tachycardia appears to be less important. There is no association between the induced supraventricular tachycardia rate and the clinical occurrence of syncope in patients with syncope due to supraventricular tachycardia.[25] Hemodynamic changes occur with rapid atrial pacing and are associated with a decrease in the diastolic filling time and stroke volume when paced rates exceed 120 bpm.[6] However, these changes alone are not sufficient to cause syncope. Other changes in hemodynamics and autonomic output are most likely required for the occurrence of syncope during supraventricular tachycardia.

Hemodynamic Changes During Tachycardia

Ventricular Tachycardia

Syncope during ventricular tachycardia is the result of an inability to maintain an adequate blood pressure. It is postulated that syncope during ventricular tachycardia is caused by a combination of incoordinate ventricular contraction, reduced diastolic filling, atrioventricular valve regurgitation, and concurrent myocardial ischemia, and results in an inability to maintain an adequate blood pressure within the first minute of the onset of tachycardia.[13,26] Patients with inducible ventricular tachycardia, with and without syncope demonstrate no difference in resting mean arterial pressure, pulmonary capillary wedge pressure, right atrial pressure, or systemic vascular resistance index than those.[13] However, when ventricular tachycardia is induced, patients with syncope develop a significant initial drop in the mean arterial pressure to <50 mm Hg, while those who remain conscious are able to maintain a mean arterial pressure of 50 mm Hg after the onset of ventricular tachycardia.[13] After the initial drop in arterial pressure, patients with syncope demonstrate little recovery of arterial pressure. In comparison, patients without syncope have a greater initial mean arterial pressure, with a subsequent recovery of the mean arterial pressure after 1 minute of ventricular tachycardia. This results in the ability to maintain consciousness during ventricular tachycardia.[13]

Alterations in atrioventricular synchrony may contribute to hemodynamic compromise during ventricular tachycardia. Rapid ventricular rates result in the loss of normal atrioventricular synchrony. With a loss of atrioventricular synchrony, end-diastolic dimensions decrease.[27] This decrease, as well as asynchronous ventricular contraction and relaxation, abnormal atrioventricular transport, and abbreviated filling periods, contributes to hemodynamic compromise during tachycardia.[28]

The introduction of late premature ventricular depolarizations results in an alteration of ventricular contraction with a subsequent delay in myocardial diastolic relaxation.[26] As premature ventricular depolarizations become increasingly earlier, a decrease in left ventricular filling occurs along with the development of both systolic and diastolic dysfunction. A similar decrease in systolic and diastolic dysfunction occurs during sustained ventricular tachycardia.[26]

Alterations in the left ventricular ejection fraction during ventricular tachycardia have been reported, but results have not been uniform. Left ventricular ejection fraction has been measured in patients with induced ventricular tachycardia.[29] In one study, the patients had preexisting left ventricular dysfunction with an initial average ejection fraction of 0.25 during sinus rhythm. Immediately after the onset of ventricular tachycardia, the left ventricular ejection fraction dropped to an average of 0.11 in both patients with syncope, and in those without syncope. In the patients who remained hemodynamically stable, a significant rise in the ejection fraction to an average of 0.17 occurred. After termination of ventricular tachycardia, the average ejection fraction returned to baseline. In contrast, other studies have demonstrated no correlation between decreased ejection fraction and syncope from ventricular tachycardia.[13]

Other preexisting structural abnormalities of the heart, such as valvular heart disease or left ventricular outflow tract obstruction, may contribute to hemodynamic compromise during ventricular tachycardia. In a patient with severe mitral regurgitation, ventricular tachycardia at a rate of 165 bpm was associated with a mean arterial blood pressure of 43 mm Hg and syncope.[13]

Supraventricular Tachycardia

The hemodynamic effects of induced supraventricular tachycardia have been described.[30] Ventricular filling decreases secondary to rapid tachycardia rates, and the arterial pressure initially decreases. Initially, the pulmonary artery pressure is not affected, but it subsequently increases during supraventricular tachycardia. This occurs along with an increase in the right atrial pressure. At the onset of supraventricular tachycardia, the pulse pressure initially falls, then may stabilize.[31] Subsequently, the systemic vascular resistance increases and there is an increase in arterial pressure that results in a decrease in blood pressure, in stroke volume, and in cardiac output.[23,32-37] When there is hemodynamic stabilization during supraventricular tachycardia, a marked decrease in stroke volume and a modest increase in cardiac output may occur.[38] In contrast, hemodynamic deterioration during supraventricular tachycardia may occur due to decreased ventricular filling secondary to shortening of diastole, in addition to atrioventricular valvular regurgitation and changes in atrioventricular synchrony.[21,22,30,39] Large "a" waves may be seen due to a loss of atrioventricular synchrony during supraventricular tachycardia.[34,35] As with ventricular tachycardia, supraventricular tachycardia in the presence of structural heart disease may result in a marked decrease in ejection fraction and stroke volume.[38]

Autonomic Alterations During Tachycardia

Ventricular Tachycardia

Alterations in autonomic activity may play an important role in the development of syncope associated with tachycardia. Ventricular tachycardia initiation produces hypotension and increased filling pressures that result in the stimulation of arterial baroreceptors and, hypothetically, cardiac mechanoreceptors may be activated by increased atrial pressure.[40] At the onset of ventricular tachycardia, severe hypotension occurs. Subsequent recovery of left ventricular systolic pressure and an increase in contractility may result in hemodynamic recovery with the development of hemodynamic stability during ventricular tachycardia.[28] During tachycardia, the diastolic pressures remain unchanged and the sinus rate increases.[28] In the presence of β-blockade, left ventricular pressure recovery that occurs after the onset of ventricular tachycardia is blunted and the left ventricular contractile state is reduced.[28] During α-blockade, a sustained fall in peak left ventricular pressures occurs. Ganglionic blockade during ventricular tachycardia demonstrates features consistent with combined effects of α- and β-blockade.[28] These data support the idea that initial hypotension occurring at the initiation of ventricular tachycardia has a baroreceptor-mediated reflex component that is triggered by the initial fall in arterial pressure.[28] Other features suggest a role for autonomic alterations during ventricular tachycardia. Such alterations include an increased contractile state and alteration of left ventricular relaxation during ventricular tachycardia.[28] Therefore, the activation of autonomic reflexes may determine the hemodynamic response to ventricular tachycardia. Hemodynamic recovery during ventricular tachycardia depends on both α-adrenergic-mediated peripheral vascular effects and β-adrenergic-augmented left ventricular contractility.[28]

Muscle sympathetic nerve response increases during ventricular tachycardia, suggesting that arterial baroreceptors continue to modulate sympathetic outflow during ventricular tachycardia. However, the pattern of sympathetic discharge is different, suggesting that sympathetic outflow is not simply an arterial baroreflex mechanism.[41] Ventricular pacing duplicates the sympathetic nerve response that occurs with ventricular tachycardia. During ventricular tachycardia, the more rapid the tachycardia rate, the greater the arterial pressure drops, and the greater the sympathetic response. It is thought that the arterial pressure drop that occurs during ventricular tachycardia results in an increase in sympathetic outflow.[41]

Changes in the sinus rate during ventricular tachycardia suggest alteration of autonomic tone. During hemodynamically stable ventricular tachycardia, the sinus rate increases.[42] Beta-blockade has no effect on the sinus rate during ventricular tachycardia, suggesting a more important role for vagal withdrawal, resulting in sinus rate increase during ventricular tachycardia as opposed to sympathetic activation.[42] During hemodynamically unstable ventricular tachycardia, significant sinus slowing occurs.[42]

Patients with left ventricular dysfunction have abnormal control of peripheral circulation during simulated orthostatic stress.[43] It appears that this abnormal control is related to selective impairment of cardiopulmonary and/or arterial baroreflexes.[43] Impairment of baroreflexes during ventricular tachycardia may contribute to hemodynamic compromise and syncope during ventricular tachycardia in patients with left ventricular dysfunction.

Supraventricular Tachycardia

An increase in sympathetic tone occurs with the onset of supraventricular tachycardia.[19-23,28] During supraventricular tachycardia, left ventricular filling is decreased by abbreviation of diastolic filling time and alteration of atrioventricular synchrony.[21,23,39,40] This sympathetic activation, seen with supraventricular tachycardia, results in venoconstriction, improved cardiac inotropy, improved diastolic relaxation, and an increase in the peripheral vascular resistance.[44] Activation of cardiac mechanoreceptors during supraventricular tachycardia results in withdrawal of sympathetic tone, enhanced vagal tone, and hypotension, with an inadequate hemodynamic response that results in syncope by a mechanism similar to vasodepressor syncope.[44-47] At the onset of supraventricular tachycardia, pulse pressure falls then stabilizes.[31] With upright posture, the fall in pulse pressure is more pronounced and compensation occurs more rapidly.

Physiological changes that occur during upright posture have been described.[48-51] With upright posture, central blood volume decreases and cardiac output may decrease by 20% to 30%. An increase in venous volume is seen in dependent limbs. Prompt vasoconstriction occurs, as does a reduction in peripheral blood flow. An increase in heart rate subsequently follows. If compensatory vasoconstriction is delayed or insufficient, arterial blood pressure can decrease, resulting in symptoms of lightheadedness and/or syncope.

Supraventricular tachycardia, induced during upright posture, may be associated with a vasodepressor response and syncope,[25] with 98% of patients experiencing reproduction of their clinical symptoms including lightheadedness, near syncope, or syncope.[52] It was observed that during upright posture, the supraventricular tachycardia rate may be increased when compared to tachycardia while supine, and it is associated with a significant decrease in blood pressure while in the upright position.[52] In a small number of patients, supraventricular tachycardia is sustained only in the upright position as opposed to being nonsustained in the supine position.[52] Tachycardia rate changes during upright posture are thought to occur as the result of increased sympathetic tone and decreased vagal tone associated with the assumption of upright posture.[52]

In patients with atrioventricular nodal tachycardia, upright posture affects dual atrioventricular nodal physiology.[53] With upright posture, shortening of the fast and slow pathway refractoriness occurs, which may facilitate initiation of supraventricular tachycardia, convert nonsustained tachycardia to sustained, and shorten the tachycardia cycle length.[53] Autonomic tone changes with upright tilt are important. Atrioventricular nodal conduction is decreased with the assumption of upright posture, and is increased with supine posture. There is also a decrease in the atrioventricular nodal refractoriness with upright posture.[31] The effects of verapamil on the atrioventricular node are diminished with upright tilt.[31]

Cerebrovascular Contribution

A reduction in cerebral blood supply during cardiac arrhythmias may result in symptoms of dizziness, in syncope, and in transient ischemic attacks.[54-61] In 1926, Banes[62] reported that paroxysmal atrial tachycardia could cause neurological disorders. There are also reports of hemiplegia occurring after episodes of paroxysmal supraventricular and ventricular tachycardia.[63,64] Other neurological events, such as transient neurological deficits, may occur as the result of cardiac arrhythmias.[54] It is important to recognize that coexisting cerebrovascular disease may decrease the threshold for syncope during tachyarrhythmias.

Large reductions in carotid blood flow can be demonstrated during a variety of tachyarrhythmias.[1] Frequent premature atrial contractions or premature ventricular contractions may decrease carotid blood flow by 7% to 12%. Carotid blood flow during paroxysmal supraventricular tachycardia is associated with a 14% reduction in flow, with atrial fibrillation causing a 23% reduction. The greatest reduction in carotid blood flow, a 40% to 70% reduction, occurs during ventricular tachycardia.

An abrupt decrease in cerebral blood flow of approximately 30% occurs during ventricular stimulation and is accompanied by a simultaneous decrease in the mean arterial blood pressure. As ventricular pacing rates increase, the peak flow velocity in the carotid arteries incrementally decreases.[65] Animal studies have been performed to evaluate the effect of rapid ventricular pacing on cerebrovascular blood flow.[66] During ventricular stimulation, cerebral blood volume and flow become markedly reduced. Immediately after cessation of pacing, a mild and transient reactive hyperemia occurs and may last up to 3 hours. The phenomenon of reactive hyperemia has been associated with cerebral ischemia, and occurs after termination of global or focal cerebral ischemia.[67] Changes in the autonomic nervous system during tachycardia will also be important, as the autonomic nervous system plays a major role in the autoregulation of cerebral blood flow.

Atrial Natriuretic Peptide

Atrial natriuretic peptide (ANP) may have both autonomic and direct effects on cardiac electrophysiology.[68] The role of ANP in the hemodynamic response to tachyarrhythmias is undetermined, however it is possible that its effects may contribute to the maintenance of hemodynamic stability during tachycardia.[69]

Under normal conditions, ANP is synthesized and stored in the atria. In the settings of hypoxia, ischemia, and heart failure, ANP may be synthesized and stored in the ventricles. Synthesis of ANP also occurs in the cells of the cardiac conduction system and the sinoatrial and atrioventricular nodes. Elevation of intracardiac chamber pressure results in myocyte membrane stretch, which triggers the release of ANP. ANP may act at several levels to influence cardiac electrophysiology. Autonomic effects occur via sympathoinhibitory and vagoexcitatory properties of ANP. Baroreceptor sensitization can occur as well. ANP also causes a decrease in β_1-receptor stimulation and an increase in muscarinic receptor activity. Inhibition of calcium currents (I_{CA}) can also occur in the presence of ANP.

In the setting of tachyarrhythmias, the autonomic and direct effects of ANP may produce alterations in heart rate and the hemodynamic response to tachyarrhythmias. Most of the effects are related to the sympathoinhibitory and vagoexcitatory actions of ANP. The inhibition of calcium currents will influence heart rate and refractory periods, which may influence the ability to sustain tachycardia.

Conclusions

Tachyarrhythmias, both ventricular and supraventricular, may be associated with syncope. As discussed, the development of syncope during tachycardia is a multifactorial process. Tachycardia rate and duration in conjunction with altered hemodynamics associated with tachycardia are important determinants of syncope. Other factors such as the autonomic state, presence of cerebrovascular disease or altered cerebrovascular blood flow, atrial function, and other concomitant organ system diseases may contribute to the development of syncope that is associated with tachyarrhythmias.

References

1. Corday E, Irving DW. Effect of cardiac arrhythmias on the cerebral circulation. *Am J Cardiol* 1960;6:803–808.
2. Samet P. Hemodynamic sequelae of cardiac arrhythmias. *Circulation* 1973; 47:399–407.
3. Schulze RA Jr, Strauss HW, Pitt B. Sudden death in the year following myocardial infarction: Relation to ventricular premature contractions in the late hospital phase and left ventricular ejection fraction. *Am J Med* 1977;62:192–199.
4. Vandepol CJ, Farshidi A, Spielman SR, et al. Incidence and clinical significance of induced ventricular tachycardia. *Am J Cardiol* 1980;45:725–731.
5. Berman DS, Maddahi J, Garcia EV, et al. Assessment of left and right ventricular function with multiple gated equilibrium cardiac blood pool scintigraphy. In: Berman DS, Mason DT (eds): *Clinical Nuclear Cardiology.* New York: Grune and Stratton, Inc.;1981;224.
6. Ross J, Linhart JW, Braunwald E. Effects of changing heart rate in man by electrical stimulation of the right atrium: Studies at rest, during exercise, and with isoproterenol. *Circulation* 1965;32:549–558.

7. Goldstein S, Medendorp SV, Landis JR. Analysis of cardiac symptoms preceding cardiac arrest. *Am J Cardiol* 1986;58:1195–1198.
8. Morady F, Shen EN, Bhandari A, et al. Clinical symptoms in patients with sustained ventricular tachycardia. *West J Med* 1985;142:341–344.
9. Krol RB, Morady F, Flaker GC. Electrophysiologic testing in patients with unexplained syncope: Clinical and noninvasive predictors of outcome. *J Am Coll Cardiol* 1987;10:358–363.
10. Middlekauff HR, Stevenson WG, Stevenson LW, et al. Syncope in advanced heart failure: High risk of sudden death regardless of origin of syncope. *J Am Coll Cardiol* 1993;21:110–116.
11. Buxton AE, Marchlinski FE, Blores BT, et al. Nonsustained ventricular tachycardia in patients with coronary artery disease: Role of electrophysiology study. *Circulation* 1987;75:1178–1185.
12. Sulpizi AM, Friehling TD, Kowey PR. Value of electrophysiologic testing in patients with nonsustained ventricular tachycardia. *Am J Cardiol* 1987;59:841–845.
13. Hamer AWF, Rubin SA, Peter T, et al. Factors that predict syncope during ventricular tachycardia in patients. *Am Heart J* 1984;107:997–1005.
14. Camm AJ, Lau CP. Syncope of undetermined origin: Diagnosis and management. In: Zipes DP, Rowlands DJ (eds): *Progress in Cardiology*. Philadelphia, PA: Lea and Febiger; 1988;139–156.
15. Yee R, Klein GJ. Syncope in the Wolff-Parkinson-White syndrome: Incidence and electrophysiologic correlates. *Pacing Clin Electrophysiol* 1984;7:381–388.
16. Auricchio A, Klein H, Trappe HJ. Lack of prognostic value of syncope in patients with Wolff-Parkinson-White syndrome. *J Am Coll Cardiol* 1991;17:152–158.
17. Paul T, Guccione P, Garson A Jr. Relation of syncope in young patients with Wolff-Parkinson-White syndrome to rapid ventricular response during atrial fibrillation. *Am J Cardiol* 1990;65:318–321.
18. Rinne C, Klein GJ, Sharma AD. Relation between clinical presentation and induced arrhythmias in the Wolff-Parkinson-White syndrome. *Am J Cardiol* 1987; 60:576–579.
19. Waxman MB, Cameron DA. The reflex effects of tachycardias on autonomic tone. *Ann N Y Acad Sci* 1990;601:378–393.
20. Feldman T, Carroll JD, Munkenbeck F, et al. Hemodynamic recovery during simulated ventricular tachycardia: Role of adrenergic receptor activation. *Am Heart J* 1988;115:576–587.
21. Hung J, Kelly DT, Hutton BF, et al. Influence of heart rate and atrial transport on left ventricular volume and function: Relation to hemodynamic changes produced by supraventricular arrhythmia. *Am J Cardiol* 1981;48:632–638.
22. Curry PVL. The hemodynamic and electrophysiological effects of paroxysmal tachycardia. In: Narula OS (ed): *Cardiac Arrhythmias: Electrophysiology, Diagnosis, and Management*. Baltimore: Williams and Wilkins; 1979;364–381.
23. McIntosh HD, Morris JJ. The hemodynamic consequences of arrhythmias. *Prog Cardiovasc Dis* 1966;8:330–363.
24. Lloyd EA, Hauer RN, Zipes DP, et al. Syncope and ventricular tachycardia in patients with ventricular preexcitation. *Am J Cardiol* 1983;52:79–82.
25. Leitch JW, Klein GJ, Yee R, et al. Syncope associated with supraventricular tachycardia: An expression of tachycardia rate or vasomotor response? *Circulation* 1992;85:1064–1071.
26. Saksena S, Ciccone JM, Craelius W, et al. Studies on left ventricular function during sustained ventricular tachycardia. *J Am Coll Cardiol* 1984;4:501–508.
27. Gomes JA, Damato AN, Akhtar M, et al. Ventricular septal motion and left ventricular dimensions during abnormal ventricular activation. *Am J Cardiol* 1977;39:641–650.

28. Feldman T, Carroll JD, Munkenbeck F. Hemodynamic recovery during simulated ventricular tachycardia: Role of adrenergic receptor activation. *Am Heart J* 1988;115:576–587.
29. Sharma AD, Purves P, Yee R. Hemodynamic effects of intravenous procainamide during ventricular tachycardia. *Am Heart J* 1990;119:1034–1041.
30. Goldreyer BN, Kastor JA, Kershbaum KL. The hemodynamic effects of induced supraventricular tachycardia in man. *Circulation* 1976;54:783–789.
31. Curry PVL, Rowland E, Fox KM, et al. The relationship between posture, blood pressure and electrophysiological properties in patients with paroxysmal supraventricular tachycardia. *Arch Mal Coeur Vaiss* 1978;71:293–299.
32. Stewart HJ, Deitrick JE, Crane NF, et al. Studies of the circulation in the presence of abnormal cardiac rhythms: Observations relating to rhythms associated with a rapid ventricular rate and to rhythms associated with a slow ventricular rate. *J Clin Invest* 1938;17:449–463.
33. Lequime J. Circulatory disturbances in pathological conditions with high heart rate. *Cardiologia* 1941;5:105–112.
34. Ferrer MI, Harvey RM, Weiner HM, et al. Hemodynamic studies in two cases of Wolff-Parkinson-White syndrome with paroxysmal av nodal tachycardia. *Am J Med* 1949;6:725–733.
35. Saunders DE, Ord JW. The hemodynamic effects of paroxysmal supraventricular tachycardia in patients with the Wolff-Parkinson-White syndrome. *Am J Cardiol* 1962;9:223–236.
36. Benchimol A, Ellis JG, Dimond EG, et al. Hemodynamic consequences of atrial and ventricular arrhythmias in man. *Am Heart J* 1965;70:775–787.
37. Ferrer MI. Hemodynamic effects of prolonged supraventricular tachycardia in normal heart. *N Y State J Med* 1970;70:2120–2124.
38. Swiryn S, Pavel D, Byrom E. Assessment of left ventricular function by radionuclide angiography during induced supraventricular tachycardia. *Am J Cardiol* 1981;47:555–561.
39. Sganzerla P, Fabbiocchi F, Grazi S, et al. Electrophysiologic and haemodynamic correlates in supraventricular tachycardia. *Eur Heart J* 1989;10:32–9.
40. Bishop VS, Malliani A, Thoren P. In: Shepherd JT, Abboud FM, Geiger SR (eds): *Handbook of Physiology: The Cardiovascular System.* Baltimore: Williams and Wilkins; 1983;497–556.
41. Smith ML, Ellenbogen KA, Beightol LA, et al. Sympathetic neural responses to induced ventricular tachycardia. *J Am Coll Cardiol* 1991;18:1015–1024.
42. Huikuri HV, Zaman L, Castellanos A, et al. Changes in spontaneous sinus node rate as an estimate of cardiac autonomic tone during stable and unstable ventricular tachycardia. *J Am Coll Cardiol* 1989;13:646–652.
43. Ferguson DW, Abboud FM, Mark AL. Selective impairment of baroreflex-mediated vasoconstrictor responses in patients with ventricular dysfunction. *Circulation* 1984;69:451–460.
44. Waxman MB, Sharma AD, Cameron DA, et al. Reflex mechanisms responsible for early spontaneous termination of paroxysmal supraventricular tachycardia. *Am J Cardiol* 1982;49:259–272.
45. Oberg B, Thoren P. Increased activity in left ventricular receptors during hemorrhage or occlusion of caval veins in the cat: A possible cause of the vaso-vagal reaction. *Acta Physiol Scand* 1972;85:164–173.
46. Almquist A, Goldenberg IF, Milstein S, et al. Provocation of bradycardia and hypotension by isoproterenol and upright posture in patients with unexplained syncope. *N Engl J Med* 1989;320:346–351.
47. Abboud FM. Ventricular syncope: Is the heart a sensory organ? *N Engl J Med* 1989;320:390–392.

48. Robinson BF, Epstein SE, Beiser GD, et al. Control of heart rate by the autonomic nervous system: Studies in man on the interrelation between baroreceptor mechanisms and exercise. *Circ Res* 1966;19:400–411.
49. Wang Y, Marshall RJ, Sheppherd JT. The effect of changes in posture and of graded exercise on stroke volume in man. *J Clin Invest* 1960;39:1051–1061.
50. Loeppky JA, Greene ER, Hoekenga DE, et al. Beat-to-beat stroke volume assessment by pulsed Doppler in upright and supine exercise. *J Appl Physiol* 1981;50:1173–82.
51. Rushmer RF. Effects of posture. In: Rushmer RF (ed): *Structure and Function of the Cardiovascular System, 2nd Ed.* Philadelphia: WB Saunders Co.; 1976;217–246.
52. Hammill SC, Holmes DR, Wood DL, et al. Electrophysiologic testing in the upright position: Improved evaluation of patients with rhythm disturbances using a tilt table. *J Am Coll Cardiol* 1984;4:65–71.
53. Mann DE, Reiter MJ. Effects of upright posture on atrioventricular nodal reentry and dual atrioventricular nodal pathways. *Am J Cardiol* 1988;62:408–412.
54. Lavy S, Stern S. Transient neurological manifestations in cardiac arrhythmias. *J Neurol Sci* 1969;9:97–102.
55. McHenry LC Jr, Fazekas JF, Sullivan JF. Cerebral hemodynamics of syncope. *Am J Med Sci* 1961;241:173–178.
56. Corday E, Bazika V, Lang TW, et al. Detection of phantom arrhythmias. *JAMA* 1965;193:417–421.
57. McAllen PM, Marshall J. Cardiac dysrhythmia and transient cerebral ischemic attacks. *Lancet* 1973;2:1212–1214.
58. Reed RL, Siekert RG, Merideth J. Rarity of transient focal cerebral ischemia in cardiac dysrhythmia. *JAMA* 1973;223:893–895.
59. Stern S, Ben-Shachar G, Tzivoni D, et al. Detection of transient arrhythmias by continuous long-term recording of electrocardiograms of active subjects. *Isr J Med Sci* 1970;6:103–112.
60. Van Durme JP. Cardiac dysrhythmia and transient cerebral ischemic attacks. *Lancet* 1973;2:210.
61. Walter PF, Reid SD Jr, Wenger NK. Transient cerebral ischemia due to arrhythmia. *Ann Intern Med* 1970;72:471–474.
62. Barnes AR. Cerebral manifestations of paroxysmal tachycardia. *Am J Med Sci* 1926;171:489–495.
63. Corday E, Rothenberg SF, Putnam TJ. Cerebral vascular insufficiency; An explanation of some types of localized cerebral encephalopathy. *Arch Neurol Psych* 1953;69:551–570.
64. Corday E, Rothenberg S, Weiner SM. Cerebral vasucular insufficiency: An explanation of the transient stroke. *Arch Int Med* 1956;98:683–690.
65. Benchimol A, Baldi J, Desser KB. The effects of ventricular tachycardia on carotid artery blood flow velocity. *Stroke* 1974;5:60–67.
66. Kobari M, Fukuuchi Y, Tomita M, et al. Cerebral microcirculatory changes during and following transient ventricular tachycardia in cats. *J Neurol Sci* 1992; 111:153–157.
67. Gourley JK, Heistad DD. Characteristics of reactive hyperemia in the cerebral circulation. *Am J Physiol* 1984;246:H52–H58.
68. Clemo HF, Baumbarten CM, Ellenbogen KA. Atrial natriuretic peptide and cardiac electrophysiology: Autonomic and direct effects. *J Cardiovasc Electrophysiol* 1966;7:149–162.
69. Ellenbogen KA, Rogers R, Walsh M, et al. Increased circulatory atrial natriuretic factor (ANF) release during induced ventricular tachycardia. *Am Heart J* 1988;116:1233–1238.

Use of Electrophysiological Studies in Syncope:

Practical Aspects for Diagnosis and Treatment

Edward A. Telfer, MD and Brian Olshansky, MD

Introduction

The cause of syncope can be difficult to determine with certainty. Despite a careful history and physical examination, and even with properly directed noninvasive testing, the etiology can remain unidentified in almost 50% of syncope patients.[1] The prognosis for the majority of patients can be favorable,[2-6] but it varies widely depending on underlying (and causative) or concomitant diagnoses, specifically cardiac causes.

Cardiac arrhythmias, often a suspected and serious cause of syncope, are generally transient, difficult to record and diagnose, and represent a potentially life-threatening situation. Underlying structural cardiac disease is not always a prerequisite for arrhythmic syncope. Even for patients with cardiac disease in whom an arrhythmia is suspected as the cause of syncope, the etiology can be difficult to diagnose with absolute certainty unless electrocardiographic assessment, hemodynamic monitoring, and direct observation are all present at time of syncope. Clinical variability in presentation further confounds the diagnosis. Empirical therapy directed against suspected or potential arrhythmic cause of syncope can, ironically, worsen the prognosis without necessarily treating the arrhythmia or the syncope effectively.

From Grubb BP, Olshansky B (eds.). *Syncope: Mechanisms and Management.* Armonk, NY: Futura Publishing Co., Inc.; © 1998.

Syncope that is undiagnosed despite an extensive noninvasive evaluation is a large problem. It often requires more than diagnostic acumen to determine that the cause is self-limited and benign, and it clearly is not always associated with a good outcome. The mortality may approach 30% in the first year after presentation if syncope is due to a cardiovascular cause such as ventricular tachycardia, and if structural heart disease is present.[1,6]

This chapter focuses on the practical use of electrophysiological (EP) studies to evaluate and treat patients with otherwise undiagnosed syncope. Illustrative case examples are included.

Background

Almost 30 years ago, it was discovered that endocardial catheters could be placed in the heart and used to record, pace, and deliver premature extrastimuli from the atria and the ventricles (EP studies). Initial application of this technique was used to assess conduction through the heart.[7,8] Later, the EP study was used on patients with known tachycardias to reproduce reentrant supraventricular tachycardias[9-11] (excluding, perhaps, atrial flutter and fibrillation, for which the technique has questionable efficacy) and ventricular tachycardia.[10-13] EP studies were found particularly sensitive (90% to 95%) in initiating "clinical" (spontaneous) sustained monomorphic ventricular tachycardia in patients with coronary artery disease. Sustained monomorphic ventricular tachycardia was rarely induced at EP study in patients without spontaneous sustained ventricular tachycardia. Vandepol et al[12] and others[13] showed that the test was less sensitive (about 50%) in reproducing nonsustained ventricular tachycardia in patients who had spontaneous nonsustained ventricular tachycardia.

EP studies have also been used as a method of evaluating conduction, pathological and normal, through the atrioventricular (AV) node and His-Purkinje system.[8,9,14-16] Sinus node function has been assessed at EP study in patients with known sinus node dysfunction as well.[17-24] Several techniques are described.

Approximately 15 years ago, the use of EP studies expanded to assess the *potential* risk of arrhythmia in patients with suspected, but not clinically documented, arrhythmias.[25] This application included the attempt to identify arrhythmias in patients with syncope of unknown origin.[26-41] In these early investigations, the patient population enrolled in the studies comprised those with undiagnosed syncope as the only criteria for study. Patients were not specifically selected or targeted with any specific diagnoses in mind. Various types of arrhythmias, including nonsustained and sustained ventricular tachycardia, ventricular fibrillation, polymorphic ventricular tachycardia, and supraventricular arrhythmias, were induced and correlated to syncope. It was recognized that abnormalities discovered at EP study did not convincingly reproduce the patient's clinical syncopal episodes. However, it was hypothesized that the observed abnormalities of conduction and induced tachycardias were related to the patient's syncope.

Induction techniques and the specificity of the EP study were assessed further in the mid-1980s to determine the potential clinical significance of the arrhythmias initiated.[41–50] Techniques used to perform EP studies were also assessed in greater detail. Stimulation protocols, patient recruitment, even the definitions of abnormal responses were highly variable, making comparison between different investigations difficult. As experience with EP studies in syncope patients grew, a consensus emerged concerning reasonable stimulation protocols and definitions of induced arrhythmia abnormalities.[9] Investigators became more sophisticated in the interpretation of EP study results. In addition, an attempt to correlate the prognosis to EP study results was undertaken.[41,51-54] Treatment based on the EP study results was evaluated to determine whether the test had utility in directing therapy. Several reports show that treatment of abnormalities observed at EP study resulted in a better prognosis and/or a reduction in the rate of recurrent syncope,[41,51-57] (Chapter 2: Table 15).

Teichman et al[58] popularized the notion of quantifying the severity of abnormalities observed from normal to minor ("borderline") to "clearly abnormal" findings. The diagnostic yield of EP studies was 36% if only "clearly abnormal" results were considered, but when "borderline" abnormalities were combined with "clearly abnormal" results, the diagnostic yield rose to 75%.

The diagnostic yield of arrhythmia abnormalities found at EP study varied tremendously between investigations (see Chapter 2, Table 14). This was likely related to patient selection, stimulation protocols, and definition of electrophysiological abnormalities. Despite these issues, the most common abnormality of clinical significance noted was induction of sustained monomorphic ventricular tachycardia. This finding suggests a potential cause of syncope and provides predictive data regarding the risk of cardiac death.

Some patient subgroups clearly did not benefit from EP study, indicating that the electrophysiological results were nondiagnostic. Identification of these patients became important so that the risk and expense of EP study could be avoided. Krol et al[59] found that the predictors of an abnormal study (ventricular tachycardia in 71%) included: left ventricular ejection fraction ≤40%, bundle branch block, presence of coronary artery disease, history of remote myocardial infarction, use of class I antiarrhythmic drugs, injury related to loss of consciousness, and male sex. Predictors of nondiagnostic study included: left ventricular ejection fraction ≥40%, absence of structural heart disease, a normal 12-lead ECG, and normal 24-hour ambulatory monitoring. The probability of a normal EP study increased with the number and duration of the syncopal episodes. While these predictors are generally accurate, 1) not all reports show the same results (for example, injury that does not clearly predict a poor prognosis or an arrhythmic etiology of syncope, but this point is controversial)[59,60] and 2) a positive study could still occur without any of the above predictors. In fact, 35% of all positive EP studies occurred in patients with left ventricular ejection fraction (LVEF)≥40%.

Krol et al[59] had restrictive definitions of an abnormal EP study: 1) sinus node recovery time ≥3 seconds; 2) HV interval ≥100 ms; 3) infra-Hisian block during atrial pacing; 4) monomorphic ventricular tachycardia; 5) supraventricular tachycardia associated with hypotension. The "clearly abnormal" EP study results remain the accepted standard.

Kushner et al[61] and others[52] found that patients with normal or less serious and specific abnormalities than defined by Krol et al had a good prognosis independent of the frequency of recurrent syncope. Some investigators have even suggested that there is a reduction in syncope recurrence even if the EP study is nondiagnostic (a placebo effect of the EP study, perhaps).[62] The nondiagnostic EP study has other important implications: a patient with coronary artery disease with impaired LV function and syncope who has a negative EP study has a good long-term prognosis.

Other investigators have identified a high incidence of inducible ventricular tachycardia in syncope patients with bundle branch block.[28,32] The expected cause of syncope (in this example, infra-Hisian block) may instead be only a predictor for other potentially life-threatening arrhythmic problems including ventricular tachycardia.

EP studies have continued to emerge over the past decade as a common diagnostic tool for syncope patients. At Loyola University Medical Center, about 20% of our primary EP studies are performed to assess patients with otherwise undiagnosed syncope.

According to recent ACC/AHA guidelines, syncope in association with suspected heart disease and no other apparent cause is considered a "class I" indication for EP study.[63] The EP study may help to provide a potential cause of syncope in this group of patients.

Electrophysiological Study Protocols

The EP study in an invasive but relatively low-risk procedure requiring placement of venous sheaths through which electrode catheters are placed in order to determine sinus node function and conduction properties through the heart, as well as to determine the presence of inducible supraventricular and ventricular arrhythmias.[64] The procedure takes approximately 1 to 3 hours. Each EP study protocol has been well tested for its sensitivity and specificity in specific pathological conditions and in normals. A consensus on a "standard" EP test for syncope has now been reached.[63,65]

After catheters are placed in the heart, conduction intervals are measured. Then sinus node recovery time is measured by rapid pacing of the atria followed by abrupt termination and measurement of the time it takes for the sinus node to "recover." Atrioventricular conduction is determined by a progressively shorter fixed rate and by ramp pacing to assess AV nodal and His-Purkinje conduction. The presence of conduction block below the His bundle is distinctly abnormal and indicative of the need for a pacemaker.

Single extrastimuli are then introduced at two or more cycle lengths in the high right atrium. Then single, double, and triple premature extrastimuli are introduced at two or more paced cycle lengths in the ventricle at two sites (generally at the apex and outflow tract of the right ventricle). There are several acceptable and well-tested protocols used to attempt to induce tachycardias. Isoproterenol can be given, and may be helpful, to attempt to induce both supraventricular tachycardia and ventricular tachycardia, but it should be reserved for patients for whom EP studies without isoproterenol infusion are nondiagnostic and in whom there is little risk of exacerbating severe ischemia.[66] The sensitivity and specificity of isoproterenol in this setting is unknown.

Procainamide infusion of up to 15 mg/kg can be used as a conduction "stress test" in patients suspected of having infra-Hisian block (ie, those with bundle branch block, bifasicular block, or a prolonged HV interval). Procainamide can further impair conduction though the His-Purkinje system. Patients who show infra-Hisian block become pacemaker dependant in short order and do not tend to have recurrent syncope after pacemaker implantation.[67] Procainamide can also be used to facilitate induction of bundle branch reentry ventricular tachycardia when it is suspected but cannot be induced with extra stimuli (including long-short coupling interval) alone. Drugs including atropine, adenosine, and β-blockers may also have utility in conjunction with pacing maneuvers.

Expected Yield of Electrophysiological Studies

The yield expected from an EP study is variable and dependent upon anticipated abnormalities and patient risk factors (see Table 1).[68] Some

_____ **Table 1** _____

**Data Acquired During
an Electrophysiological Study**

Sinus node function
AV nodal function
His-Purkinje conduction properties
Induction of supraventricular tachycardia
Induction of ventricular tachycardia

AV = atrioventricular.

findings, such as severe sinus node disease, are generally independent of left ventricular function, but can be anticipated by noninvasive monitoring. Unequivocally abnormal findings (ie, symptomatic sinus node recovery time ≥3 seconds) are quite specific for serious sinus node dysfunction, but are rare findings in syncope patients (see Chapter 2: Table 13, Figure 4). While the EP study techniques are specific to reproduce serious sinus node dysfunction, the technique is unreliable in syncope patients to detect sinus node dysfunction as the cause of syncope.[69,70]

Fujimura et al[69] describe an alarmingly high incidence of "missed" conduction and sinus node disease in syncope patients using EP studies. In this study, they identified 21 patients with either intermittent AV block (13 patients) or sinus pauses (8 patients) associated with syncope, who then underwent EP study prior to the implantation of a permanent pacemaker. For the patients with documented sinus node disease, only 3 of the 8 (sensitivity=37.5%) had evidence of sinus node disease at EP study. Three of these same eight patients with documented sinus node disease as a cause of syncope demonstrated other abnormalities at EP study, including dual AV nodal physiology, atrial flutter, and sustained monomorphic ventricular tachycardia. Only two of the 13 patients with documented intermittent AV block demonstrated evidence of AV block at EP study (sensitivity=15.4%). These same 13 patients displayed other abnormalities including inducible atrial fibrillation with rapid ventricular response associated with hypotension.

Similarly, Kahn et al[70] found a high incidence of intermittent sinus arrest and AV block in recurrent syncope patients who had previously undergone a negative tilt table test and a nondiagnostic EP study using implanted long-term ambulatory monitors. In this study, 5 of 16 patients demonstrated sinus arrest associated with syncope, and 2 of 16 patients demonstrated AV block associated with syncope. Interestingly, no patient suffered any complication or sequelae from the time of the initial nondiagnostic EP study to the time that the diagnosis was established by the subcutaneous long-term ambulatory monitor.

Severe conduction system disease is most commonly found in patients with some type of advanced conduction delay on noninvasive monitoring and 12-lead ECG. Severe infra-Hisian conduction delay or block is rare in patients without a wide QRS (QRS duration≥120 msec) or AV block (first-degree or higher). Syncope patients with bifascicular block have been described as having a high incidence of sustained monomorphic ventricular tachycardia, making the EP study as useful for excluding coexisting ventricular tachycardia as it is for confirming infra-Hisian block in this group.[28]

Patients with a history of supraventricular tachycardia who later develop syncope should, in general, undergo EP studies. The same holds true for patients with documented or suspected preexcitation on a 12-lead ECG.[40] The situation is less clear-cut for patients with atrial fibrillation or atrial flutter discovered on noninvasive monitoring, if a direct association with syncope is lacking. Atrial fibrillation can rarely cause syncope due to alterations in ventricular response, but the yield of the EP study tends to be low unless there is an additional coexisting reason to perform it. Reproduction of a suspected tachycardia-bradycardia syndrome is sometimes accomplished in atrial flutter patients, given that atrial flutter is often terminated with pacing maneuvers. Once in sinus rhythm, an assessment of underlying sinus node function and AV nodal conduction properties is possible. Termination of atrial fibrillation is occasionally successful with antiarrhythmic drug infusion, but it generally requires electrical cardioversion. However, the pause that occasionally follows electrical cardioversion provides almost no diagnostic information. Atrial fibrillation and atrial flutter are both associated with an increased risk of thromboembolic events, especially around the time of cardioversion (by whatever means). The risk of thromboembolic events must be weighed when making the decision to perform an EP study, especially if either atrial fibrillation or atrial flutter is the only reason that the study is performed. Since atrial flutter can also be "cured" with current radiofrequency ablation techniques (without concurrent need for a permanent pacemaker), the yield of the EP study is perhaps higher for atrial flutter than it is for atrial fibrillation.

The yield of the EP study for sustained monomorphic ventricular tachycardia is most dependent on ventricular function and the type of underlying heart disease (see Table 5). For patients with ventricular dysfunction, the etiology of heart disease is vital for determining the expected yield of EP studies.[10-12,71-75] The yield is highest for patients who have a history of distant myocardial infarction associated with left ventricular dysfunction (LVEF ≤35%).[59] Patients with a history of distant myocardial infarction but with preserved left ventricular function (LVEF ≥40%) associated with late potentials on a signal-averaged ECG may also have a high incidence of inducible sustained monomorphic ventricular tachycardia.[76-78] The diagnostic yield of ventricular stimulation protocols is lower in patients with left ventricular dysfunction on the basis of a dilated or nonischemic cardiomyopathy than in those with a history of distant myocardial infarction. The potential for inducible sustained monomorphic ventricular tachycardia cannot be dismissed in patients with nonischemic or dilated cardiomyopathy; however, an EP study may be negative in a patient with dilated cardiomyopathy and syncope, but the risk of death can remain high.[79]

In patients without ventricular dysfunction, ventricular stimulation has an extraordinarily low yield and, in general, should not be performed unless there is some specific reason to expect that syncope is due to ventricular tachycardia. Examples include syncope patients in whom right ventricular dysplasia or sarcoid associated cardiomyopathy is *strongly* suspected.

Interpretation of Electrophysiological Study Results: Goals

Several important questions arise for syncope patients who undergo EP study and have an arrhythmia found: 1) Is the arrhythmia clinically relevant? 2) Is the arrhythmia the cause of syncope? 3) How can the arrhythmia be treated? 4) Will treatment prevent recurrent syncope? 5) What is the implication of multiple arrhythmia abnormalities at testing? 6) Is a well-tolerated but abnormal arrhythmia the cause of syncope? 7) What are the prognostic implications of abnormal results? While there are no tacit answers to these questions, clinical acumen in light of the test results is always the key to proper and effective long-term treatment. The next several sections attempt to clarify and answer these questions.

Interpretation of the Electrophysiological Study: The Level of Uncertainty

The presence of an arrhythmic problem as assessed by the EP study in a syncope patient can be difficult to correlate with the clinical situation. Abnormal results must be interpreted in the context of the individual patient. Nondiagnostic responses to programmed stimulation, such as ventricular fibrillation, result in syncope in the electrophysiology laboratory. Conversely, the absence of syncope during an induced monomorphic tachycardia is not an appropriate reason to dismiss the tachycardia as clinically irrelevant.

Leitch et al[80] examined the changes in vasomotor tone imposed by inducing supraventricular tachycardia in patients on a tilt table in the supine and the passive head-up position. Seven of 22 patients developed syncope in the head-up position. The mean supraventricular tachycardia rate was identical to that of the 15 patients who did not develop syncope. It was hypothesized that syncope was related to inadequate compensation of "vasomotor factors" rather than to tachycardia rate. Waxman[81,82] described the autonomic responses imposed by an abrupt increase in heart rate imposed by the initiation of supraventricular tachycardia (see Figure A). From these data, it is clear that body position, autonomic tone, and vasoregulatory factors, all of which are patient dependant, can precipitate syncope when syncope is present. Since the vast majority of EP studies are performed in sedated and supine patients, reproduction of syncope cannot be used as a confirmatory marker that the observed or induced abnormality is clinically relevant.

There is no reason to suspect that any evaluation, including EP study, should completely clarify syncope in all instances.[68] The endpoints are not always clear. For example, what is the significance of reproducibly inducible nonsustained monomorphic ventricular tachycardia? Some nonsustained

MECHANISM OF SPONTANEOUS TERMINATION OF PSVT

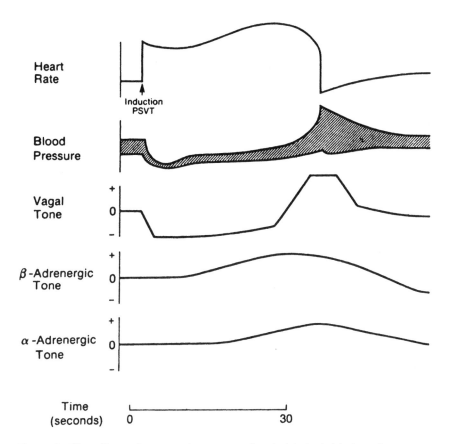

Figure A. The effects of autonomic tone associated with the initiation of supraventricular tachycardia. Reprinted with permission from Reference 82.

monomorphic ventricular tachycardia can be self terminating and still result in hemodynamic intolerance and syncope. Such a response to ventricular stimulation may be labeled "nonspecific" in the electrophysiology laboratory.[44–46] The prognostic implications of inducible nonsustained monomorphic ventricular tachycardia are unknown and will likely remain so. Alternatively, induced sustained monomorphic ventricular tachycardia may not be the cause of syncope, but the weight of available data suggest that its induction, in general, is associated with a poorer prognosis.[83–86] The ultimate prognostic implications of inducible sustained monomorphic ventricular tachycardia are also intertwined with other factors such as left ventricular function and the nature of the structural heart disease, if any.

As protocols become more aggressive, the potential for nonspecific responses increases.[41-46,48] Nonsustained polymorphic ventricular tachycardia is not uncommon during EP study of syncope patients, but probably has much less significance than nonsustained monomorphic ventricular tachycardia. Sustained polymorphic ventricular tachycardia, a potentially abnormal response to stimulation, may have clinical significance. Polymorphic ventricular tachycardia is the most common response, with short coupling intervals for premature extrastimuli, and it is most likely to occur with triple extrastimuli at intervals close to the ventricular refractory period. Polymorphic ventricular tachycardia may occasionally be an ominous marker if it is sustained and if it occurs with two or fewer ventricular extrastimuli not close to the ventricular refractory period, but evidence supporting this is scant. It may, on occasion, be a cause of syncope. It has been suggested that one possible way to enhance the specificity of EP study in patients with induced polymorphic Ventricular tachycardia is to repeat the stimulation protocol after procainamide infusion. If a slower monomorphic ventricular tachycardia is then induced, the specificity of the abnormal response is likely more clinically relevant.[83] Ventricular fibrillation induction is a nonspecific EP study finding in a syncope patient because ventricular fibrillation causes death, not syncope, unless promptly electrically defibrillated. Only rarely has ventricular fibrillation been found to be a cause of syncope.[87]

If a ventricular tachycardia or supraventricular tachycardia is initiated, it is obviously abnormal; but is it the cause of syncope? Supraventricular tachycardia can be autonomically mediated with respect to rate and hemodynamic response.[81-83] The induction of supraventricular tachycardia occurs in approximately 13% of syncope patients referred for EP study, but it is highly unlikely in a general patient population without symptoms. Supraventricular tachycardia is more likely the cause of syncope if the rate is fast or if the tachycardia is poorly tolerated. Simultaneous atrial and ventricular activation can worsen hemodynamic tolerance of a tachycardia even at slower rates. Ventricular tachycardia is population dependant, but is a very likely cause of syncope if no other abnormality is found at testing.

EP studies can provide the diagnosis of the arrhythmic cause that may have been associated with hypotension and collapse in a clinical setting, independent of whether syncope is precipitated during the procedure. Sympathetic tone and postural position affect the ability of patients to compensate for alterations in cardiac output that are associated with an arrhythmia. Most EP studies are performed in the supine position, while most arrhythmic syncope occurs nonsupine. The abrupt change in heart rate at initiation of a tachycardia is associated with hypotension with release of parasympathetic tone and gradual increase in sympathetic tone as time progresses (Figure A). Overshoot in sympathetic tone can lead to increase in parasympathetic tone and accentuated antagonism, stopping the tachycardia.[82,83] This is one way that supraventricular tachycardia can cause syncope but stop spontaneously. The abrupt change in heart rate resulting in hypotension can be enhanced by orthostatic positional change. Even a non-sustained ventricular tachycardia, not associated with syncope in the electrophysiology laboratory, may clinically result in syncope. The EP study is not focused on recreating syncope in the electrophysiology laboratory, but is instead focused on trying to diagnose a potential arrhythmic cause of syncope. Noninvasive data (telemetry, electrocardiogram, echocardiogram, signal-averaged electrocardiogram) help the electrophysiologist interpret the EP study more accurately.[88–92] The use of newer noninvasive tests, such as T wave alternans, heart rate variability, and QT dispersion, is emerging. Presently, these additional noninvasive tests cannot be incorporated effectively into algorithms to evaluate syncope.

Interpretation of the Electrophysiological Study: Prognostic Implications

Electrophysiological abnormalities have been identified in 12% to 70% of patients with otherwise unexplained syncope, with sustained monomorphic ventricular tachycardia the most common abnormality (see Chapter 2). Studies are performed not only with the hope of identifying abnormalities that would lead to therapy for the prevention of recurrent syncope, but also with the expectation of determining prognosis. Therapy directed to treat the underlying abnormality (most commonly sustained monomorphic ventricular tachycardia) has been associated with a reduction in the risk of death and recurrent syncope in some, but not all, studies.[41,51,52,54] In high-risk patients treatment may alter the course, but no randomized prospective trials have been performed.

Analysis of the Electrophysiologic Study Versus Electrocardiographic Monitoring (ESVEM) trial[93] (in the context of syncope) is illustrative. Based on retrospective analysis of this prospective study, no statistically significant difference was found in the incidence of arrhythmic death and cardiac arrest between the four defined subgroups. In other words, patients that presented with a diagnosis of syncope, but without documented tachycardia, and who met the inclusion criteria ($\geq$10 PVC/hr* and induced sustained monomorphic ventricular tachycardia) carried a prognosis similar to patients with documented ventricular tachycardia (with or without syncope) or ventricular fibrillation/cardiac arrest. The incidence of arrhythmic death in the syncope alone group at 1 year was 24%, and not signifi-

---

*PVC = premature ventricular contraction.

cantly different from the 20% mortality found in those patients who had survived a prior cardiac arrest. By the fourth year, the mortality in the syncope group was 37%. It is not clear if syncope imparts an excess risk of death, but patients with sustained monomorphic ventricular tachycardia, PVCs, a decreased left ventricular ejection fraction, and syncope are at a particularly high risk.

The finding that syncope alone in patients with inducible ventricular tachycardia and frequent ventricular ectopy on Holter monitoring carries a mortality comparable to that of cardiac arrest survivors is not only interesting, but it is also of substantial clinical importance. Based on these results, it appears that syncope in the face of organic heart disease and inducible ventricular tachycardia when frequent ectopy is present is associated with a substantial mortality. Until more data are available, an aggressive approach to treatment of the underlying ventricular arrhythmias appears to be warranted in syncope patients who fulfill ESVEM inclusion criteria.

Based on a consensus of the present data, it appears that patients with unexplained syncope found to have inducible ventricular tachycardia at EP study appear to have a poorer prognosis when compared with those without inducible ventricular tachycardia.[84–86]

Treatment guided by EP study diagnoses of syncope patients is associated with an improved prognosis in several small uncontrolled trials, with no prospective controlled trials presently available. A normal or nondiagnostic study carries a favorable prognosis. Alternatively, syncope has been associated with a poor prognosis independent of etiology or results of EP studies in some groups (eg, severe cardiomyopathy patients, particularly patients with nonischemic cardiomyopathy). Data conflict on these issues. It is very possible that patients with advanced heart disease can develop syncope from profound but transient hemodynamic collapse. This may be related to autonomic failure, aggressive vasodilator therapy, or even temporary electromechanical dissociation without even the presence of an arrhythmia. Death in these patients may be by a similar nonarrhythmic mechanism that would not be expected to be diagnosed at EP testing.

Using the Electrophysiological Study to Direct Therapy

Fortunately, the EP study can be used to assess prognostic implications of syncope, and it can also help to direct therapy. Studies such as those by Olshansky et al,[41] Krol et al,[59] and Kurshner et al[61] are most useful for defining the electrophysiologically related results for which treatment is indicated. Thus, certain abnormalities found at EP study may require treatment independent of whether they caused syncope. If findings are definitive and indicate high risk for arrhythmic death, treatment should be offered to prevent syncope*and* to prevent arrhythmic cardiac death independent of the true cause of syncope (Table 2). There are "borderline" abnormalities found at EP study that may require treatment, but experience (and the literature) suggests that it is safe to withhold treatment until the situation is better clarified.[52,61] In other words, borderline abnormalities may reflect the true cause of syncope but have less prognostic meaning; immediate treatment is less pressing (Table 3). In such cases, further diagnostic tests or a period of observation may be indicated. Normal or nondiagnostic test results suggest that an arrhythmic cause of syncope is unlikely.

The use of the EP study results in order to guide therapy is disease- and stimulation protocol-specific. For example, the absence of inducible sustained monomorphic ventricular tachycardia has little meaning in patients with dilated cardiomyopathy or long QT interval syndrome (Tables 3,4, and 5).

_____ Table 2 _____

Definite Abnormality (Treatment Indicated)

Sustained monomorphic ventricular tachycardia with hypotension
Rapid supraventricular tachycardia with marked hypotension
AV block in the His-Purkinje system (intra- or infra-His) at an atrial cycle length
    <320 ms (not pseudo infra-Hisian block) ± procainamide infusion
Symptomatic sinus node recovery time (>3 seconds)

AV = atrioventricular.

_____ Table 3 _____

Borderline Abnormality (Treatment May be Needed)

Nonsustained monomorphic ventricular tachycardia with hypotension
AV nodal refractory period >600 ms
HV >100 ms (very rare) ± procainamide infusion
Supraventricular tachycardia rate >180 beats/minute without hypotension
Sinus node recovery time >2 seconds without symptoms

_____ Table 4 _____

Nondiagnostic Findings (Treatment Generally not Needed)

Polymorphic ventricular tachycardia without other supportive history
Sinus node recovery time <2 seconds without symptoms
No induced tachycardia

—— **Table 5** ——

Utility of Specific Protocols Within an EP Study

Atrial stimulation likely to be very useful
1) Chronotropic incompetence proven or suspected
2) Tachycardia-bradycardia syndrome suspected by monitoring
3) Bundle branch block on ECG
4) Supraventricular tachycardia suspected by history or on monitoring
5) Second-degree heart block or higher

Atrial stimulation protocols may be useful
1) Asymptomatic sinus pauses
2) To assess coexisting sinus node or conduction system disease in patient with impaired ventricular function and suspected VT

Atrial stimulation protocols are unlikely to be useful
1) As part of routine protocol to replace the role of noninvasive monitoring
2) Chronic atrial fibrillation (except for measurement of HV interval)

Ventricular stimulation protocols are likely to be very useful
1) Structural heart disease, LVEF >0.4, and an abnormal SAECG
2) LVEF <0.40, coronary artery disease but no acute MI
3) Bundle branch block and suspected structural heart disease
4) Idiopathic ventricular tachycardia suspected by monomorphic ectopy on monitoring
5) Recurrent syncope in a patient already treated for ventricular tachycardia

Ventricular stimulation protocols may be useful
1) Long QT (to assess response to epinephrine and monophasic action potentials)
2) Dilated cardiomyopathy
3) Palpitations with syncope early after cardiac surgery and myocardial infarction
4) Syncope associated with use of antiarrhythmic drugs
5) Recurrent, undiagnosed syncope
6) Sarcoid cardiomyopathy
7) Right ventricular dysplasia

Ventricular stimulation protocols not useful and may be counterproductive
1) Hypertrophic cardiomyopathy without documented arrhythmia
2) Structurally normal heart when specific, occult cardiac disease is not strongly suspected

EP = electrophysiological; VT = ventricular tachycardia; HV = His-ventricular; LVEF = left ventricular ejection fraction; SAECG = signal-averaged electrocardiogram; MI = myocardial infarction.

It is clear that interpretation of the EP study requires thorough understanding of the technique, its strengths, and its limitations. The answers to questions raised in interpreting abnormal responses are specific only to each particular patient subgroup. The strategy of using the results of the EP study to guide therapy, while limited, provides a necessary framework to further care for the individual patient.

Interpretation of Electrophysiological Study Results: Clinical Examples

The several clinical examples that follow illustrate the complexity of interpreting EP study results in syncope patients. The cases are chosen deliberately for their complexity, and may not necessarily be indicative of the routine syncope patient. It should be noted, however, that the EP study may raise more questions than it answers.

Clinical Example 1: A 55-year-old male truck driver with nonischemic cardiomyopathy presents with one episode of syncope to an emergency room. He has had an intermittent "unusual feeling" (Figure 1A). Lidocaine is given and the unusual feeling resolves. At EP study, no ventricular tachycardia is induced with up to three ventricular extrastimuli at two sites. Isoproterenol infusion with rapid pacing precipitates prolonged episodes of ventricular tachycardia lasting up to 16 seconds associated with hypotension (Figure 1B). Radiofrequency ablation successfully treats the ventricular tachycardia originating from the right ventricular outflow tract. He is discharged, off of all antiarrhythmic therapy, and has no recurrent symptoms.

Comments: This case illustrates several points. 1) The 12-lead ECG during symptoms provided the diagnosis of right ventricular outflow tract ventricular tachycardia Had that information not been available, the diagnosis may have been missed at EP study because isoproterenol may not have been given, or the result may have been dismissed as nonspecific. 2) Syncope in patients with left ventricular dysfunction has been associated with a poor prognosis. Given the low sensitivity and specificity of EP studies for patients with dilated cardiomyopathy, the patient may have been offered an empirical therapy such as an implantable defibrillator. Fortunately, during his study, he had very long runs of ventricular tachycardia observed before and during EP study.

Clinical Example 2: A 70-year-old man with a history of myocardial infarction and impaired left ventricular function develops recurrent, otherwise unexplained, syncope. An EP study is positive for sustained monomorphic ventricular tachycardia. An implantable cardioverter defibrillator (ICD) is implanted and programmed appropriately. He has received apparently "appropriate" ICD shocks, associated with near syncope. Subsequently, he develops atrial fibrillation, is admitted to the hospital, and placed on amiodarone. He undergoes a noninvasive EP study through his defibrillator, along with defibrillation threshold testing, prior to discharge on amiodarone. Two years later, he develops recurrent syncope. An EP study is again performed noninvasively via

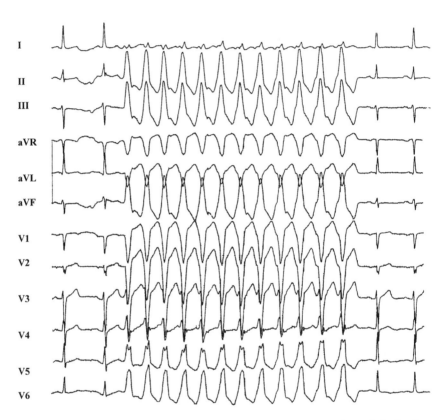

Figure 1A. A 12-lead ECG for a patient with syncope who experienced similar but more intense symptoms of palpitations prior to syncope. The morphology is consistent with right ventricular outflow tract ventricular tachycardia.

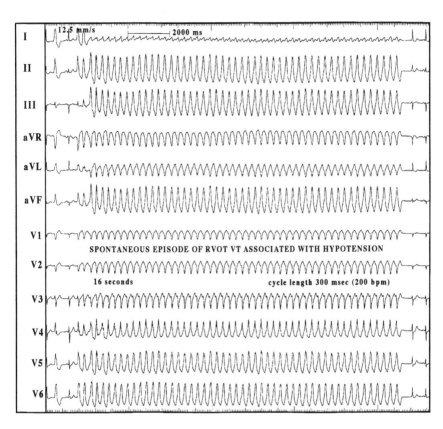

Figure 1B. A diagnosis of right ventricular outflow tract ventricular tachycardia is confirmed at EP study. Salvos of prolonged but self-terminating VT are associated with hypotension but not syncope during the study. The tissue responsible for tachycardias is successfully ablated using radiofrequency ablation techniques.

the ICD. Sustained monomorphic ventricular tachycardia is induced below the programmed rate cut off of the ICD (Figure 2). Since the ICD has been reconfigured to detect and treat the slower but recurrent poorly tolerated ventricular tachycardia, he has no recurrent syncope. *Comments*: Several points are apparent: 1) An ICD can treat induced arrhythmias and abort syncope in syncope patients. 2) EP studies can be performed without catheters directly via the ICD. 3) Subsequent syncopal episodes in patients who appear to have been effectively treated in the past need further evaluation. The cause of recurrent syncope may represent a failure of the previously effective therapy, or the patient may have developed syncope from a different etiology. 4) Ventricular tachycardia can result in hemodynamic collapse and syncope, independent of the rate. 5) ICDs may also prevent death in such patients, independent of the ability to prevent recurrent syncope.

Clinical Example 3: A 74-year-old man with a recent history of chest discomfort develops palpitations associated with near syncope and syn-

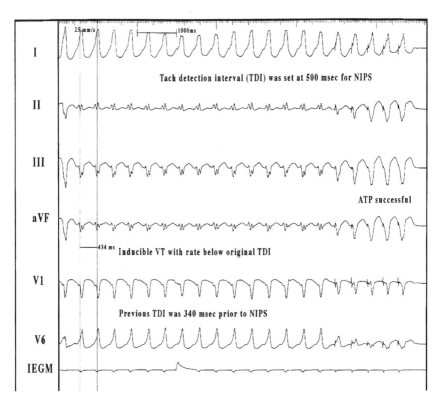

Figure 2. Induction of ventricular tachycardia in a patient who had been previously successfully treated for ventricular tachycardia associated with syncope with an implantable defibrillator. After presenting with recurrent syncope, he is found to have a slower morphology of ventricular tachycardia with a rate that is below the previous cut-off of the device.

cope. The ECG is normal. There is normal systolic function on an echo-cardiogram. Less intense palpitations occur without other symptoms during a 12-lead ECG (Figure 3A). A cardiac catheterization demonstrates a critical lesion in a large ramus intermedius branch, for which he undergoes angioplasty associated with dissection and stent placement, but the artery remains patent. He continues to have near-incessant nonsustained ventricular tachycardia similar to that seen in Figure 3A with near syncope. β-blockers suppress the ventricular tachycardia but render him dependent on a temporary pacemaker. An EP study without β-blockers is negative for sinus node dysfunction and sustained ventricular tachycardia, but reproduces the clinical arrhythmia (nonsustained ventricular tachycardia). Figure 3B demonstrates the effect of spontaneous nonsustained ventricular tachycardia on his arterial pressure.

Comments: This case illustrates several points: 1) The EP study can reproduce the clinical arrhythmia even though sustained ventricular tachycardia cannot be induced. 2) Nonsustained ventricular tachycardia can result in syncope. 3) While ablation of the tachycardia origin is possible, the EP study is inadequate to guide medical therapy. 4) Prog-

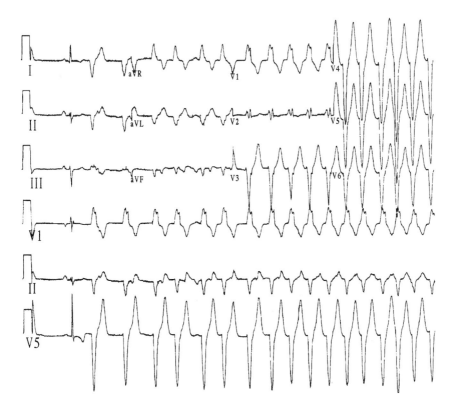

Figure 3A. A 12-lead ECG of a man who presents with recent onset syncope and near syncope.

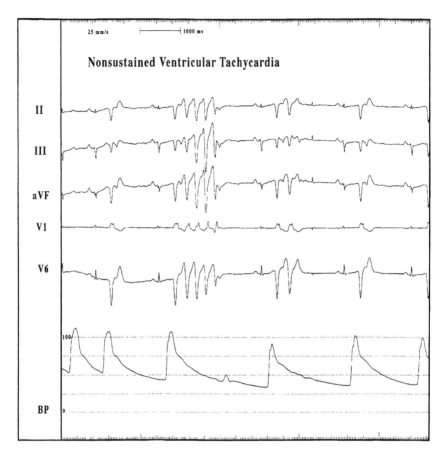

Figure 3B. Nonsustained ventricular tachycardia associated with a fall in perfusion pressure in a syncope patient. Blood pressure (BP) is measured from a radial artery catheter.

nosis, based on left ventricular function, is good. 5) An ICD would not prevent recurrent symptoms and in this patient's circumstances may result in multiple shocks due to nonsustained ventricular tachycardia.

Clinical Example 4: A 63-year-old man has a history of angina. He has one episode of syncope and is found to have atrial flutter with a left bundle branch block (LBBB) and a controlled ventricular response. The duration of the atrial flutter and LBBB are unknown. He has a witnessed but undocumented cardiac arrest (requiring electrical cardioversion of ventricular fibrillation) while in the hospital, not associated with chest pain. During resuscitation, he converts to sinus rhythm with a first-degree block and a LBBB. He is found to have critical three-vessel coronary artery disease and left ventricular dysfunction and therefore undergoes coronary artery bypass graft surgery. At EP study, the baseline HV interval is 67 msec, (Figure 4A). He develops infra-Hisian

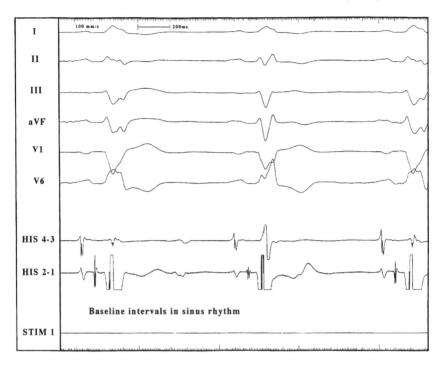

Figure 4A. Baseline His bundle electrogram (His 4–3 and His 2–1) during sinus rhythm. The HV interval is slightly abnormal at 67 msec.

block with atrial pacing at 460 msec (Figure 4B). He has inducible atrial flutter, which is associated with prolonged infra-Hisian block lasting several seconds (Figures 4C and 4D). Sustained ventricular tachycardia cannot be induced.

Comments: This patient has several potential etiologies for syncope. Infra-Hisian block precipitated by paroxysmal atrial flutter is the most likely. Alternatively, the patient may have had a self-limited ischemia-mediated episode of ventricular tachycardia. It is not unusual for cardiac arrest to be predated by one or more episodes of syncope. The patient was treated with a combination of amiodarone and a dual-chamber pacemaker with mode-switching capabilities. In several months of follow-up he has done well, without cardiac arrest or recurrent syncope. Also, this patient underwent cardiac catheterization after the cardiac arrest. Syncope without cardiac arrest is a very poor indication for cardiac catheterization unless the diagnosis of critical aortic stenosis is to be confirmed.

Clinical Example 5: A 37-year-old man with treated non-Hodgkin's lymphoma complicated by pericarditis has unexplained syncope. On admission, he is in atrial flutter with a controlled ventricular response at rest, raising suspicion that a rapid response to atrial flutter may have precipitated syncope. Despite a normal two-dimensional echocardio-

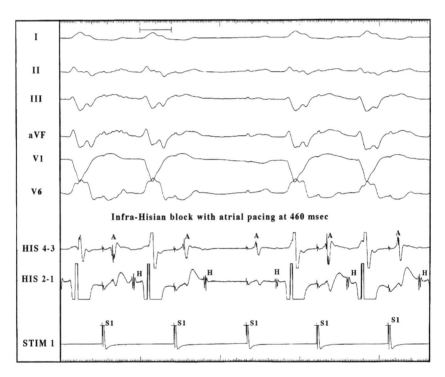

Figure 4B. Atrial pacing (STIM 1) at 460 msec induces block below the level of the His bundle.

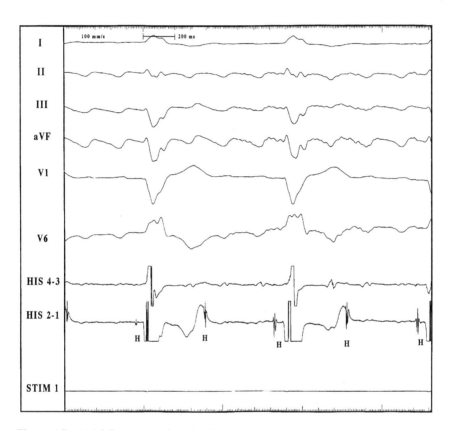

Figure 4C. Atrial flutter is induced with rapid atrial pacing. This is associated with 2:1 infra-Hisian block. There are two His bundle electrograms (see HIS 4–3 and His 2–1) for every conducted QRS complex.

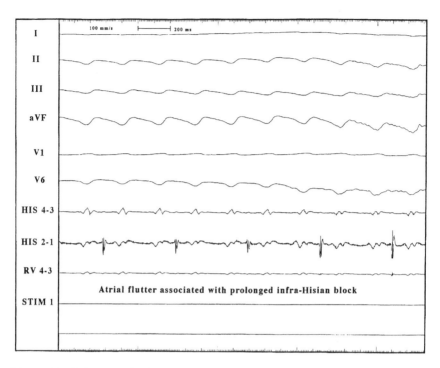

Figure 4D. Subsequently, the patient develops ventricular asystole associated with complete infra-Hisian block (see HIS 2–1). The rhythm is atrial flutter with complete AV block. Ventricular pacing is instituted within a matter of seconds.

gram, an EP study is performed to treat his atrial flutter and assess other arrhythmic causes. Atrial flutter terminates during radio frequency ablation. (Figure 5A). He has a 6.3 second pause prior to the first junctional beat and a 39 second sinus node recovery time. The sinus node recovery time and the corrected sinus node recovery time are both abnormal (Figure 5B). The patient was treated with a rate responsive, dual-chamber permanent pacemaker, with mode-switching capabilities. He has not had recurrent syncope.

Comments: This patient probably had syncope due to the tachycardia-bradycardia syndrome. In this example, EP study was very useful even though the heart was grossly normal by echocardiographic criteria. At study, the abnormal sinus node recovery time did not mimic the duration of the pause that occurred at the termination of atrial flutter. If the patient had presented in sinus rhythm, it is conceivable that a diagnosis of atrial flutter associated with the tachycardia-bradycardia syndrome may not have been considered. Because his heart was "normal," EP study may not have been considered, or the sinus node abnormality may have been considered borderline. Noninvasive monitoring may similarly have been able to demonstrate sinus node dysfunction, but perhaps at the cost of recurrent syncope.

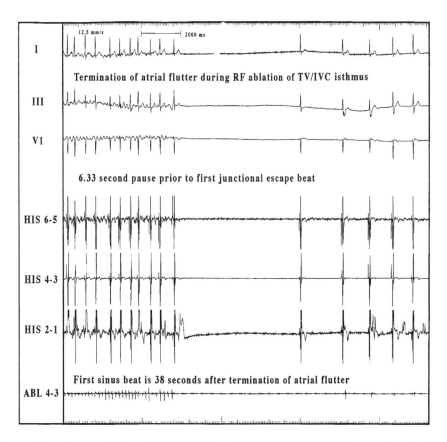

Figure 5A. A 37-year-old man presents with new onset syncope and is found to be in atrial flutter associated with a controlled ventricular response. After successful termination of atrial flutter during radiofrequency ablation, a prolonged pause is noted with a delay of 6.3 seconds prior to the first junctional beat. Analysis suggests that the first sinus depolarization occurred 38 seconds after the termination of atrial flutter.

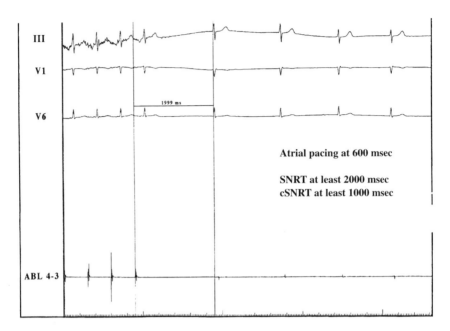

Figure 5B. Sinus node recovery times are clearly abnormal, but not to the degree seen after the termination of atrial flutter. Sinus node recovery time is at least 2000 msec. The corrected sinus node recovery time (cSNRT) is at least 1000 msec. The upper limit of normal for the cSNRT is 545 msec.

Clinical Example 6: A 77-year-old man experiences syncope while driving, and drives his car into a river. Although he has no cardiac history, he does have hypertension and diabetes mellitus. Telemetry reveals nonsustained ventricular tachycardia (Figure 6A). He is found to have significant coronary artery disease and moderate left ventricular dys-

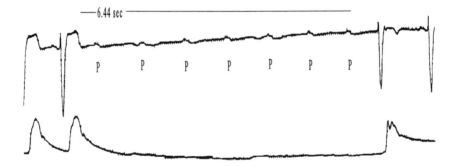

Figure 6A. High-degree heart block (top tracing) associated with a decrease in the arterial blood pressure (lower tracing) in a man who presents with new onset syncope. He also demonstrates nonsustained ventricular tachycardia on telemetry.

function at cardiac catheterization. Both the referring cardiologist and the patient wish to avoid coronary artery bypass graft surgery, so the patient is treated medically for ischemia. At EP study, the HV interval is 70 msec (Figure 6B). With the infusion of procainamide 15 mg/kg, his HV interval prolongs to 100 msec (Figure 6C). Atrial pacing after procainamide induces 2:1 infra-Hisian block (Figure 6D). He does not have monomorphic ventricular tachycardia induced. A permanent pacemaker is placed. He remains asymptomatic, but he becomes pacemaker dependent.

Comments: Atrioventricular block was shown conclusively on telemetry. The arterial pressure showed an immediate drop in blood pressure after the first dropped QRS complex. The referring physician performed cardiac catheterization prior to consulting us. We would not have automatically performed cardiac catheterization, but we used the information given to us. Because he had left ventricular dysfunction associated with nonsustained ventricular tachycardia in the setting of coronary artery disease, it was necessary for coexisting ventricular tachy-

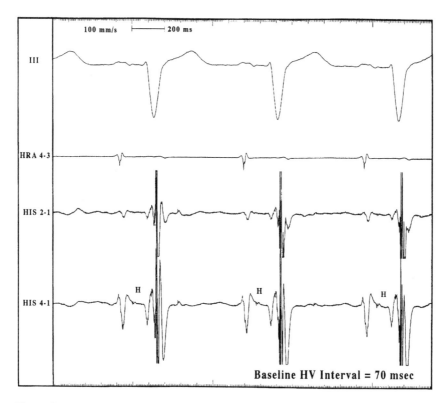

Figure 6B. Baseline HV interval in sinus rhythm is 70 msec in a patient who presents with syncope and is found to have the telemetry findings shown in Figure 6A. Atrial pacing is associated with block above the level of the His bundle. HRA = high right atrial position; HIS = His bundle position.

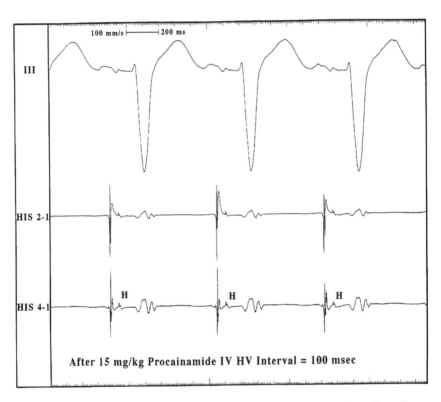

Figure 6C. This tracing represents conduction seen in the His bundle catheter (HIS) for the same patient shown in Figure 6A and Figure 6B. The HV interval prolongs to 100 msec after the infusion of 15 mg/kg of procainamide.

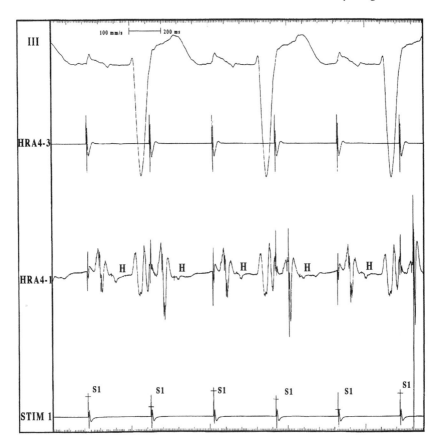

Figure 6D. In the same patient shown in Figures 6A, 6B, and 6C, atrial pacing results in 2:1 infra-Hisian block after infusion of 15 mg/kg of procainamide.

cardia to be excluded. The EP study revealed a baseline HV of 70 msec. The HV lengthened to 100 msec on procainamide. Infra-Hisian block was demonstrable only with procainamide. Despite the noninvasive evidence of AV block, it took a provocative maneuver (procainamide) to demonstrate infra-Hisian block.

Clinical Example 7: A 69-year-old man with a history of a nonischemic cardiomyopathy is admitted with syncope. At EP study, multiple morphologies of sustained monomorphic ventricular tachycardia are reproducibly induced. An arterial sheath is placed with the hope of finding a well-tolerated predominant morphology that is suitable for ablation. Figure 7A reveals a beat-to-beat alteration in arterial blood pressure associated with a "slow" ventricular tachycardia. The tachycardia terminates spontaneously with an immediate improvement in blood pressure (Figure 7B). A second, faster ventricular tachycardia is associated with electromechanical dissociation (Figure 7C). The patient is treated with amiodarone and an ICD.

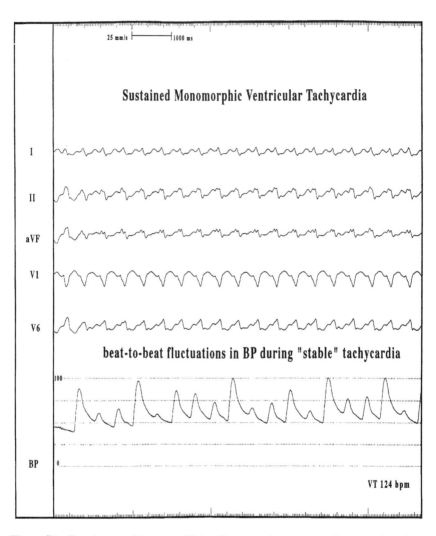

Figure 7A. Despite a stable rate of "slow" ventricular tachycardia, there is a fluctuation of the arterial blood pressure and therefore hemodynamic impairment in a patient with syncope that had been presumed to be secondary to this ventricular tachycardia.

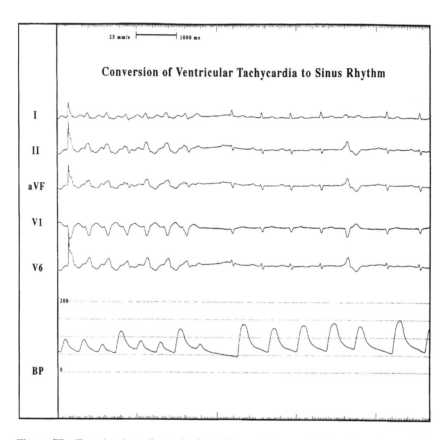

Figure 7B. Termination of ventricular tachycardia is associated with an immediate improvement in the blood pressure. The fluctuations in beat-to-beat arterial pressure also improve.

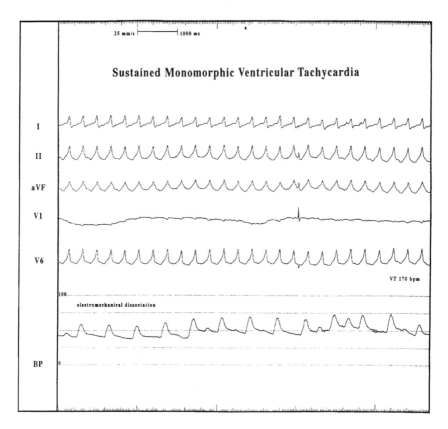

Figure 7C. A faster ventricular tachycardia in the same patient shown in Figure 7A and Figure 7B results in electrical-mechanical dissociation without alterations in the rate of the ventricular tachycardia.

> *Comments*: Even though this patient had a nonischemic cardiomyopathy, he had inducible sustained monomorphic ventricular tachycardia. Although bundle branch reentry can occur commonly in this population, it was not present here. While it is less common to be able to induce sustained monomorphic ventricular tachycardia in these patients, the response is still very specific.

The Role of the Electrophysiological Study in Frequent Recurrent Syncope

In the 50% of patients for whom no obvious cause of syncope is found, the syncope itself appears to be self limited and often benign. Many patients appear to have spontaneous resolution of syncope. Noninvasive monitoring can help to identify those patients in whom the EP study will provide a high yield (Tables 6 and 7). In this group, the EP study should be performed

_____ Table 6 _____

Variables Associated With an Abnormal EP Study

Presence of structural heart disease
Previous myocardial infarction
Late potentials present on signal-averaged ECG
Bifasicular block present on 12-lead ECG
Preexcitation present on 12-lead ECG
Noninvasive monitoring suggestive of sinus node dysfunction
Noninvasive monitoring suggestive of fixed AV block
Older age
History of supraventricular tachycardia

_____ Table 7 _____

Strong Indications for EP Study in Syncope Patients
(High Utility†)

Previous myocardial infarction associated with left ventricular dysfunction
Bifasicular block on 12-lead ECG
Preexcitation on 12-lead ECG
Late potentials present on signal-averaged ECG
Previous history of supraventricular tachycardia
Noninvasive monitoring suggests, but does not convincingly demonstrate,
   sinus node dysfunction
Noninvasive monitoring suggests, but does not convincingly demonstrate,
   AV block
To exclude coexisting ventricular tachycardia
To reassess previously effective antiarrhythmic therapy

Other Indications for EP Study in Syncope Patients
(Variable Utility‡)

Frequent recurrent syncope in low yield patients
Long QT interval syndrome
Dilated cardiomyopathy
Hypertrophic cardiomyopathy

† The EP study is generally indicated, with results influencing therapy.
‡ The EP study may be useful in some circumstances, but should be interpreted with caution.
AV = atrioventricular.

early into the work-up. Still, there is a group of patients who have frequent recurrent episodes of syncope and who have undergone repeated noninvasive evaluations, for whom all noninvasive parameters are normal. In this small group, an EP study can be offered later into a diagnostic work-up. Data from both Krol et al[59] and Krahn et al[70] suggest that the EP study will occasionally find surprising and possibly clinically important abnormalities even in "low-yield" patients. However, when performing and interpreting results in "low-yield" patients, one should be extremely careful to ensure that any abnormality discovered is clinically relevant.

Unusual Indications for Electrophysiological Studies in Syncope

There are other unusual reasons to consider EP studies. Ventricular stimulation protocols may occasionally be useful in conjunction with the infusion of epinephrine in patients who are suspected of having the long QT interval syndrome to assess the effects of pacing rate and epinephrine dose on the QT_C interval.[94–95]

Patients with hypertrophic cardiomyopathy can develop syncope as part of their clinical syndrome, of which sustained monomorphic ventricular tachycardia is an occasional cause.[96] Also in these patients, an outflow tract gradient may potentially be reduced by dual-chamber pacing with a short atrioventricular interval. If obstruction is the cause of syncope, testing the influence of atrioventricular pacing may have some benefit, although the use of pacing in this patient population is still highly controversial.[97–99]

In patients with syncope and relative bradycardia, the hemodynamic effects of atrioventricular sequential pacing can be assessed to see if the patient will benefit from a dual-chamber pacemaker. In other patients with paroxysmal bradycardia, it may not be clear if the sinus node dysfunction is due to intrinsic sinus node disease or to a reflex neurocardiogenic cause. In these cases, the EP study may help to differentiate one cause from the other. Some investigators advocate a role for dual-chamber pacing for some patients with neurocardiogenic syncope.[100,101] The placement of temporary atrial and a ventricular pacing wires during a tilt table test may provide insight into the utility of dual-chamber pacing as therapy for selected patients.

Clinical Example 8: The patient is a 54-year-old male with recurrent syncope. It has been determined that he has deglutition syncope any time he drinks excessively cold liquids. He also has carotid hypersensitivity. An EP study is performed to assess the benefit of dual-chamber pacing and single-chamber pacing to prevent hemodynamic collapse. (Figure 8A). During carotid massage in the electrophysiology lab, the patient becomes asystolic (Figure 8B). With ventricular pacing he remains hypotensive (Figure 8C), but with atrioventricular sequential pacing his systolic blood pressure remains intact (Figure 8D). He undergoes the implantation of a DDD pacemaker. Subsequently to this, he remains asymptomatic with no recurrent syncope with carotid massage or while drinking cold liquids.

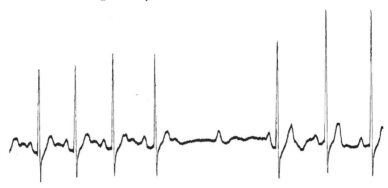

SWALLOWING COLD WATER

Figure 8A. In a patient who presents with recurrent syncope, after swallowing cold water, slowing of the sinus rate precedes AV block.

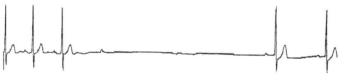

Left Carotid Massage

Right Carotid Massage

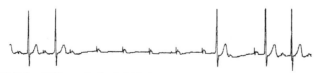

Right Carotid Massage During Atrial Pacing

Figure 8B. Carotid sinus massage is associated with long sinus pauses. Atrial pacing demonstrates concurrent high-degree block in the AV node.

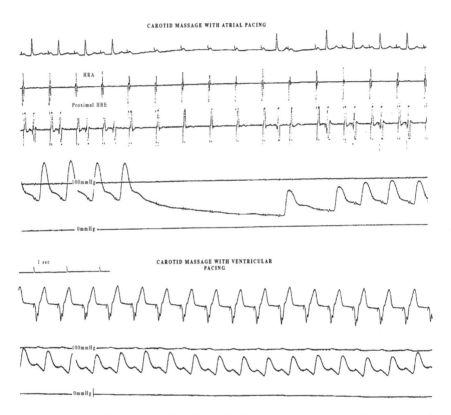

Figure 8C. The effects of atrial and ventricular pacing on the blood pressure with carotid sinus massage.

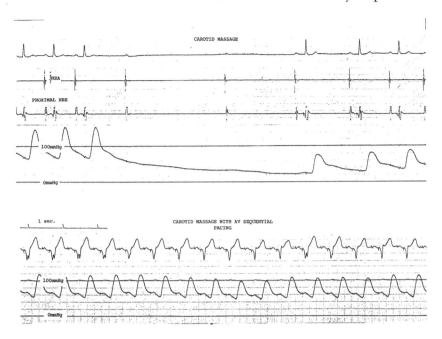

Figure 8D. Temporary AV sequential pacing during carotid sinus massage virtually normalizes the arterial blood pressure. This effect is more pronounced than the effect of ventricular pacing as shown in Figure 8C.

Conclusions

EP studies clearly have a role in the management of patients with syncope. Use of EP studies, guided by information collected during the history, physical examination, and noninvasive testing, provides supportive information that is not easily available by any other means. While the EP study is an important method to diagnose arrhythmias and help guide therapy, it has several noteworthy limitations. In essence, the EP study provides additional supportive data regarding the diagnostic cause of syncope. It is useful only in this regard.

The greatest yield of the EP study is in patients with impaired left ventricular function, structural heart disease and other suggestive findings, or history of serious arrhythmia problems. For this population, the EP study can help to direct further appropriate arrhythmia management decisions to reduce the risk of recurrent syncope and to reduce the risk of death.

References

1. Kapoor WN, Karpf M, Wienand S, et al. A prospective evaluation and follow-up of patients with syncope. *N Engl J Med* 1983;309:197–204.
2. Silverstein MD, Singer DE, Mulley AG, et al. Patients with syncope admitted to medical intensive care units. *JAMA* 1982;248:1185–1189.
3. Savage DD, Corwin L, McGee DL, et al. Epidemiologic features of isolated syncope: The Framingham study. *Stroke* 1985;16:626–629.
4. Kapoor WN, Hanusa BH. Is syncope a risk factor for poor outcomes? Comparison of patients with and without syncope. *Am J Med* 1996;100:646–655.
5. Eagle KA, Block HR, Cook EF, et al. Evaluation of prognostic classifications for patients with syncope. *Am J Med* 1985;79:455–460.
6. Kapoor WN. Evaluation and outcome of patients with syncope. *Medicine* 1990;69:160–175.
7. Scherlag BJ, Lau SH, Helfant RH, et al. Catheter technique for recording His bundle activity in man. *Circulation* 1969;39:13–18.
8. Rosen K, Ehsani A, Rahimtoola S. H-V intervals in left bundle-branch block. *Circulation* 1972;46:717–723.
9. Rosen K, Mehta A, Miller RA. Demonstration of dual atrioventricular nodal pathways in man. *Am J Cardiol* 1974;33:291–294.
10. Josephson ME. *Clinical Cardiac Electrophysiology: Techniques and Interpretations 2nd Ed.* Philadelphia: Lea & Febiger; 1993.
11. Fisher JD, Role of electrophysiologic testing in the diagnosis and treatment of patients with known and suspected bradycardias and tachycardias. *Prog Cardiovasc Dis* 1981;24:25–90.
12. Vanderpol CJ, Farshidi A, Spielman S, et al. Incidence and clinical significance of induced ventricular tachycardia. *Am J Cardiol* 1980;45:725–731.
13. Wellens HJ, Schuilenburg RM, Durrer D. Electrical stimulation of the heart in patients with ventricular tachycardia. *Circulation* 1972;45:216–226.
14. Dhingra RC, Wyndham C, Bauernfeind R, et al. Significance of block distal to the His bundle induced by atrial pacing in patients with chronic bundle branch block. *Circulation* 1979;60:1455–1464.
15. Dhingra RC, Palileo E, Strasberg B, et al. Significance of the HV interval in 517 patients with chronic bifasicular block. *Circulation* 1981;64:1265–1271.
16. McAnulty JH, Rahimtoola SH. Bundle branch block. *Prog Cardiovasc Dis* 1983;26:333–354.
17. Narula O, Samet P, Javier R. Significance of the sinus-node recovery time. *Circulation* 1972;45:140–158.
18. Mandel W, Hayakawa H, Danzig R, et al. Evaluation of sino-atrial node function in man by overdrive suppression. *Circulation* 1971;44:59–66.
19. Rosen KM, Loeb HS, Sinno MZ, et al. Cardiac conduction in patients with symptomatic sinus node disease. *Circulation* 1971;43:835–844.
20. Scheinman MM, Strauss HC, Abbott JA, et al. Electrophysiologic testing in patients with sinus pauses and/or sinoatrial exit block. *Eur J Cardiol* 1978;51–60.
21. Gupta PK, Lichstein E, Chadda KD, et al. Appraisal of sinus nodal recovery time in patients with sick sinus syndrome. *Am J Cardiol* 1974;34:265–270.
22. Strauss HC, Bigger JT, Saroff AL, et al. Electrophysiologic evaluation of sinus node function in patients with sinus node dysfunction. *Circulation* 1976;53:763–776.
23. Gang ES, Reiffel JA, Livelli FD Jr. Sinus node recovery times following the spontaneous termination of supraventricular tachycardia and following atrial overdrive pacing: A comparison. *Am Heart J* 1983;105:210–215.

24. Breithardt G, Seipel L, Loogen F. Sinus node recovery time and calculated sinoatrial conduction time in normal subjects and patients with sinus node dysfunction. *Circulation* 1977;56:43–50.
25. Gann D, Tolentino A, Samet P. Electrophysiologic evaluation of elderly patients with sinus bradycardia: A long term follow-up study. *Ann Intern Med* 1979;9:24–29.
26. DiMarco JP, Garan H, Harthorne JW, et al. Intracardiac electrophysiologic techniques in recurrent syncope of unknown origin. *Ann Intern Med* 1981; 95:542–548.
27. Hess DS, Morady F, Scheinman MM. Electrophysiologic testing in the evaluation of patients with syncope of undetermined origin. *Am J Cardiol* 1982; 50:1309–1315.
28. Ezri M, Lerman BB, Marchlinski FE, et al. Electrophysiologic evaluation of syncope in patients with bifascicular block. *Am Heart J* 1983;106:693–697.
29. Akhtar M, Shenasa M, Denker S, et al. Role of cardiac electrophysiology studies in patients with unexplained recurrent syncope. *Pacing Clin Electrophysiol* 1983;6:192–201.
30. Morady F, Shen E, Schwartz A, et al. Long-term follow-up of patients with recrrent unexplained syncope evaluated by electrophysiologic testing. *J Am Coll Cardiol* 1983;2:1053–1059.
31. Scharma AD, Klein GJ, Milstein S. Diagnostic assessment of recurrent syncope. *Pacing Clin Electrophysiol* 1984;7:749–759.
32. Morady F, Higgins J, Peters RW, et al. Electrophysiologic testing in bundle branch block and unexplained syncope. *Am J Cardiol* 1984;54:587–581.
33. Morady F. The evaluation of syncope with electrophysiologic studies. *Cardiol Clin* 1986;4:515–526.
34. DiMarco JP. Electrophysiologic studies in patients with unexplained syncope. *Circulation* 1987;75(suppl III):140–143.
35. McAnulty JH. Syncope of unknown origin: The role of electrophysiologic studies. *Circulation* 1987;75(suppl III);144–145.
36. Click RL, Gersh BJ, Sugrue DD, et al. Role of invasive electrophysiologic testing in patients with symptomatic bundle branch block. *Am J Cardiol* 1987;59:817–823.
37. Nelson SD, Kou WH, de Buitleir M, et al. Value of programmed ventricular stimulation in presumed carotid sinus syndrome. *Am J Cardiol* 1987; 60:1073–1077.
38. Andrews NP, Fogel RI, Evans IJ, Prystowski EN. Implantable defibrillator event rates in patients with syncope of unknown origin and induced sustained ventricular tachycardia: Comparison with patients with documented ventricular tachycardia. *J Am Coll Cardiol* 1997;29(suppl A):257A.
39. Kapoor WN, Hammill SC, Gersh BJ. Diagnosis and natural history of syncope and the role of invasive electrophysiologic testing. *Am J Cardiol* 1989;63:730–734.
40. Paul T, Guccione P, Garson A. Relation of syncope in young patients with Wolff-Parkinson-White syndrome to rapid ventricular response during atrial fibrillation. *Am J Cardiol* 1990;65:318–321.
41. Olshansky B, Mazuz M, Martins JB. Significance of inducible tachycardia in patients with syncope of unknown origin: A long-term follow-up. *J Am Coll Cardiol* 1985;5:216–223.
42. Platia EV, Greene HL, Vlay SC, et al. Sensitivity of various extrastimulus techniques in patients with serious ventricular arrhythmias. *Am Heart J* 1983; 106:698–703.
43. Brugada P, Abdollah H, Heddle B, et al. Results of a ventricular stimulation protocol using a maximum of 4 premature stimuli in patients without

documented or suspected ventricular arrhythmias. *Am J Cardiol* 1983;52: 1214–1218.

44. DiCarlo LA, Morady F, Schwartz AB, et al. Clinical significance of ventricular fibrillation-flutter induced by ventricular programmed stimulation. *Am Heart J* 1985;109:959–963.

45. Platia EV, Reid PR. Nonsustained ventricular tachycardia during programmed stimulation: Criteria for a positive test. *Am J Cardiol* 1985;56:79–83.

46. Wellens HJ, Brugada P, Stevenson WG. Programmed electrical stimulation of the heart in patients with life-threatening ventricular arrhythmias: What is the significance of induced arrhythmias and what is the correct stimulation protocol? *Circulation* 1985;72:216–227.

47. Morady F, DiCarlo L, Winston S, et al. A prospective comparison of triple extrastimuli and left ventricular stimulation in studies of ventricular tachycardia induction. *Circulation* 1984;70:52–57.

48. Kou WH, de Buitleir M, Kadish AH, Morady F. Sequelae of nonsustained polymorphic ventricular tachycardia induced during programmed ventricular stimulation. *Am J Cardiol*1989;64:1148–1151.

49. Morady F, Shapiro W, Shen W, et al. Programmed ventricular stimulation in patients without spontaneous ventricular tachycardia. *Am Heart J* 1984;107: 875–882.

50. Meinertz T, Treese N, Kasper W, et al. Determinants of prognosis in idiopathic dilated cardiomyopathy as determined by programmed electrical stimulation. *Am J Cardiol* 1985;56:337–341.

51. Bass EB, Elson JJ, Fogoros RN, et al. Long-term prognosis of patients undergoing electrophysiologic studies for syncope of unknown origin. *Am J Cardiol* 1988;62:1186–1191.

52. Doherty JU, Pembrook-Rogers D, Grogan EW, et al. Electrophysiologic evaluation and follow-up characteristics of patients with recurrent unexplained syncope and presyncope. *Am J Cardiol* 1985;55:703–708.

53. Moazez F, Peter T, Simonson J, et al. Syncope of unknown origin: Clinical, noninvasive, and electrophysiologic determinants of arrhythmia induction and symptom recurrence during long-term follow-up. *Am Heart J* 1991;121:81–88.

54. Kall JG, Olshansky B, Wilber, DJ. Sudden death and recurrent syncope in patients presenting with syncope of unknown origin: Predictive value of electrophysiologic testing. *Pacing Clin Electrophysiol* (Abstr) 1991;14:714A.

55. Sra JS, Anderson AJ, Sheikh SH, et al. Unexplained syncope evaluated by electrophysiologic studies and head-up tilt testing. *Ann Intern Med* 1991;114:1013–1019.

56. Muller T, Roy D, Talajic M, et al. Electrophysiologic evaluation and outcome of patients with syncope of unknown origin. *European Society of Cardiology* 1991;20:139–143.

57. Englund A, Bergfeldt L, Rehnqvist N, et al. Diagnostic value of programmed ventricular stimulation in patients with bifascicular block: A prospective study of patients with and without syncope. *J Am Coll Cardiol* 1995;26:1508–1515.

58. Teichman, SL, Felder SD, Matos JA, et al. the value of electrophysiologic studies in syncope of undetermined origin: Report of 150 cases. *Am Heart J* 1985;110:469–479.

59. Krol RB, Morady F, Flaker GC, et al. Electrophysiologic testing in patients with unexplained syncope: Clinical and noninvasive predictors of outcome. *J Am Coll Cardiol* 1987;10:358–363.

60. Day SC, Cook EF, Funkenstein H, Goldman L. Evaluation and outcome of emergency room patients with transient loss of consciousness. *Am J Med* 1982;73:15–23.

61. Kushner JA, Kou WH, Kadish AH, Morady F. Natural history of patients with unexplained syncope and a nondiagnostic electrophysiology study. *J Am Coll Cardiol* 1989;14:391–396.
62. Scheinman MM, personal communication.
63. Zipes DP, DiMarco JP, Gillette PC, et al. Task force on practice guidelines (Committee on clinical intracardiac electrophysiologic and catheter ablation procedures). *J Am Coll Cardiol* 1995;26:555–573.
64. Horowitz LN, Kay HR, Kutalek SP, et al. Risks and complications of clinical electrophysiologic studies: A prospective analysis of 1,000 consecutive patients. *J Am Coll Cardiol* 1987;9:1261–1268.
65. Brooks R, Garan H, Ruskin JN. Evaluation of the patient with unexplained syncope. In: Zipes DP (ed): *Cardiac Electrophysiology: From Cell to Bedside*. Philadelphia, PA: W.B. Saunders Co.; 1990:646–666.
66. Olshansky B, Martins JB. Isoproterenol facilitation of ventricular tachycardia induction during extrastimulus testing predicts effective chronic therapy with beta adrenergic blockade. *Am J Cardiol* 1987;59:573–577.
67. Wilber DW, Kall J, Olshansky B, Scanlon P. Pacing induced infra-His block in patients with syncope of unknown origin: Incidence and clinical significance. *Pacing Clin Electrophysiol* (Abstr) 1990;13:562A.
68. Klein GJ, Gersh BJ, Yee R. Electrophysiological testing: The court of final appeal for the diagnosis of syncope? *Circulation* 1995;92:1332–1335.
69. Fujimura O, Yee R, Klein GJ, et al. The diagnostic sensitivity of electrophysiologic testing in patients with syncope caused be transient bradycardia. *New Engl J Med* 1989;321:1703–1707.
70. Krahn AD, Klein GJ, Norris C, et al. The etiology of syncope in patients with negative tilt table and electrophysiologic testing. *Circulation* 1995;92:1819–1824.
71. Middlekauff H, Stevenson W, Stevenson L, et al. Syncope in advanced heart failure: High risk of sudden death regardless of origin of syncope. *J Am Coll Cardiol* 1993;21:110–116.
72. Middlekauff HR, Stevenson WG, Saxon LA. Prognosis after syncope: Impact of left ventricular function. *Am Heart J* 1993;125:121–127.
73. Brembilla-Perrot B, Donetti J, Terrier de la Chaise A, et al. Diagnostic value of ventricular stimulation in patients with idiopathic dilated cardiomyopathy. *Am Heart J* 1991;121:1124–1131.
74. Olhausen KV, Stienen U, Schwarz F, et al. Long-term prognostic significance of ventricular arrhythmias in idiopathic dilated cardiomyopathy. *Am J Cardiol* 1988;61:146–151.
75. Poll DS, Marchlinski FE, Buxton AE, et al. Usefulness of programmed stimulation in idiopathic dilated cardiomyopathy. *Am J Cardiol* 1986;112:992–997.
76. Gang ES, Peter T, Rosenthal PT, et al. Detection of late potentials on the surface electrocardiogram in unexplained syncope. *Am J Cardiol* 1986;58:1014–1020.
77. Winters SL, Stewart D, Targonski A, et al. Signal averaging of the surface QRS complex predicts inducibility of ventricular tachycardia in patients with syncope of unknown origin: A prospective study. *J Am Coll Cardiol* 1987;10:775–781.
78. Kuchar DL, Thornburn CW, Sammel NL. Signal averaged electrocardiogram for evaluation or recurrent syncope. *Am J Cardiol* 1986;58:949–953.
79. Tchou P, Krebs AC, Sra J, et al. Syncope: A warning sign of sudden death in idiopathic dilated cardiomyopathy patients. *J Am Coll Cardiol* (Abstract) 1991;17:196A.

80. Leitch JW, Klein GJ, Yee R, et al. Syncope associated with supraventricular tachycardia: An expression of tachycardia rate or vasomotor response? *Circulation* 1992;85:1064–1071.

81. Waxman MB, Wald RW, Cameron D. Interactions between the autonomic nervous system and tachycardias in man. *Cardiol Clin* 1982;1:143–185.

82. Waxman MB, Sharma AD, Cameron DA, et al. Reflex mechanisms responsible for early spontaneous termination of paroxysmal supraventricular tachycardia. *Am J Cardiol* 1982;49:259–272.

83. Buxton AE, Josephson ME, Marchlinski FE, et al. Polymorphic ventricular tachycardia induced by programmed stimulation: Response to procainamide. *J Am Coll Cardiol* 1993;21:90–98.

84. Morady F, DiCarlo L, Winston S, et al. Clinical features and prognosis of patients with out of hospital cardiac arrest and a normal electrophysiologic study. *J Am Coll Cardiol* 1984;4:39–44.

85. Wilber DJ, Garan H, Finkelstein D, et al. Out-of-hospital cardiac arrest: Use of electrophysiologic testing in the prediction of long-term-outcome. *N Engl J Med* 1988;318:19–24.

86. Wyndham CR. Role of invasive electrophysiologic testing in the management of life-threatening ventricular arrhythmias. *Am J Cardiol* 1988;62:13I–17I.

87. Masrani K, Cowley D, Bekheit S, et al. Recurrent syncope for over a decade due to idiopathic ventricular fibrillation. *Chest* 1994;106:1601–1603.

88. Prystowsky EN, Knilans TK, Evans JJ. Diagnostic evaluation and treatment strategies for patients at risk for serious cardiac arrhythmias: Part 1: Syncope of unknown origin. *Modern Concepts of Cardiovascular Disease* American Heart Association; 1991;60:49–54.

89. Manolis AS, Linzer M, Salem D, et al. Syncope: Current diagnostic evaluation and management. *Ann Med* 1990;112:850–863.

90. Denes P, Uretz E, Ezri MD, et al. Clinical predictors of electrophysiologic findings in patients with syncope of unknown origin. *Arch Intern Med* 1988; 148:1922–1928.

91. Bachinsky WB, Linzer M, Weld L, et al. Usefulness of clinical characteristics in predicting the outcome of electrophysiologic studies in unexplained syncope. *Am J Cardiol* 1992;69:1044–1049.

92. Lacroix D, Dubuc M, Kus T, et al. Evaluation of arrhythmic causes of syncope: Correlation between Holter monitoring, electrophysiologic testing, and body surface potential mapping. *Am Heart J* 1991;122:1346–1354.

93. Olshansky B, Hahn E, Hartz V, and the ESVEM Investigators. Is Syncope in the ESVEM trial a marker of cardiac arrest of all-cause mortality? *Circulation* 1994;90:I-456A.

94. Bhandari AK, Shapiro WA, Morady F, et al. Electrophysiologic testing in patients with the long QT syndrome. *Circulation* 1985;71:63–71.

95. Jackman WM, Friday KJ, Anderson JL, et al. The long QT syndromes: A critical review, new clinical observations and a unifying hypothesis. *Prog Cardiovasc Dis* 1988;31:115–172.

96. Fananapazir L, Chang AC, Epstein SE, McAreavey D. Prognostic determinants in hypertrophic cardiomyopathy: Prospective evaluation of a therapeutic strategy based on clinical, Holter, hemodynamic, and electrophysiological findings. *Circulation* 1992;86:730–740.

97. Fananapazir L, Epstein ND, Curiel RV, et al. Long-term results of dual-chamber (DDD) pacing in obstructive cardiomyopathy: Evidence for progressive symptomatic and hemodynamic improvement and reduction of left ventricular hypertrophy. *Circulation* 1994;90:2731–2742.

98. Nishimura RA, Hayes DL, Ilstrup DM, et al. Effect of dual-chamber pacing on systolic and diastolic function in patients with hypertrophic cardiomyopathy: Acute Doppler echocardiographic and catheterization hemodynamic study. *J Am Coll Cardiol* 1996;27:421–430.

99. Betocchi S, Losi MA, Boccalatte M, et al. Effects of dual-chamber pacing in hypertrophic cardiomyopathy on left ventricular outflow tract obstruction and on diastolic function. *Am J Cardiol* 1996;77:498–502.

100. Sra JS, Jazayeri MR, Avitall B, et al. Comparison of cardiac pacing with drug therapy in the treatment of neurocardiogenic (vasovagal) syncope with bradycardia or asystole. *N Engl J Med* 1993;328:1085–1090.

101. Benditt DG, Petersen M, Lurie KG, et al. Cardiac pacing for prevention of recurrent vasovagal syncope. *Ann Intern Med* 1995;122:204–209.

Neurological and Related Causes of Syncope:

The Importance of Recognition and Treatment

David Robertson, MD and Thomas L. Davis, MD

Introduction

Twenty-five percent of young healthy adults experience syncope (transient loss of consciousness) at least once, usually as an emotional faint with a well-recognized precipitating stimulus. This type of syncope requires no medical work-up. Syncope in the absence of a precipitating stimulus is far less common and must be evaluated.[1-11] Syncope is usually due to seizures or inadequate central nervous system (CNS) bloodflow (if one considers the latter in the broad sense of embracing hypotension, arrhythmias, etc.). It is therefore important to try to determine right at the outset if a syncopal episode is due to seizures or inadequate CNS bloodflow. Some helpful distinguishing features are noted in Table 1. A third diagnostic category, atypical syncope, includes miscellaneous causes such as hypoglycemia and emboli, psychogenic and vestibular.

When a healthy subject stands, systolic blood pressure usually falls approximately 10 mm Hg and diastolic pressure increases 5 mm Hg. Heart rate rises 5 to 20 beats per minute. Within 20 minutes of standing, about 15% of plasma volume exits from the vasculature. A fall in blood pressure (BP) of 20/10 or greater in the first 3 to 5 minutes of upright posture is called orthostatic hypotension. When orthostatic symptoms occur with less

From Grubb BP, Olshansky B (eds.). *Syncope: Mechanisms and Management.* Armonk, NY: Futura Publishing Co., Inc.; © 1998.

_____ **Table 1** _____

Differential Diagnosis of Syncope: Seizures vs Hypotension

Observation	Seizures	Inadequate Perfusion
1) Onset	Sudden	More gradual
2) Duration	Minutes	Seconds
3) Jerks	Frequent	Rare
4) Headache	Frequent (after)	Occasional (before)
5) Confusion afterwards	Frequent	Rare
6) Loss of sphincter control	Frequent	Rare
7) Eye deviation	Horizontal	Vertical (or no deviation)
8) Tongue biting	Frequent	Rare
9) Prodrome	Aura	Dizziness
10) EEG	Often abnormal	Usually normal

EEG = electroencephalogram.

than a 20/10 fall in BP, it is called orthostatic intolerance. The most common symptoms of orthostatic hypotension are dizziness, dimming of vision, and discomfort in the neck, shoulders, or head. With orthostatic intolerance, the most common symptoms are tachycardia, palpitations, weakness, and anxiety. Orthostatic hypotension and orthostatic intolerance are most pronounced (and hence most easily detected) in the hour after the patient has ingested a large breakfast.

Many years ago, studies in healthy subjects demonstrated that cessation of carotid and vertebral blood flow for 5 to 6 seconds caused eyes to fix in midposition; this was followed in 1 to 2 seconds by complete loss of consciousness.[12] With immediate restoration of blood flow, many subjects were unaware of their loss of consciousness. A remembered loss of consciousness usually implies the equivalent of 10 seconds of complete loss of brain circulation.

Videometric studies of 56 episodes of transient cerebral hypoxia in normal subjects provide further information on the clinical characteristics of syncope as defined by loss of postural balance in a setting of loss of consciousness.[13] In these studies syncope tended to last 12 seconds. Myoclonus occurred in 90% of subjects, starting about 2.6 seconds after loss of consciousness and lasting 6.6 seconds. Most subjects had bilateral synchronous and asynchronous jerking. Forty percent of individuals had a short duration low-pitched vocalization, usually starting 2 seconds after loss of consciousness.

During loss of consciousness, the electroencephalogram (EEG) demonstrated high-amplitude theta and delta waves, which attenuated in half of cases, leaving a flat EEG. After a few seconds, the slow waves reappeared, passing into alpha activity as consciousness returned.

Orthostatic hypotension as a cause of syncope is relatively common. In our 600-bed hospital, we see approximately 150 new cases of orthostatic hypotension each year. Among 68 consecutive patients seen for orthostatic hypotension at Vanderbilt, half had a primary dysautonomia and half had a secondary dysautonomia. Primary dysautonomia includes multiple system atrophy (Shy-Drager syndrome) and pure autonomic failure. Secondary dysautonomia includes amyloidosis, diabetes mellitus, and malignancy (especially bronchogenic carcinoma).

Patients with orthostatic intolerance are much more commonly seen than patients with orthostatic hypotension. Causes of orthostatic intolerance include partial dysautonomia (often associated with mitral valve prolapse, hypovolemia, and tachycardia on standing), diuretic abuse, dumping syndrome, deconditioning, and drug ingestion. Partial dysautonomia usually occurs in young women following a viral infection or a major weight loss. It is the most common dysautonomia.

There is currently great investigative interest in partial dysautonomia (see chapters 4 and 10). It is likely, in fact, that a large number of unusual medical problems derive from this fundamental pathophysiology (Table 2). Many new insights into this disorder are emerging. Some patients with orthostatic intolerance have reduced cerebral blood flow in the upright posture, even when blood pressure does not fall.[14,15] Reduced tone in the leg vasculature has been observed.[16] These patients have excessive dynamic orthostatic hypovolemia.[17] They also have pharmacological evidence of de-

_____ **Table 2** _____

**Diagnostic Categories Used to Describe
Orthostatic Intolerance**

Hyperadrenergic orthostatic hypotension
Orthostatic tachycardia syndrome
Postural orthostatic tachycardia syndrome
Postural tachycardia syndrome
Hyperadrenergic postural hypotension
Sympathotonic orthostatic hypotension
Hyperdynamic β-adrenergic state
Idiopathic hypovolemia
Orthostatic tachycardia plus
Sympathicotonic orthostatic hypotension
Mitral valve prolapse syndrome
Soldier's heart
Vasoregulatory asthenia
Neurocirculatory asthenia
Irritable heart
Orthostatic anemia
Chronic fatigue syndrome

nervation of the lower extremity in that there is hypersensitivity of both α_1- and β_1-adrenoreceptors.[18] Some of these patients have a subtly reduced plasma renin activity, which leads to reduced aldosterone levels.[19] These changes in the renin-aldosterone axis lead to an impaired ability to retain sodium in the upright posture.[20] Taken together, it is clear that a constellation of effects resulting from a partially reduced sympathetic function leads to hypovolemia and impairment in vascular responsiveness to upright posture, which leads directly to the orthostatic intolerance with orthostatic tachycardia seen in many young patients who present with syncope.[21–23]

Neurological Diseases Associated with Hypotension (Table 3)

Multiple System Atrophy (Shy-Drager Syndrome)

Multiple system atrophy is a degenerative disorder, with neuronal loss and gliosis in many central nervous system areas.[24–27] Depending on which brain area manifests initial clinical symptoms, the disorder may be given different names. When it begins with imbalance, incoordination, and dysarthria, it is often called olivopontocerebellar atrophy (OPCA). When rigidity and bradykinesia out of proportion to tremor occur initially, it is sometimes called striatonigral degeneration (SND). When autonomic failure dominates the initial presentation, it is often called the Shy-Drager syndrome (SDS). The term "multiple system atrophy" (MSA) can be used to describe any or all of these features.

Most people develop MSA after age 40, and twice as many men as women are affected. Patients usually have autonomic symptoms first. Genitourinary dysfunction is the most frequent initial complaint in women and impotence is the most frequent initial complaint in men. Orthostatic hypotension is common and may present with dizziness, dimming of vision, head or neck pain, yawning, temporary confusion, slurred speech, and, if the hypotension is severe, syncope. Because of autonomic failure, patients respond in an exaggerated fashion to drugs that raise or lower blood pressure. They are also very susceptible to postprandial hypotension.

When the disorder presents with nonautonomic features, imbalance due either to cerebellar or parkinsonian abnormalities is the most common feature. Patients sometimes complain of stiffness, clumsiness, or a change in handwriting at the onset of MSA.

MSA may progress rapidly. With involvement of cerebellar, extrapyramidal, and pyramidal systems, the movement disorder usually constitutes the most profound disability. Vocal cord paralysis may lead to hoarseness and stridor. A neurogenic and obstructive mixed form of sleep apnea occurs. Patients survive an average of 9 years after the onset of the illness.

_____ **Table 3** _____

Differential Diagnosis of Neurological Causes of Syncope

Neurological Diseases Associated With Hypotension
A. Degenerative disease
  1. Multiple system atrophy (Shy-Drager syndrome)
  2. Pure autonomic failure
  3. Parkinson's disease
B. Peripheral neuropathy
  1. Diabetes mellitus
  2. Amyloidosis
  3. Alcoholic neuropathy
  4. Prophyria
  5. Guillain-Barré syndrome
  6. Sjögren's syndrome
  7. Dopamine-hydroxylase deficiency
  8. Monoamine oxidase deficiency
  9. Lisker's syndrome
  10. Anand's syndrome
C. Spinal cord lesions
  1. Subacute combined degeneration (B_{12} deficiency) (pernicious anemia)
  2. Syringomyelia

Conditions Leading to Isolated Cerebral Ischemia
A. Atherosclerosis
B. Takayasu's disease
C. Subclavian steal syndrome (Millikan-Siekert Syndrome)
D. Innominate artery syndrome

Paroxysmal Disorders
A. Seizures
  1. Generalized
    a. absence
    b. atonic
    c. tonic
    d. tonic-clonic
  2. Partial complex
    a. frontal
    b. temporal
B. Disorders of presumed central dysregulation
  1. Bruns' syndrome
  2. Autonomic epilepsy
  3. Baroreflex failure
  4. Penfield's syndrome
  5. Wallenberg's syndrome
  6. Williams-Bashore syndrome
C. Paroxysmal reflex activation
  1. Bezold-Jarisch reflex activation
  2. Carotid sinus syncope
  3. Weisenburg's syndrome (glossopharyngeal neuralgia)
  4. Cough syncope

continues

—— Table 3   Continued ——————————————————————

Differential Diagnosis of Neurological Causes of Syncope

Paroxysmal Disorders Continued
  5. Defecation syncope
  6. Diver's syncope
  7. Breath holding spells
   a. cyanotic type
   b. Pallor type

Neurohumoral Disorders
  A. Allgrove's syndrome
  B. Ulick's syndrome
  C. Verner-Morrison syndrome
  D. Streeten's syndrome (hyperbradykininism)
  E. Mastocytosis
  F. Pheochromocytoma
  G. Hyperepinephrinemia

Miscellaneous Hemodynamic Disorders
  A. Analbuminemia
  B. Bouveret's syndrome
  C. McKittrick-Wheelock syndrome
  D. Schroeder's syndrome
  E. Short's syndrome
  F. Roenheld's syndrome
  G. Supine hypotension syndrome

Nonsyncopal Entities
  A. Bárány syndrome (benign postitional vertigo)
  B. Cataplexy
  C. Gélineau's syndrome (narcolepsy)

Approximately 10% to 20% of patients diagnosed with Parkinson's disease in the United Kingdom are found at autopsy to have MSA. This suggests that clinical differentiation of Parkinson's disease and MSA is extremely difficult. MSA should be suspected in patients believed to have Parkinson's disease when 1) disability progresses rapidly, 2) patients are poorly responsive to levodopa, 3) autonomic features such as urinary retention or incontinence or orthostatic hypotension are pronounced, and 4) rigidity and bradykinesia are out of proportion to tremor.

The diagnosis is usually made on clinical grounds, but desperate patients sometimes seek more invasive evaluation. Routine CSF and EEG analysis are nonrevealing. CT scanning sometimes reveals cerebellar and brainstem atrophy. A T2 weighted MRI may show an abnormal decrease in putaminal signal intensity. PET scanning reveals regional reductions in glucose metabolism in proportion to degenerative involvement.

For many years, only neuronal loss and gliosis had been noted in MSA. Recently, glial cytoplasmic inclusions have been discovered in involved CNS sites.[28,29] These inclusions are sometimes in neurons, but are particularly prominent in oligodendroglial cells. It is noteworthy that Lewy bodies are absent in MSA. The irregularly shaped glial cytoplasmic inclusions in MSA are very different from the round target-shaped Lewy bodies seen in Parkinson's disease. Both Lewy bodies and glial cytoplasmic inclusions contain ubiquitin.

In MSA, there is loss of function of both the sympathetic and parasympathetic nervous systems. Many neurotransmitters in the brain are reduced in MSA. The ultimate cause of MSA remains unknown. Antibodies in cerebrospinal fluid from patients with MSA have been shown to react specifically with the rat locus ceruleus, suggesting an immunologic basis for the degenerative process, but the true significance of this remains unknown.

Therapy for MSA remains inadequate. This movement disorder tends to respond more favorably to anticholinergic drugs than to dopaminergic drugs, but both should be tried with the recognition that the dopaminergic drugs may reduce blood pressure in some individuals. The orthostatic hypotension can be managed through the judicious use of fludrocortisone, midodrine, and epoetin alfa (recombinant erythropoietin). (See Table 4).

The neuropathology of multiple system atrophy was described in 1960 by George Milton Shy (1919–1967), a neurologist in Bethesda, MD and Phildelphia, PA and Glenn Albert Drager (1917–1968), a neurologist in Bethesda, MD and Houston, TX.[30]

Pure Autonomic Failure (Bradbury-Eggleston Syndrome, Idiopathic Orthostatic Hypotension, Idiopathic Autonomic Failure)

Pure autonomic failure is much less common than multiple system atrophy. It is usually unassociated with any central neurological involve-

_____ **Table 4** _____

General Therapeutic Measures for Syncope

1) Avoid diet and cold preparations containing sympathomimetic amines
2) Place head of bed on shock blocks and give bedtime snack
3) Increase salt intake and avoid excessive physical exertion after meals
4) Support garments **that come to the waist** are helpful, especially in winter
5) Air conditioning in summer
6) Swimming (orthostatic hypotension) or running (orthostatic intolerance)
7) Take plenty of fluids (eg, coffee, tea, tomato juice) with meals
8) Fludrocortisone
9) Midodrine
10) Epoetin alfa

ment. Both sympathetic and parasympathetic systems are involved. Presentation includes the Bradbury-Eggleston triad (orthostatic hypotension, impotence, and anhidrosis), nocturia, constipation, urinary retention, anemia, and orthostatic headache.[31–34] Low levels of plasma noradrenaline and its metabolites are seen. There is hypersensitivity to pressor and depressor stimuli. The prognosis in pure autonomic failure is much brighter than in multiple system atrophy. Many patients survive for decades, and most learn to accommodate to their abnormalities in autonomic function.

Samuel Bradbury (1883–1947) was an internist in New York and Philadelphia. Cary Eggleston (1884–1958) was an internist and President of the US Pharmacopeial Convention.[30]

Parkinson's Disease[35,36]

Patients with Parkinson's disease may have autonomic failure with orthostatic hypotension, presumably due to a defect in the central engagement of the autonomic nervous system. Lewy bodies have been reported in sympathetic ganglion cells as well as in the involved structures in the brains of patients with Parkinson's Disease. It is difficult to know how much autonomic failure may occur in Parkinson's disease. Although many such cases are reported in the literature, few have confirmation by autopsy that the disorder truly was Parkinson's disease. It seems likely that many cases of multiple system atrophy were misdiagnosed as Parkinson's disease in the era before careful autopsies differentiating the two syndromes were able to be carried out. Nevertheless, it seems clear that some autonomic failure, usually relatively mild, does occur in Parkinson's disease. This is suggested by relatively low plasma renin activity, as well as a tendency for therapy with levodopa/carbidopa and dopamine agonists to bring out or worsen orthostatic hypotension in patients with Parkinson's disease.

James Parkinson (1755–1824) was a physician and political activist in London, England.

Peripheral Neuropathy

Diabetes Mellitus

Diabetic dysautonomia of mild degree is extremely common in diabetics, and correlates with duration of illness and patient age.[37,38] It is known that hyperglycemia, per se, worsens the dysautonomia.

While all organ systems innervated by autonomic nerves are affected in diabetes, it is the cardiovascular and adrenomedullary abnormalities that have the greatest influence on orthostatic tolerance. One of the earliest signs of insipient abnormalities in cardiovascular regulation is the disappearance of the respiratory variation in heart rate. With more serious involvement, symptoms of orthostatic intolerance associated with postural tachycardia may supervene. As the disorder becomes more severe, outright orthostatic hypotension initially with tachycardia, but ultimately with limited increase in heart rate, may be seen.

In addition, cardiac denervation syndrome, a near total loss of innervation of the heart, leads to greatly increased risk including sudden death, cardiomyopathy, painless myocardial ischemia, poor anesthesia outcome, and complications of pregnancy. Extrasystoles that would be inconsequential in normal subjects may be quite symptomatic in patients with diabetic dysautonomia because these patients may have marginal orthostatic tolerance to begin with. Syncope may therefore occur in such patients at a relatively higher blood pressure than would be seen in many other dysautonomic syndromes.

Amyloidosis

Amyloidosis is caused by the deposition of a homogeneous protein of polypeptide fibrils arranged in pleated sheets.[39–41] The deposits may be widespread and can cause considerable injury in many different tissues. The clinical presentation reflects the organs predominantly involved. A common clinical triad of systemic amyloidosis is a) small fiber neuropathy, b) autonomic neuropathy, and c) carpal tunnel syndrome. Autonomic failure occurs commonly in immunoglobulin-derived amyloidosis and in hereditary systemic amyloidosis. Nerve injury is probably due to the physical pressure exerted by amyloid deposits on neuronal structure. Additional prominent target organs include the heart, the kidney, the liver, the tongue, and the intestine. Diagnosis is by abdominal fat aspiration and/or rectal biopsy with green birefringence under polarized light after Congo red staining.

It is extremely difficult to treat the orthostatic hypotension of amyloidotic dysautonomia. Patients often seem very resistant to pressor agents, whether fludrocortisone or α_1-adrenoreceptor agonists. The reason for this poor response is not entirely clear, but does not appear to be commonly due to antibody binding to the relevant receptor sites.

Management of patients with amyloidotic dysautonomia is particularly difficult because amyloid deposition in the cardiac conduction fiber system can lead to benign and malignant arrhythmias, complicating the assessment of whether orthostatic hypotension or ventricular tachycardia underlies the symptomatic syncopal attacks patients may describe.

Alcohol Neuropathy[42-44]

Alcohol neuropathy is a mixed sensory and motor neuropathy. The onset often occurs as a burning on the soles of feet with prominent dysesthesia. Deep tendon reflexes may be absent. Vagal involvement is particularly likely to occur, and in the severest cases can even include hoarseness. Severe orthostatic hypotension from alcohol neuropathy is uncommon, but the irregular fluid balance encountered in alcoholic patients may lead to hypovolemia that exacerbates the autonomic impairment and makes the orthostatic hypotension a greater problem. Hypothermia and hypotension due to sympathetic trunk degeneration have also been seen.

Porphyria[45,46]

Acute hepatic porphyrias are autosomal dominantly inherited disorders, which may occur as severe life-threatening motor and autonomic neuropathy, abdominal pain, and neuropsychiatric manifestations. They occur in 1/80,000 people. Symptoms of an acute attack include nausea, abdominal pain, vomiting, discomfort in the limbs, urinary frequency, abnormal behavior, and in some cases, convulsions. Cerebrospinal fluid is typically normal.

Autonomic disturbances, when they occur, typically appear early in the course of acute attacks. Sinus tachycardia and blood pressure lability are particularly common. Chronic mild hypertension between attacks is sometimes seen. The combination of abdominal pain and orthostatic hypotension may suggest an addisonian crisis in some individuals if the correct diagnosis is not made. It is rare for severe incapacitating orthostatic hypotension with early syncope to develop in patients with porphyria.

Guillain-Barré Syndrome (Acute Idiopathic Demyelinating Polyradiculopathy)[47,48]

When sought carefully, autonomic abnormalities are common in the Guillain-Barré syndrome.[49,50] The full gamut of autonomic failure may appear in severely affected patients. The most common cardiovascular abnormalities encountered in the Guillain-Barré syndrome include sinus tachycardia, worsened dramatically by upright posture, and occasionally more serious arrhythmias of either supraventricular or ventricular origin. Sometimes paroxysmal hypertension is also seen, and abnormalities of afferent baroreflex pathways have also been encountered. Hypotension, both supine and orthostatic, can be seen. Significant orthostatic hypotension probably occurs in approximately 25% of patients, and is most likely due to demyelination of peripheral sympathetic pathways. In such cases, most autonomic function tests are abnormal. Autonomic involvement tends to improve when the muscle symptoms improve. There is a highly variable prognosis, with children usually having milder illness than adults.

Georges Guillain (1876-1961) was a Professor of Neurology in Paris, France, and Jean Alexander Barré (1880-1967) was a Strasbourg neurologist.

Sjögren's Syndrome (Keratoconjunctivitis Sicca)[51]

Symptoms of Sjögren's syndrome include dryness of the eyes, ears, nose, mouth, and vagina, sometimes with associated renal tubular acidosis, mononeuritis multiplex, achlorhydria, and associated autoimmune disorders. Dysautonomia of mild degree is relatively common, either from ganglionitis or cumulative mononeuritis multiplex lesions involving autonomic areas. Over a period of years, the clinical picture may be dominated by the loss of sensory function including proprioceptive reflexes, and autonomic impairment. Cases of severe orthostatic hypotension occasionally develop. The most common presentation of autonomic impairment in Sjögren's syndrome is orthostatic tachycardia in the setting of orthostatic intolerance.

Henrik Samuel Conrad Sjögren (1899-1973) was an ophthalmologist in Stockholm and Göteberg, Sweden.

Dopamine-β-Hydroxylase (DBH) Deficiency

DBH deficiency is extremely rare, but it is important to recognize because it is so easily treated.[52-55] Fewer than 20 patients with DBH deficiency have been recognized so far. They have presented with lifelong orthostatic hypotension, ptosis of the eyelids, nasal stuffiness, and in males, retrograde ejaculation. There is often a history of stillbirth among siblings. The diagnosis is made by the absence or near absence of norepinephrine and its metabolites in blood, cerebrospinal fluid, and urine. Dopamine and its metabolites are elevated. A dopamine/norepinephrine ratio in blood of 1 is highly suggestive of DBH deficiency, and a ratio of 10 is pathognomonic. Hypomagnesemia, hyperprolactinemia, and atrial fibrillation are sometimes seen.

Monoamine Oxidase Deficiency

Monoamine oxidase deficiency was originally described in association with Norrie's syndrome, an X-linked disorder due to one or more gene deletions near MAO A and MAO B.[56] Absence of the Norrie disease gene leads to an X-linked congenital blindness, sometimes accompanied by mild mental retardation and progressive hearing loss. Patients with both Norrie syndrome and monoamine oxidase deficiency seem to differ from Norrie patients primarily in that they have severe mental retardation, flushing, hypotension, seizures, and poor growth. These individuals are noncommunicative and may have hypertensive crises in response to dietary tyramine intake. The full clinical spectrum of monoamine oxidase deficiency in its pure form remains inadequately understood.[57-59]

The urine, cerebrospinal fluid (CSF), and plasma demonstrate very low levels of methoxyhydroxyphenylglycol (MHPG), the deaminated norepinephrine metabolite, as well as elevated levels of normetanephrine, and very high levels of phenylethylamine.[60] When the chromosomal deletion spares the monoamine oxidase A gene, the phenotype is not associated with any obvious symptoms. Males who have complete loss of monoamine oxidase A may demonstrate aggressiveness with stress, sensitivity to dietary amines, and a shortened life span owing to cardiovascular complications.

Lisker's Syndrome[61]

Lisker's syndrome is a slowly progressing distal muscle weakness and atrophy that starts in childhood and advances to autonomic dysfunction characterized by excessive sweating, distal cyanosis in cold weather, and ultimately orthostatic hypotension and achalasia by the third decade of life. An abnormality in cholinergic innervation has been proposed as the etiology. Nonspecific demyelinization has been observed in some patients with this disorder. The precise nature and cause of this disorder and its relation to other disorders remains to be elucidated.

Anand's Syndrome

A single case of Anand's syndrome is reported in a 30-year-old woman with undetectable plasma norepinephrine, epinephrine, dopamine and DBH in a setting of life-long severe orthostatic hypotension.[62] A biopsy reveals absent tyrosine hydroxylase and neuropeptide Y in sympathetic neurons and absence of substance P and calcitonin gene-related peptide (CGRP) in sensory neurons. Sural nerve biopsy also shows loss of myelinated fibers. The constellation of changes and the relative dearth of nerve growth factor (NGF) in tissue suggests a syndrome due to loss of the trophic action of NGF.

Spinal Cord Lesions

Subacute Combined Degeneration (Vitamin B$_{12}$ Deficiency)

Vitamin B$_{12}$ deficiency may occasionally present with subacute combined degeneration of the spinal cord, with or without macrocytic anemia.[63,64] There may be paresthesias of hands and feet together with unsteadiness of gait. There may also be mental slowing, depression, hallucinations, and presence of a positive Romberg sign. Deep tendon reflexes may be decreased. Visual loss is rare. When there is autonomic involvement, it may appear as orthostatic hypotension, which has occasionally been severe.

Acute worsening by nitrous oxide anesthesia ("anesthesia paresthetica") may occur.

Syringomyelia

In syringomyelia, there is development of a long cystic cavity within the substance of the spinal cord. While it sometimes extends over only a few segments, it may extend far up and down the cord. When it involves the medulla, it is referred to as syringobulbia. In some cases, the cavity involves the anterior horns of the gray matter. The cavity wall usually demonstrates only gliosis. While primary syringomyelia seems to be a developmental abnormality, secondary syringomyelia may develop in response to tumor, trauma, or ischemia of the spinal cord. Patients present with loss of temperature and pain, but with intact proprioception. The lower motor neuron weakness can be characterized by flaccid paralysis, atrophy, and fasciculations. Horner's syndrome due to sympathetic nerve damage is sometimes seen in the setting of syringomyelia, and orthostatic hypotension may occur if there is more widespread sympathetic involvement.

Conditions Leading to Isolated Cerebral Ischemia

Atherosclerosis

Atherosclerosis may involve any artery in the central nervous system. When this involvement crucially impairs blood flow to the brain, syncope may result.[65] One of the most insidious forms of atherosclerosis is vertebrobasilar insufficiency. Involvement of the vertebrobasilar system leads to vertigo, lightheadedness, memory change, syncope, aphasia and/or dysphasia. Patients with these syndromes are particularly liable to neurological symptoms in the face of influences that reduce overall blood pressure, in which case cerebral blood flow may be particularly compromised.

Takayasu's Disease (Pulseless Disease)

Takayasu's disease is a large vessel vasculitis that usually affects the aortic arch but may also involve the lower portions of the aorta.[66] It is the cause of 30% of cases of renovascular hypertension in Japan, but it appears to be much less common in the United States. Takayasu's arteritis may respond to glucocorticoids, cytotoxic agents, and in appropriate circumstances, surgical intervention.

Mikoto Takayashu (1860-1938) was a professor of ophthalmology in Kanazawa, Japan.

Subclavian Steal Syndrome (Millikan-Siekert Syndrome)

In basilar artery insufficiency due to subclavian steal, exercise of the left arm precipitates neurological symptoms including syncope, facial paresthesia, headache, and transient blindness. Subclavian steal syndrome is due to reversed blood flow from the vertebrobasilar system into the subclavian system.[67]

Innominate Artery Syndrome

Innominate artery syndrome is the partial occlusion of the innominate artery, usually by atherosclerosis. It may lead to lightheadedness, memory change, syncope, diplopia, visual impairment, seizures, and motor/sensory involvement. This disorder can be ruled out by careful monitoring of blood pressure in all extremities.

Paroxysmal Disorders

Seizures

Seizure is a rare cause of syncope.[68,69] In most cases, seizure remains a historical diagnosis. The presence of a prolonged aura or of postictal confusion helps to confirm the diagnosis of seizure. The diagnostic yield of a single interictal EEG in known epileptics is only about 50%, while 1% to 2% of asymptotic adults have EEG findings that may suggest seizure. For these reasons, standard EEG should not be part of the routine evaluation of syncope.

Absence Seizures

Typical absence seizures occur in young children may be precipitated by hyperventilation; they usually improve with age. Absence seizures are sudden in onset and usually last 5 to 6 seconds. They interrupt activity such as chewing, walking, and talking and they are not followed by postictal confusion. The patient is usually unaware of having had a seizure. In some cases, tone may be lost and the patient may fall. The EEG is characterized by generalized three-per-second spike and slow wave activity.

Atonic Seizures

Atonic seizures (drop attacks) usually begin in childhood; new onset atonic seizures in adults are extremely rare. The episodes are characterized by the abrupt loss of tone. This usually lasts only a few seconds. Patients are at high risk for injury due to the suddenness of the fall (rarely seen in cardiogenic causes of syncope). Loss of consciousness is very brief and may not be noticed by the patient or a witness. There is little if any postictal confusion.

Akinetic Seizures

Like atonic seizures, akinetic seizures are of abrupt onset, brief, and without postictal confusion. Although patients with atonic seizures remain motionless and have impaired consciousness, tone is preserved.

Partial-Complex Seizures

Of all the partial-complex seizure types, frontal lobe seizures are the most likely to be misdiagnosed as cardiogenic syncope.[70] All frontal lobe seizures may begin abruptly, be brief in duration, and be associated with little postictal confusion. Although they may cause loss of tone and consciousness, stereotypies, complex motor gestures, or hallucinations may provide historical clues to their epileptic origin. Unlike the generalized seizures discussed above, frontal lobe seizures are commonly of adult onset.

Disorders of Presumed Central Dysregulation

Bruns' Syndrome

In Bruns' syndrome there is sudden development of neurological symptoms, usually on extension of the neck.[71,72] Symptoms include amaurosis fugax, flashes of light, irregular breathing, and occasionally apnea and syncope. Vertigo, headache, and vomiting commonly occur. The etiology is most commonly an organic lesion of the fourth ventricle, usually a tumor or cyst, which obstructs flow of cerebrospinal fluid or disturbs the vestibular nuclei. It is noteworthy that some of the most important structures involved in cardiovascular regulation occur in close proximity to the fourth ventricle. These structures include the nucleus of the solitary tract (NTS), and the area postrema; the glossopharyngeal and vagal afferents conveying baroreflex and cardiopulmonary input impinge on the nucleus of the solitary tract near this site.

L. von Bruns (1858-1916) was a neurologist in Hannover, Germany.

Autonomic Epilepsy

Autonomic epilepsy is a rare and poorly characterized syndrome characterized by transient paroxysms of hypertension, tachycardia, and flushing.[73] Pheochromocytoma must be ruled out in these patients. Autonomic epilepsy closely resembls baroreflex failure. Plasma catecholamines rise to high levels during spells. Clonidine therapy is helpful. The seizure focus appears to be in the temporal lobe.

Baroreflex Failure

Baroreflex failure is a poorly described heterogeneous condition whose clinical manifestation depends on the distribution, severity, and duration of the insult.[74-80] It is usually due to trauma, tumor, or surgery in the brainstem, neck, or chest. With acute complete baroreflex denervation, blood pressure and heart rate rise precipitously with wakefulness, anxiety, and stress. Blood pressures of 280/160 mm Hg may be seen. On the other hand, during sedation or sleep, blood pressure may decline well into the normal range. Orthostatic hypotension is not marked in such presents, if it is present at all. With chronic baroreflex failure, some orthostatic hypotension is occasionally seen.[81,82] Clonidine may have a marked vasodepressor effect in these patients who also have baroreflex failure. The plasma norepinephrline is often in the 1000 to 2000 pg/mL range during hypertensive episodes. With unilateral baroreflex involvement, little or no clinical abnormalities are seen, but when the right vagus nerve is damaged, tachycardia may occur because of loss of parasympathetic tone in the sinoatrial node.

Penfield's Syndrome[83]

Penfield's syndrome occurs in males, starting in childhood, in whom seizures have an autonomic character: facial congestion, salivation, sweating, tearing, apparent exothalmos, tachycardia, hyperventilation, restlessness, and hypertension. Third ventricle tumor is reported to induce the disorder. It is similar to autonomic epilepsy.

Wallenberg's Syndrome[84]

Wallenberg's syndrome is a thrombosis of the posterior inferior cerebellar artery. This generally involves the dorsolateral medulla and presents with vertigo, vomiting, dysphagia, diplopia, and loss of temperature sensitivity on the ipsilateral side of the face with contralateral hypoesthesia for pain and temperature in the extremities and trunk. In the setting of Wallenberg's syndrome there is ipsilateral ptosis and enophthalmos together with miosis. In some individuals, following this lesion, we have observed chronic orthostatic hypotension.

A. Wallenberg (1862-1949) was a German neurologist.

Williams-Bashore Syndrome[85]

There is a single case report of Williams-Bashore syndrome in a 50 year old who had frequent (up to multiple times daily) episodes of lightheadedness without premonitory signs. Between attacks (which lasted minutes to hours), blood pressure was normal. During the attack, noradrenaline fell and bradycardia and hypotension were marked. There was no evidence of damage to carotid sinus or glossopharyngeal nerve (see Carotid Sinus Syncope and Weisenburg's Syndrome).

Paroxysmal Reflex Activation

Bezold-Jarisch Reflex Activation

Bezold-Jarisch reflex activation is characterized by bradycardia, hypotension, and nausea elicited by reflex receptors in the left ventricle, particularly in the inferior distribution of that chamber.[86,87] The reflex can be elicited by enhanced contractility and by stretch of receptors. This reflex probably accounts for the bradycardia and hypotension sometimes encountered in acute inferior myocardial infarction, in aortic stenosis, and in coronary artery spasm in the distribution of the inferior left ventricular wall. The hypotension seen with veratrum alkaloids may also depend on this reflex.

A. von Bezold (1836-1868) was a professor of physiology in Würzburg, Germany. A. Jarisch (1850-1902) was a professor of dermatology in Graz, Austria.

Carotid Sinus Syncope

This disorder is also called glossopharyngeal syncope or Weiss-Baker syndrome.[88] Hypotension and bradycardia are induced by neck pressure, a tight collar, turning of the head, shaving, swallowing, or they can occur spontaneously. The clinical picture may be dominated by the hypotension, the bradycardia, or by both. The form in which bradycardia predominates may be improved by a demand pacemaker. Approximately 20% of patients with carotid sinus syncope ultimately require surgical denervation of the nerve. Occasionally, symptoms of headache, dizziness, vertigo, paresthesias, homonymous hemianopsia, and hemiplegia are said to occur in the absence of measured blood pressure or heart rate changes; it is usually referred to as the Weiss-Baker syndrome, but the validity of this presentation is not established.[89]

Weisenburg's Syndrome (Glossopharyngeal Neuralgia)

Weisenburg's syndrome is commonly referred to as glossopharyngeal neuralgia.[90] In this disorder, severe paroxysmal pain occurs, beginning in the tonsillar region, lateral pharynx, or base of the tongue, and radiating deeply into the ear. It may be elicited by eating or talking. It results in sinus bradycardia and hypotension, sometimes with recurrent episodes of syncope. (See Williams-Bashore Syndrome).

Cough Syncope

Cough syncope is also called Charcot's vertigo,[91] tussive syncope, and laryngeal epilepsy. In cough syncope, sudden syncope without sequelae occurs during a paroxysm of heavy coughing. A burning or tingling of the larynx may precede the cough. It most typically occurs in obese individuals and those with emphysema or bronchial asthma. Convulsions occur in less than 10% of cases.

Defecation Syncope[92]

Defecation syncope is sinus bradycardia, often associated with AV block or hypotension on sudden decompression of the rectum or during removal of an impaction. It is described primarily in elderly and bedfast patients.

Diver's Syncope[93]

Diver's syncope is the loss of consciousness during diving. It is probably related to the diving reflex, which may sometimes elicit bradycardia or heart block. This reflex can be tested by placing a cold wet face cloth over the forehead while monitoring heart rate and blood pressure.

Breath-Holding Spells

Breath-holding spells represent an involuntary response to an adverse stimuli.[94] They represent a familial disorder that occurs in almost 5% of children. Episodes usually begin before age 18 months, but can have an onset as late as 3 years of age. The spells spontaneously end by age 8. Cyanotic and pallid types have been described.

Cyanotic Breath-Holding Spells

Cyanotic breath-holding spells are typically provoked by anger, frustration, or fear. The child abruptly stops breathing in expiration (usually while crying), and cyanosis rapidly develops. This is followed by loss of tone and consciousness. There is no effective medical treatment for these spells, but it is important to explain to the parents that the episodes are benign and will eventually resolve.

Pallid Breath-Holding Spells

Pallid breath-holding spells represent a reflex asytole that is usually provoked by an unexpected painful event. Instead of crying, the patient becomes pallid and loses tone and consciousness. Following a spell, the child often falls asleep and is normal upon awakening. As with the cyanotic type, there is no effective treatment for pallid breath-holding spells, and the episodes resolve spontaneously with age.

Neurohumoral Disorders

Allgrove's Syndrome[95]

The full syndrome is a familial glucocorticoid deficiency, achalasia, and alacrima, with addisonian symptoms and achalasia that tend to develop later in life. Inheritance is recessive. In patients with Allgrove's syndrome there is an absent zona fasciculata in the adrenal, but the zona glomerulosa is essentially normal.

Ulick's Syndrome

Ulick's syndrome is a form of aldosterone deficiency that occurs primarily in Iranian Jews.[96,97] In Ulick's syndrome there is autosomal recessive inheritance presenting as hypotension that is life threatening to children, but which may resolve into postural hypotension in adults. This is due to deficiency of 18-dehydrogenase.

Verner-Morrison Syndrome[98]

This disorder presents as watery diarrhea associated with an islet cell tumor and electrolyte abnormalities. It is sometimes called pancreatic cholera. It may occur with bronchogenic carcinoma or MEN I. Secretion of vasoactive intestinal polypeptide (VIP) is usually etiologic. In 84% of cases, the origin is the pancreas. A metabolic acidosis is usually present in Verner-Morrison syndrome.

Hyperbradykininism (Streeten's Syndrome)[99]

In hyperbradykininism lightheadedness and an orthostatic fall in pulse pressure are attended by tachycardia, purplish discoloration of legs on standing, and erythema of face and neck. High blood levels of bradykinin are described. Improvement is reported with fludrocortisone, cyproheptadine, and propranolol.

Mastocytosis[100–101]

This disorder is due to an increased numbers of mast cells or an increased responsiveness of mast cells. Release of histamine and prostaglandin D_2 dominate the clinical picture. Characteristic chronic skin changes (erythematous acneform papular lesions) are seen in a minority of patients, but red flushing and urticaria are common during attacks. Palpitations with or without chest pain, headaches, nausea, vomiting, diarrhea, and dyspnea may occur. Perhaps 25% of cases are familial (autosomal dominant). Some patients have severe attacks with hypotension that must be treated by epinephrine infusion, but increases in blood pressure are also seen. During severe attacks, disturbances in mental status may seem out of proportion to the hypotension. Sometimes enough heparin is released to raise the partial thromboplastin time.

Pheochromocytoma[102–104]

Pheochromocytoma is a catecholamine-producing tumor of chromaffin origin. In its most common manifestation, pheochromocytoma is characterized by paroxysmal hypertension, sweating, palpitations, and headache. In addition, significant numbers of patients experience weight loss, nausea, tremor, abdominal discomfort, chest pain, hyperglycemia, pallor during attacks, and anxiety. Approximately 4% of patients present with orthostatic hypotension. This presents a diagnositc problem because most physicians do not consider pheochromocytoma in their differential diagnosis of syncope. It is important to recognize that some individuals will have profound orthostatic hypotension with no evidence of elevated blood pressure in spite of having pheochromocytoma with substantial levels of plasma and urinary associated with elevated catecholamines and their metabolites. This has been seen in patients, both young and old, with pheochromocytoma. It may be more common in those producing predominantly epinephrine.

Among patients with hypertension, orthostatic fall in blood pressure is particularly common in patients with pheochromocytoma. With treatment using metyrosine or phenoxybenzamine, this orthostatic fall in blood pressure may become extremely symptomatic. Orthostatic hypotension usually limits the amount of phenoxybenzamine we are able to give to patients with pheochromocytoma. Inasmuch as blood volume is usually reduced in pheochromocytoma, vigorous volume replacement and liberal salt intake will attenuate symptomatic orthostatic hypotension in pheochromocytoma patients receiving phenoxybenzamine or metyrosine.

Pheochromocytoma is also seen in von Recklinghausen's disease and von Hippel-Lindau disease. Approximately 5% of patients with pheochromocytoma have neurofibromatosis (von Recklinghausen's disease). Among all patients with von Recklinghausen's disease, only approximately 1% have pheochromocytoma. There is also an increased incidence of renovascular hypertension in von Recklinghausen's disease (due to neurofibromatous infiltration of renal artery or external impingement). The neurofibromatosis may involve peripheral nerves, central nervous system neurons, or visceral nerves; neurofibromas may undergo malignant sacromatous degeneration.

Hyperepinephrinemia[105]

Patients with hyperepinephrinemia present with palpitations, nervousness, weakness, lightheadedness, hot sensation, pallor, and tremors. Three of five reported cases had orthostatic hypotension. Supine blood pressure in these patients ranged from 100/64 to 166/82 with heart rate from 68 to 100 bpm. Plasma epinephrines ranged from 0.3 to 4.2 nmol/L. Pheochromocytoma was ruled out. β-blockade was helpful, as was unilateral adrenalectomy in two patients with adrenal cysts.

Miscellaneous Hemodynamic Disorders

Analbuminemia[106]

This uncommon disorder is characterized by defective synthesis of albumin, probably with autosomal recessive inheritance. Affected individuals have mild persistent edema, sometimes associated with hypotension and mild diarrhea. Protein electrophoresis shows absence of the albumin band, and serum osmolality is reduced by 50%.

Bouveret's Syndrome[107]

This disorder is more commonly, and perhaps more usefully, called idiopathic paroxysmal atrial tachycardia. The initial attack usually occurs in the second to fourth decades of life. Onset is usually sudden, and is occasionally precipitated by emotion, alcohol, caffeine, or sleep deprivation. There may be pain in the throat, anxiety, dyspnea, sweating, gastrointestinal symptoms, and during or following the attack, polyuria. The disorder is occasionally associated with biliary tract disease. Its incidence is relatively high in patients with orthostatic intolerance, or at least its hemodynamic consequences are more serious in this popoulation.

McKittrick-Wheelock Syndrome[108]

Also called colonic villous adenoma, this disorder is characterized by severe dehydration and electrolyte imbalance. BUN may reach 200 mg/dL, but it often returns to near normal with fluid replacement. Orthostatic hypotension may occur and is usually profound.

Schroeder's Syndrome[109]

Schroeder's syndrome is a hyponatremia syndrome in congestive heart failure patients who are treated with excessive diuresis. It is manifested by thirst, anorexia, nausea, orthostatic hypotension, and syncope. Oliguria is common. Schroeder's syndrome is now less common than it was in the past because of improved pharmacology for heart failure.

Short's Syndrome[110]

Short's syndrome is a bradycardia-tachycardia syndrome. It is a result of an abnormal sinus node that is susceptible to excessive suppressive influence of ectopic atrial activity. It usually occurs in women over age 60. More than half of these patients may experience syncope.

Roenheld's Syndrome[111]

Roenheld's syndrome is postprandial angina. Following food ingestion, patients with this disorder may experience chest pain with associated ST-T wave changes. Tachycardia or bradycardia may occur. Atropine is said to be therapeutic, and caffeine has been found to be beneficial.

Supine Hypotension Syndrome

This is an inferior vena cava syndrome. It occurs in the last month of pregnancy in as many as 10% of pregnant women. In supine hypotension syndrome there is a sudden fall in systolic blood pressure, accompanied by nausea and vomiting on assumption of the supine position. This is associated with tachycardia and is believed to be due to compression of the inferior vena cava by the pregnant uterus, which decreases venous return and hence decreases cardiac output.

Nonsyncopal Entities

Bárány Syndrome (Benign Positional Vertigo)[112,113]

Bárány syndrome is a paroxysmal positional vertigo. Periodic recurrences of paroxysms of vertigo occur when the patient is moved from sitting to recumbency or from recumbency to sitting. The paroxysm of vertigo causes the patient to wish to return to the previous posture, at which time nystagmus occurs for 10 to 15 seconds. Repetition of the maneuver leads to extinction for a period of time. There are no hearing abnormalities associated with this disorder. The condition is benign if falling injuries are avoided. Nevertheless, the first attack is often very frightening to the patient.

Robert Bárány (1876-1936) was a Viennese physician who pioneered the use of syringing ears to induce nystagmus; He was a Nobel Laureate and ultimately a professor of otology in Uppsala, Sweden.

Cataplexy

Cataplexy is muscular hypotonia and partial paralysis that affects primarily the face, jaw, and neck muscles, but also the truncal and limb muscles. Cataplexy is frequently seen in narcolepsy. Cataplectics may fall suddenly, injure themselves, and be unable to open their eyes, speak, or move. Respiration and consciousness, however, are not usually compromised. Laughter, anger, fright, joy, and coughing are common precipitants of cataplexy.

Gélineau's Syndrome (Narcolepsy)[114–117]

Narcolepsy, or Gélineau's syndrome, is characterized by sudden episodes of sleep-like state. Such bouts of excessive sleepiness last from a few seconds to over 30 minutes. Patients may fall asleep in highly inappropriate circumstances such as while driving or while speaking. In approximately 75% of cases, there is associated loss of muscle control, called cataplexy, which may cause the whole body to become flaccid or in some cases only cause the head to nod. Hypnogogic hallucinations, both visual and auditory, may be present. In approximately 60% of patients, there are bouts of sleep paralysis, during which the patient is unable to move for several minutes at the time of entry into sleep or awakening from sleep. Narcolepsy occurs with an incidence of 1/2000. Onset is usually between puberty and age 25. The disease tends to progress. Diagnosis is extremely difficult. While it was once believed that the disease was more common in men than women, recent studies seem to suggest a more nearly equal incidence between the genders. The social problems associated with narcolepsy are considerable. Recent research has focused on an autoimmune etiology in addition to a genetic component. Identical twins have only 20% coincidence of narcolepsy. It has been suggested that the human leukocyte antigen gene may be involved in the disorder.

Therapy is usually at least partially successful for 75% of patients. Amphetamine agents such as methylphenidate and dextroamphetamine, with or without antidepressant agents, are sometimes used. Modafinil (Cephalon, Inc.) is an experimental drug that appears to be of benefit with fewer side effects than the stimulant agents.

J.B.E. Gélineau (1859-?) Was a French physician.

References

1. Benarroch EE. Central nervous system disorders. In: Robertson D, Polinsky RJ, Low P (eds): *Primer on the Autonomic Nervous System*. San Diego: Academic Press; 1996;229–233.
2. Mosqueda-Garcia R. Central autonomic regulation. In: Robertson D, Polinsky RJ, Low P. (eds): *Primer on the Autonomic Nervous System.*San Diego: Academic Press; 1996;3–25.
3. Talman WT. Cardiovascular regulation and lesions of the central nervous system. *Ann Neurol* 1983;18:1–12.
4. Low P (ed): *Evaluation and Management of Clinical Autonomic Disorders*. Boston: Little, Brown; 1992.
5. Bannister R, Mathias CJ (eds): *Autonomic Failure, 3rd Edition*. New York: Oxford University Press; 1992;1–953.
6. Korczyn AD. *Handbook of Autonomic Nervous System Dysfunction* New York: Marcel Dekker Inc.; 1995;1–567.
7. Gowers WR. *Epilepsy and Other Chronic Convulsive Diseases: Their Causes, Symptoms and Treatments*. New York: William Wood and Company; 1881;1–255.
8. Gowers WR. *The Border-Land of Epilepsy*. Philadelphia: P. Blakiston's Son & Co.; 1907;1–121.
9. Sharpey-Schafer EP. Emergencies in general practice: Syncope. *Br Med J* 1956;1:506–509.
10. Van Lieshout JJ, Wieling W, Karemaker JM, Eckberg DL. The vasovagal response. *Clin Sci* 1991;81:575–586.
11. Grubb BP, Temesy-Armos P, Hahn H, Elliott L. Utility of upright tilt-table testing in the evaluation and management of syncope of unknown origin. *Am J Med* 1991;90:6–10.
12. Rossen R, Kabat H, Anderson JP. Acute arrest of cerebral circulation in man. *Arch Neurol Psychiatr* 1943;50:510–528.
13. Lempert T, Bauer M, Schimdt D. Syncope: A videometric analysis of 56 episodes of transient cerebral hypoxia. *Ann Neurol* 1994;36:233–237.
14. Grubb BP, Samoil D, Kosinsky DJ, et al. Cerebral Syncope: Loss of consciousness associated with cerebral vasoconstriction in the absence of systemic hypotension. *Pacing Clin Electrophyiol* (in press).
15. Jacob G, Atkinson D, Shannon JR, et al. Evidence of cerebral blood flow abnormalities in idiopathic hyperadrenergic state. Submitted, 1996.

16. Streeten DHP, Scullard TF. Excessive gravitational blood pooling caused by impaired venous tone is the predominant non-cardiac mechanism of orthostatic intolerance. *Clin Sci* 1996;90:277–285.
17. Jacob G, Ertl AC, Robertson RM, Robertson D. Dynamic orthostatic hypovolemia. *J Invest Med* (in press).
18. Jacob G, Costa F, Furlan R, et al. Adrenoreceptor function in orthostatic intolerance. *J Invest Med* (in press).
19. Jacob G, Mosqueda-Garcia R, Ertl A, et al. Hyporeninemic hypovolemia: An etiology of orthostatic hypotension. *Clin Auton Res* 1995;5:319.
20. Jacob G, Mosqueda-Garcia R, Ertl AC, et al. Hyporeninemia: A novel form of orthostatic intolerance. *J Invest Med* (in press).
21. Low PA, Schondorf R. Postural tachycardia syndrome. In: Robertson D, Low PA, Polinsky RJ (eds): *Primer on the Autonomic Nervous System*. San Diego: Academic Press; 1996;279–283.
22. Fouad FM. Idiopathic hypovolemia. In: Robertson D, Low PA, Polinsky RJ (eds): *Primer on the Autonomic Nervous System*. San Diego: Academic Press; 1996;286–289.
23. Coghlan HC. Orthostatic intolerance: Mitral valve prolapse. In: Robertson D, Low PA, Polinsky RJ (eds): *Primer on the Autonomic Nervous System* San Diego: Academic Press; 1996;283–286.
24. Shy GM, Drager GA. A neurological syndrome associated with orthostatic hypotension. *Arch Neurol* 1960;2:522–527.
25. Oppenheimer D. Neuropathology and neurochemistry of autonomic failure. A. Neuropathology of autonomic failure. In: Bannister R (ed): *Autonomic Failure*. London: Oxford University Press; 1988;451–463.
26. Polinsky RJ. Shy-Drager syndrome. In: J. Jankovic J, Tolosa E (eds): *Parkinson's Disease and Movement Disorders, 2nd Edition*. Baltimore: Williams and Wilkins; 1993;191–204.
27. Polinsky RJ. Neurochemical and pharmacological abnormalities in chronic autonomic failure syndromes. In: Low P (ed): *Evaluation and Management of Clinical Autonomic Disorders*. Boston: Little, Brown; 1992;537–549.
28. Papp MI, Kahn JE, Lantos PL. Glial cytoplasmic inclusions in the CNS of patients with multiple system atrophy (striatonigral degeneration, olivopontocerebellar atrophy and Shy-Drager syndrome). *J Neurol Sci* 1989;94:79–100.
29. Tamaoka A, Mizusawa H, Mori H, Shoji S. Ubiquitinated αB-crystallin in glial cytoplasmic inclusions from the brain of a patient with multiple system atrophy. *J Neurol Sci* 1995;129:192–198.
30. Robertson D. Introduction. In: Robertson D, Biaggioni I (eds): *Disorders of the Autonomic Nervous System*. London: Harwood Academic Press; 1995;1–8.
31. Bradbury S, Eggleston C. Postural hypotension: Report of three cases. *Am Heart J* 1925;1:73–86.
32. Freeman R. Pure autonomic failure. In: Robertson D, Biaggioni I. (eds): *Disorders of the Autonomic Nervous System*. London: Harwood Academic Press; 1995;83–105.
33. Ziegler M, Lake C, Kopin I. The sympathetic nervous system defect in primary orthostatic hypotension. *N Engl J Med* 1977;296:293–297.
34. Onrot J, Goldberg MR, Hollister AS, et al. Management of chronic orthostatic hypotension. *Am J Med* 1986;80:454–464.
35. Parkinson J. *An Essay on the Shaking Palsy*. London: Sherwood Neely-Jones; 1817.
36. Davis TL. Parkinson's disease. In: Robertson D, Low PA, Polinsky RJ (eds): *Primer on the Autonomic Nervous System*. San Diego: Academic Press; 1996;219–221.
37. Pfeifer M. Diabetic autonomic failure. In: Robertson D, Low PA, Polinsky RJ (eds): *Primer on the Autonomic Nervous System*. San Diego: Academic Press; 1996;260–266.

248 • SYNCOPE: MECHANISMS AND MANAGEMENT

38. Ward J, Goto Y, (eds): *Diabetic Neuropathy.* New York: Wiley; 1990.
39. Benson MD. Amyloidosis. In: Scriver CR, Beaudet AL (eds): *The Molecular and Metabolic Basis of Inherited Disease, 7th Edition.* New York: McGraw-Hill; 1995.
40. Haan J, Peters WG. Amyloid and peripheral nervous system disease. *Clin Neurol Neurosurg* 1994;96:1–9.
41. Niklasson U, Olofsson BO, Bjerle P. Autonomic neuropathy in familial amyloidotic polyneuropathy. *Acta Neurol Scand* 1989;79:182–187.
42. Novak DJ, Victor M. The vagus and sympathetic nerves in alcoholic polyneuropathy. *Arch Neurol* 1974;30:273–284.
43. Charness ME, Simon RP, Greenberg DA. Ethanol and the nervous system. *N Engl J Med* 1989;321:442–454.
44. Low PA, McLeod JG. The autonomic neuropathies. In: Low PA (ed): *Clinical Autonomic Disorders.* Boston: Little, Brown; 1993;395–422.
45. Desnick RJ, Anderson K. Heme biosynthesis and its disorders: The porphyrias and sideroblastic anemias. In: Hoffman R, Ben EJ, Shattil Sj, et al (eds): *Hematology, Basic Principals and Practice.* New York: Churchill Livingstone; 1991;350–367.
46. Harati Y, Low PA. Autonomic peripheral neuropathies: Diagnosis and clinical presentation. In: Appel SH (ed): *Current Neurology.* Chicago: Year Book Medical Publishers; 1990;105–176.
47. Landry JBO. Note sur la paralysie ascendante aigue. *Gaz Hebd Med Chir* 1859;6:472–474 and 486-488.
48. Guillain G, Barré JA, Strohl A. Le réflexe médico-plantaire: Étude de ses caracteres graphiques et de son temps perdu. *Bull Soc Med Hop Paris* 1915-1916;40:1459–1462.
49. Zochodne DW. Autonomic involvement in Guillain-Barré syndrome. A review. *Muscle Nerve* 1994;17:1154–1155.
50. Tuck RR, McLeod JG. Autonomic dysfunction in Guillain-Barré syndrome. *J Neurol Neurosurg Psychiatry* 1981;44:983–990.
51. Sjögren HSC. Zur Kenntnis der Keratoconjunctivitis sicca. *Acta Ophthal* (Kbn) 1933;(suppl II):1–151.
52. Robertson D, Goldberg MR, Hollister AS, et al. Isolated failure of autonomic noradrenergic neurotransmission: Evidence for impaired beta-hydroxylation of dopamine. *N Engl J Med* 1986;314:1494–1497.
53. Man in't Veld AJ, Boomsma F, Moleman P, Schalekamp MADH. Congenital dopamine-β-hydroxylase deficiency: A novel orthostatic syndrome. *Lancet* 1987;1:183–187.
54. Robertson D. Genetics and molecular biology of hypotension. *Curr Opinion in Neurol* 1994;3:13–24.
55. van den Meiracker AH, Boomsma F, Man in't Veld AJ. Dopamine-β-hydroxylase deficiency. In: Robertson D, Low PA, Polinsky RJ (eds): *Primer on the Autonomic Nervous System.* San Diego: Academic Press; 1996;205–208.
56. Sims K, de la Chappelle A, Norio R, et al. Monoamine oxidase deficiency in males with an X chromosome deletion. *Neuron* 1990;2:1069–1076.
57. Hsu Y-PP, Powell JF, Sims KB, Breakefield XO. Molecular genetics of the monoamine oxidases. *J Neurochem* 1989;53:12–18.
58. Brunner HG, Nelen M, Breakefield XO, et al. Abnormal behavior associated with a point mutation in the structural gene for monoamine oxidase A. *Science* 1993;262:578–580.
59. Brunner HG, Nellen MR, van Zandvoort NGGM, et al. X-linked borderline mental retardation with prominent behavioral disturbance: Phenotype, genetic localization and evidence for disturbed monoamine metabolism. *Am J Hum Gene* 1993;52:1032–1039.

60. Murphy DL, Sims KB, Karoum F, et al. Marked amine and amine metabolite changes in Norrie disease patients with an X chromosomal deletion affecting monoamine oxidase. *J Neurochem* 1990;54:242–247.

61. Lisker R, Garcia G, de la Rosa-Laris C, et al. Peripheral motor neuropathy associated with autonomic dysfunction in two sisters: New hereditary syndrome? *Am J Med Genet* 1981;9:255–259.

62. Anand P, Rudge P, Mathias CJ, et al. New autonomic and sensory neuropathy with loss of adrenergic sympathetic function and sensory neuropeptides. *Lancet* 1991;337:1253–1254.

63. Green R, Kinsella LJ. Current concepts in the diagnosis of cobalamin deficiency. *Neurology* 1995;45:1435–1440.

64. McCombe PA, McLeod JG. The peripheral neuropathy of vitamin B_{12} deficiency. *J Neurol Sci* 1984;66:117–126.

65. Ross RR, McKusick VA. Aortic arch syndromes, diminished or absent pulses in arteries arising from the arch of the aortic. *Arch Intern Med* 1953;92:701–740.

66. Shelhamer JH, Volkman DJ, Parillo JE, et al. Takayasu's arteritis and its therapy. *Ann Int Med* 1985;103:121.

67. Millikan CH, Siekert RG. Studies in cerebrovascular disease: The syndrome of intermittent insufficiency of the basilar arterial system. *Proc Staff Meetings Mayo Clin* 1955;30:61–68.

68. Davis TL, Freemon FR. Electroencephalography should not be routine in the evaluation of syncope in adults. *Arch Intern Med* 1990;150:2027–2029.

69. Porter RJ. The absence epilepsies. *Epilepsia* 1993;34(suppl 3):S42–S48.

70. Laskowitz DT, Sperling MR, French JA, O'Connor MJ. The syndrome of frontal lobe epilepsy: Characteristics and surgical management. *Neurology* 1995; 45:780–787.

71. Bruns O. Neuropathologische Demonstrationen. *Neurol Centralbl* 1902;21:561–567.

72. Alpers BJ, Yaskin HE. The Bruns' syndrome. *J Nerv Ment Dis* 1944;100:115–134.

73. Metz SA, Halter JB, Porte D Jr, Robertson RP. Autonomic epilepsy: Clonidine blockade of paroxysmal catecholamine release and flushing. *Ann Int Med* 1978;88:189–192.

74. Hering HE. Die reflektorische Selbststeuerung des Blutdruckes vermittelst der Blutdruckzügler. *Zschr für Kreislaufforschung* 1927;19:410–415.

75. Robertson D, Goldberg MR, Hollister AS, et al. Baroreceptor dysfunction in man. *Am J Med* 1984;76:A49–A58.

76. Robertson D, Hollister AS, Biaggioni I, et al. The diagnosis and treatment of baroreflex failure. *N Engl J Med* 1993;329:1449–1455.

77. Kochar MS, Ebert TJ, Kotrly KJ. Primary dysfunction of the afferent limb of the arterial baroreflex system in a patient with severe supine hypertension and orthostatic hypotension. *J Am Coll Cardiol* 1984;4:802–805.

78. Kuchel O, Cusson JR, Larochelle P, et al. Posture- and emotion-induced severe hypertensive paroxysms with baroreceptor dysfunction. *J Hypertens* 1987;5: 227–283.

79. Aksamit TR, Floras JS, Victor RG, Aylward PE. Paroxysmal hypertension due to sinoaortic baroreceptor denervation in humans. *Hypertension* 1987;9:309–314.

80. Robertson RM. Baroreflex failure. In: Robertson D, Low PA, Polinsky RJ (eds): *Primer on the Autonomic Nervous System.* San Diego: Academic Press; 1996;197–201.

81. Eckberg D, Sleight P. *Human Baroreflexes in Health and Disease.* Oxford: Clarendon Press; 1992.

82. Persson PB, Kirchheim HR. *Baroreceptor Reflexes: Integrative Functions and Clinical Aspects.* Berlin: Springer-Verlag; 1991;1–322.

83. Penfield W. Diencephalic autonomic epilepsy. *Arch Neurol Psychiatr* 1929; 22:358–374.

250 • SYNCOPE: MECHANISMS AND MANAGEMENT

84. Wallenberg A. Acute bulbäraffection (Embolie der Art. Cerebellar post, inf. sinstr.?) *Arch Psychiatry* 1895; 27:504–540.
85. Williams RS, Bashore TM. Paroxysmal hypotension associated with sympathetic withdrawal: A new disorder of autonomic vasomotor regulation. *Circulation* 1980;62:901–908.
86. von Bezold A, Hirt L. Über die physiologischen Wirkungen des Essigsauren Veratrins. *Untersuch Physiol Lab Wuerzburg* 1867;1:73.
87. Waller A. Experimental researches on the functions of the vagus and the cervical sympathetic nerves in man. *Proc R Soc Med* 1862;11:302–315.
88. Weiss S, Baker JP. The carotid sinus reflex in health and disease: Its role in the causation of fainting and convulsions. *Medicine* 1933;12:297–354.
89. Landau WM. Neuroskepticism: Sovereign remedy for the carotid sinus syndrome. *Neurology* 1994;44:1570–1576.
90. Weisenburg TH. Cerebellopontine tumor diagnosed for six years as a tic douloureux: The symptoms of irritation of ninth and twelfth cranial nerves. *JAMA* 1910;54:1600–1604.
91. Charcot JM. Séance du 19 Novembre 1876. *Gaz Méd Paris* 1876;5:588–589.
92. Pathy MS. Defecation syncope. *Age Aging* 1978;7:233–238.
93. Weisler AM, Warren JV. Syncope: Pathophysiology and differential diagnosis. In: Hurst JW (ed): *The Heart, 6th Edition.* New York: McGraw Hill; 1986;518.
94. Lombroso CT, Lerman P. Breath holding spells (cyanotic and pallid infantile syncope). *Pediatrics* 1967;39:563–567.
95. Allgrove J, Clalyden GS, Grant DB, et al. Familial glucocorticoid deficiency with achalasia of the cardia and deficient tear production. *Lancet* 1978;1:1284–1286.
96. Royer P, Lestradet H, de Menibus CH, et al. Hyperaldosteronisme familial chronique à debut neo-natal. *Ann Paediat* 1961;8:133–138.
97. Ulick S, Gautier E, Vetter KK, et al. An aldosterone biosynthetic defect in a salt-losing disorder. *J Clin Endocrinol Metab* 1964;24:669–672.
98. Verner JV, Morrison AB. Islet cell tumor and a syndrome of refractory watery diarrhea and hypokalemia. *Am J Med* 1958;25:374–380.
99. Streeten DHP, Kerr LP, Kerry CB, et al. Hyperbradykininsim: A new orthostatic syndrome. *Lancet* 1972;2:1048–1052.
100. Roberts LJ II. Recurrent syncope due to systemic mastocytosis (clinical conference). *Hypertension* 1984;6:285–294.
101. Roberts LJ II, Oates JA. Disorders of vasodilator hormones: The carcinoid syndrome and mastocytosis. In: Wilson JD, Foster DW (eds): *Williams Textbook of Endocrinology, 8th Edition.* Philadelphia: W.B. Saunders; 1995;1619–1634.
102. Masson P, Martin J. Paraganglioma surrenal, étude d'un cas humain de tumeurs malignes de la medullo-surrenale. *Bull Assoc Fr Cancer* 1923;12:135–141.
103. Mayo C. Paroxysmal hypertension with tumour of retroperitoneal nerve: Report of a case. *JAMA* 1927;89:1047–1050.
104. Manger W, Gifford R Jr. *Pheochromocytoma.* New York: Springer-Verlag; 1977.
105. Streeten DHP, Anderson GH Jr, Lebowitz M, Speller PF. Primary hyperepinephrinemia in patients without pheochromocytoma. *Arch Int Med* 1990; 150:1528–1533.
106. Bennhold H, Peters H, Roth E. Über einem Fall von kompletter Analbuminaemie ohne wesentliche klinische Krankheitszeichen. *Verh Dsch Ges In Med Kong* 1954;60:630–634.
107. Bouveret L. De la tachycardie essentiale paroxystique. *Rev Mid* 1889;9:753–793 and 837–855.
108. McKittrick LS, Wheelock FC Jr. *Carcinoma of the Colon 3rd Edition.* Springfield: CC Thomas; 1954.

109. Schroeder HA. Renal failure associated with low extracellular sodium chloride: The low salt syndrome. *JAMA* 1949;141:117–124.

110. Short DS. The syndrome of alternating bradycardia and tachycardia. *Br Heart J* 1954;16:208–214.

111. Roenheld L. Der gastrocardiale Symptomenkomplex, eine besondere Form sogenannter Herzneurose. *Z Phys Diat Ther* 1912;16:339–349.

112. Runge H. Venous pressure during pregnancy, delivery, and puerperium. *Arch Gynäkol* 1924;122:142–157.

113. Bárány R. Vestibularapparat und Centralnerven System. *Med Klin* 1911;7:1818–1821.

114. Baloh RW, Honrubia V, Jacobson K. Benign positional vertigo: Clinical and oculographic features in 240 cases. *Neurology* 1987;37:371–378.

115. Westphal C. Eigetuemlizhe mit Einschlafen verbundene Anfaelle. *Arch Psychiat Nervenkr* 1877;7:631–635.

116. Gélineau JBE. De la narcolepsie. *Gaz Hôp Paris* 1880;53:626–628 and 635–637.

117. Sigel JM, Nienhuis R, Fahringer HM, et al. Neuronal activity in narcolepsy: Identification of cataplexy-related cells in the medial medulla. *Science* 1991;252:1315–1318.

Psychiatric Disorders in Patients with Syncope

Wishwa N. Kapoor, MD and
Herbert C. Schulberg, PhD

Syncope is difficult to evaluate because of a broad differential diagnosis and the low yield of many diagnostic tests. Studies in the 1980s showed that in approximately 34% of patients, a definitive cause of syncope could not be established.[1-3] These results led to an intensive search for etiologies in this ambiguous group and to the development of newer diagnostic modalities. In the 1990s, tilt testing, event monitoring, and electrophysiological studies are increasingly used. One clinical domain that is also receiving greater attention is the role of psychiatric illnesses in causing or predisposing to syncope. Recent studies show that 20% to 25% of the patients with unknown etiologies of syncope may have psychiatric disorders for which syncope is one of the presenting symptoms.[4-5] There are also patients diagnosed with vasovagal syncope that may have psychiatric disorders that contribute to initiation of the neurocardiogenic responses. Since psychiatric illnesses are often not recognized on general medical services (inpatient or ambulatory), syncopal patients may suffer multiple recurrences, additional costs associated with further diagnostic tests and inappropriate treatment, and disruption of their lives. This chapter reviews the association of syncope and psychiatric illnesses, and recommends evaluations of the subgroup of patients whose syncope is likely to have a psychiatric component.

From Grubb BP, Olshansky B (eds.). *Syncope: Mechanisms and Management.* Armonk, NY: Futura Publishing Co., Inc.; © 1998.

Psychiatric Illnesses and Syncope

The American Psychiatric Association's *Diagnostic and Statistical Manual of Mental Disorders, Fourth Edition* (1994),[6] includes dizziness and syncope as manifestations of somatization, generalized anxiety, and panic disorders. Major depressive disorder (MDD) has also been linked to syncope.[5] Additionally, alcohol and drug abuse and dependence disorders can include alteration or loss of consciousness.

Somatization Disorder

Patients with this disorder present with multiple unexplained physical complaints for which they often seek medical attention. The symptoms begin before 30 years of age, persist for several years, and can produce significant impairment in social, occupational, or other areas of functioning. For the DSM-IV diagnosis to be met, the patient must present at least 4 pain symptoms, 2 gastrointestinal symptoms, 1 sexual symptom, and 1 pseudoneurological symptom (Table 1). For screening purposes, detailed assessment is indicated when these symptoms are present without an evident physical basis.

A somatoform-related illness is a conversion disorder in which neurological deficit is psychologically mediated. These patients often have other manifestations of somatization disorder as well. Major depression, panic, and substance abuse are frequent concomitant additional disorders in these patients.

___ Table 1 _____

Criteria for Somatization Disorder

A. History of many physical complaints beginning before age 30, occurring over several years, and resulting in treatment being sought or significant deficits in functioning.
B. Each of the following criteria has been met:
  (1) Four pain symptoms
  (2) Two gastrointestinal symptoms
  (3) One sexual symptom
  (4) One pseudoneurological symptom
C. Either of the following:
  (1) The symptoms in Criterion B cannot be fully explained by a known general medical condition or the direct effects of a substance.
  (2) The physical complaints or degree of dysfunctioning exceed what would be expected from the general medical condition.
D. The symptoms are not intentionally produced or feigned.

From *Diagnostic and Statistical Manual of Mental Disorders, Fourth Edition*. Washington, DC: American Psychiatric Association; 1994:449–450.

Generalized Anxiety Disorder (GAD)

This disorder is characterized by excessive anxiety and worry, and three or more symptoms that affect the patient more often than not for more than 6 months and interfere with the patient's normal functioning. Table 2 presents symptoms of this disorder grouped into the several categories included within DSM-IV.

Panic Attack and Disorder

Panic attack consists of a sense of impending doom, fear, and at least four physical symptoms that develop abruptly and are often frightening to the patient (Table 3). Panic disorder is diagnosed when attacks recur and significantly disrupt the patient's life. Panic disorder often leads to agoraphobia and increasingly limited functioning.

Major Depressive Disorder (MDD)

Table 4 outlines symptoms of major depression. Physical symptoms such as fatigue, anorexia, and weight loss are increasingly recognized as important components of depression among general medical patients, and physicians need to consider these symptoms when making the diagnosis of major depression. Although DSM-IV criteria do not include syncope as an

_____ Table 2 _____

Criteria for Generalized Anxiety Disorder

A. Excessive anxiety and worry occurring more often than not for at least 6 months.
B. Difficulty controlling the worry.
C. The anxiety and worry are associated with three or more of the following six symptoms:
    (1) Restlessness or feeling on edge
    (2) Easily fatigued
    (3) Difficulty concentrating
    (4) Irritability
    (5) Muscle tension
    (6) Sleep disturbance
D. The focus of the worry is not confined to another Axis I psychiatric disorder.
E. The anxiety or symptoms produce significant deficits in functioning.
F. The disturbance is not due to direct effects of a substance or a general medical condition.

From _Diagnostic and Statistical Manual of Mental Disorders, Fourth Edition._ Washington, DC: American Psychiatric Association; 1994:435–436.

_____ Table 3 _____

Criteria for Panic Disorder Without Agoraphobia

A. Both of the following:
  (1) Recurrent unexpected panic attacks
  (2) At least one of the attacks is followed by one or more of the following:
    (a) persistent concern about additional attacks;
    (b) worry about implications of the attack; or
    (c) significant behavioral change.
B. Absence of agoraphobia
C. Attacks are not directly due to physiological effects of a substance or general medical condition.
D. The attacks are not better accounted for by another psychiatric disorder.

From *Diagnostic and Statistical Manual of Mental Disorders, Fourth Edition.* Washington, DC: American Psychiatric Association; 1994:402.

_____ Table 4 _____

Criteria for Major Depressive Episode

A. Five or more of the following symptoms, including either (1) or (2), have been present for a 2-week period.
  (1) Depressed mood
  (2) Anhedonia
  (3) Significant weight loss or gain
  (4) Insomnia or hypersomnia
  (5) Psychomotor retardation or agitation
  (6) Fatigue
  (7) Feelings of worthlessness or guilt
  (8) Diminished concentration
  (9) Recurrent thoughts of death or suicidal ideation
B. Symptoms do not meet criteria for a Mixed Episode of Bipolar Disorder.
C. Symptoms cause significant distress or impaired functioning
D. Symptoms are not due to direct effects of a substance or general medical disorder.
E. Symptoms are not better accounted for by Bereavement.

From *Diagnostic and Statistical Manual of Mental Disorders, Fourth Edition.* Washington, DC: American Psychiatric Association; 1994:327.

explicit element in the diagnosis of MDD, two studies have related depression to syncope.[4–5]

Alcohol and Substance Abuse Disorders

Alcohol abuse and alcoholism may be associated with seizure-related loss of consciousness, which may be difficult to distinguish from syncope. Alcohol may also cause orthostatic hypotension with or without an association with Wernicke's encephalopathy. Complications of alcoholism may lead to gastrointestinal bleeding, which may present with syncope.

Syncope is a well-recognized manifestation of cocaine ingestion, but sedatives, opiates, and stimulant drugs may also lead to syncope due to toxicity (eg, vomiting and dehydration), interactions with alcohol or other medications, or drug withdrawal reactions.

Stress and Syncope

The role stress plays in causing syncope has not received adequate attention. Vasovagal syncope is known to result from states of sudden apprehension and stress such as when facing fear or injury[7–8] even though the injury and stress may be trivial. Since psychological factors are so prominent in vasovagal syncope, it is sometimes referred to as "emotional fainting." For example, the exposure of healthy individuals to violent scenes has been associated with decreased heart rate and increased epinephrine levels, both of which are prevented by β-blockade.[9] Chronic stressors such as job dissatisfaction, and personality traits such as neuroticism have been suggested to play a role in vasovagal syncope.[10] Psychological coping strategies to a sudden faint sensation may also be different in people with vasovagal syncope. Suppression-type coping strategies (eg, reducing tension by not thinking about the situation) may be associated with vasovagal syncope, and may also be found among people who focus on bodily responses to acute challenge rather than the intellectual aspects of the experience.[11]

Epidemic Fainting

Syncope in large groups over a brief period of time (hours to days) has been called "epidemic fainting" and is often referred to as mass hysteria. Dizziness and fainting generally start in small groups and spread explosively among other members of the group.[12–13] The typical victims are adolescent females in a school setting. Epidemic faintness has also been reported in telephone operators, marching bands, and other groups. These epidemics are often associated with periods of uncertainty and social stress. Seeing a friend become sick has been found to predict the development of syncopal symptoms in adolescents. Fainting episodes are considered a form of transitory anxiety attack rather than acute conversion reactions. This type of mass fainting appears to represent exaggerated emotional responses and probably does not fit into a distinct disease state.

Studies of Psychiatric Illnesses in Patients with Unexplained Syncope

By use of the Diagnostic Interview Schedule (DIS), a structured interview administered to formulate DSM-III-R diagnoses, we have evaluated 414 patients with syncope to determine the prevalence of one or more of the psychiatric disorders noted above (see Table 5).[4] For the group as a whole, the highest lifetime rates were observed for MDD (9.9%), GAD (7.3%), and Alcohol Dependence (AlcDep) (6.5%). There were significant differences in the proportions of patients with psychiatric illnesses among the three categories of causes of syncope, with the highest in the syncope of unknown origin (SUO) group (24.5%) and lowest in the patients with cardiac syncope (9.7%). Patients with SUO had the highest rates for each of the eight assessed psychiatric disorders. Physicians recognized a possible psychiatric or alcohol/drug problem in only 48% of the patients found to

_____ Table 5 _____

DIS Diagnoses In Relation to the Cause of Syncope

DIS* Diagnosis	Total† (n = 414)		Unknown Cause (n = 163)	
	N	%	N	%
Any DIS Diagnosis	82	19.8	40	24.5
Somatization (SOMAT)	4	0.7	3	1.8
Panic Disorder (PD)	8	1.9	7	4.3
Generalized Anxiety Disorder (GAD)	30	7.3	14	8.6
Major Depression (MDD)	41	9.9	20	12.2
Drug Abuse (DrgAbs)	2	0.5	2	1.2
Alcohol Dependence (AlcDep)	27	6.5	15	9.2
Alcohol Abuse (AlcAbs)	2	0.5	1	0.6
Any Psychiatric Diagnosis**	58	14.0	28	17.2
Any Alcohol/Drug Diagnosis	30	7.3	15	9.2

* DIS = Diagnostic Interview Schedule;
† 114 separate psychiatric disorder were assigned to 82 patients, grouped as follows: 9 patients had 1 disorder (SOMAT-1, PD-1, GAD-14, MDD-20, DrgAbs-1, AlcAbs-2, AlcDep-20); 17 patients had 2 disorders (SOMAT + MDD-2, PD + GAD-1, PD + MDD-1, GAD + MDD-10, DrgAbs + AlcDep-1, MDD + AlcDep-2); 3 patients had 3 disorders (PD + GAD + MDD-2, SOMAT + MDD + AlcDep-1); 3 patients had 4 disorders (PD + GAD + MDD + AlcDep-3);
** Six patients had both psychiatric and alcohol/drug diagnoses.

have psychiatric illness. Recognition was better for patients experiencing multiple psychiatric disorders.

Linzer et al[5] studied 72 patients with unexplained syncope who were referred to psychiatrists. A psychiatric diagnosis was made in 17 patients (24%): panic disorder in 9, major depression in 6 and major depression and panic attack in 2. There was symptomatic improvement among those who complied with treatment of the psychiatric illness.

Correlates of Psychiatric Disorders in Patients with Syncope

Syncopal patients with psychiatric disorders are more likely to be younger females who have had a higher number of syncopal events in the last year, who experience more prodromal symptoms, and who have a larger number of other complaints.[4] In our study, multivariate predictors of psychiatric diagnoses were 1) four or more syncopal events in the past year and 2) prodromal symptoms prior to syncopal events. Two multivariate predictors of alcohol/drug diagnoses were also noted: 1) male gender and 2) age <65 years.

Outcomes of Patients with Syncope and Psychiatric Illness

In our study, the 1-year recurrence rate of syncope in patients without psychiatric illness was 15.0%, a rate not significantly different from that found in patients with only alcohol/drug disorders (5.0%).[4] However, patients with one psychiatric disorder had a 26% syncope recurrence rate and those with two or more psychiatric disorders had a 50% recurrence rate. There were no significant differences in recurrence rates when specific psychiatric disorders were compared. Age, gender, number of prior syncopal episodes, presence of psychiatric diagnosis, and unknown etiology of syncope were significantly associated with recurrences at 1 year. A psychiatric diagnosis was an independent risk factor for recurrent syncope.

Mechanism of Syncope in Psychiatric Illness

There are at least four potential mechanisms through which psychiatric disorders are related to syncope. First, psychiatric disorders may be comorbid with but have no role in causing syncope. Previous studies report a prevalence of 6% to 10% for MDD and 1% to 10% for PD in medical patients seen in primary care centers.[14] The rates of these psychiatric disorders in patients with known organic causes of syncope (cardiac and noncardiac) are similar, suggesting a baseline prevalence of psychiatric disorders in these medical patients. However, the rates of these psychiatric disorders were higher in patients with syncope of unknown cause. This argues against a simple comorbid relationship, as does our finding of a higher risk of recurrence of syncope at follow-up among patients with syncope of unknown cause.

Second, psychiatric disorders may cause syncope. Clinically, in patients with cardiac and noncardiac causes, a direct causative role for psychiatric disorders is difficult to postulate except for patients who have had vasovagal syncope that is known to be precipitated by fear, stress, anxiety, and emotional distress. However, in patients with syncope of unknown origin, psychiatric disorders are likely to be causal, since syncope is a known manifestation of these psychiatric disorders and comprises a criterion symptom in DSM-IV as described above. The high rate of syncopal recurrence at follow-up in this group is also consistent with the postulation of a causative role for psychiatric disorders.

Third, there may be a complex interaction between syncope and psychiatric disorders. Stress and psychological factors have been associated with provocation of ventricular and supraventricular arrhythmias, and the occurrence of sudden death and myocardial infarction.[15] It is possible that psychiatric disorders in patients with underlying heart disease predispose these patients to arrhythmias and syncope. However, in patients with syncope of unknown origin (most of whom do not have heart disease), it is more difficult to postulate such a link because arrhythmias and myocardial infarction are not found on evaluation. Furthermore, low mortality in patients with psychiatric disorders serves as an argument against a predisposition to major ventricular arrhythmias in these patients.

Finally, it is possible that syncope causes psychiatric disorders. This pattern is unlikely in patients with somatization disorder. However, GAD, PD, and MDD may develop in patients who suffer recurrent syncopal spells with elusive etiology and who react with intense worry, apprehension, fears of death, or chronic feeling of sadness and hopelessness. Although this causal mechanism cannot be directly verified or excluded, a previous report that syncope resolves with treatment of MDD and PD[5] strongly argues against the fact that syncope leads to psychiatric disorders.

Given the presently available evidence, the relationship of syncope and psychiatric disorders cannot be definitively specified. Future studies are needed to define causal directions and to investigate the pathophysiological mechanisms for syncope.

Testing for Psychiatric Syncope

Open-mouthed hyperventilation for 3 minutes has been used to reproduce symptoms similar to syncopal episodes.[16] In one study, the hyperventilation test had a positive predictive value of 59% for psychiatric causes of syncope (panic disorder and major depression). Experience with this bedside maneuver in evaluating syncope is limited, however, at this time. Patient responses to upright tilt testing have also been used to make a diagnosis of psychiatric or psychogenic syncope.[17] Positive responses to upright tilt testing consist of reproduction of syncope in association with hypotension and/or bradycardia. A psychosomatic response consisting of no hemodynamic alterations in a patient who develops loss of consciousness during tilt testing has also been described. Normal electroencephalogram (EEG) and cerebral blood flow have been found in several evaluated patients. Somatoform disorders are most commonly found in these patients.

Although tilt testing may provide valuable information regarding possible psychogenic syncope, the sensitivity of this test for the diagnosis of psychiatric illnesses that cause syncope is not known. Therefore, this test should not be widely used to screen for psychiatric disorders, because a careful clinical interview and psychiatric consultations are the more established means of diagnosing DSM-IV disorders. Nevertheless, tilt testing may elucidate the mechanism of syncope in known psychiatric disorders since panic, anxiety, and major depression may cause syncope by precipitating neurocardiogenic responses.

Approach to the Evaluation of Patients with Syncope

The clinical assessment and electrocardiogram (ECG) comprise the initial step in evaluating patients with syncope. This assessment may lead to a definitive diagnosis. Under such circumstances, treatment can be planned and initiated. In other instances, the clinical assessment may not be diagnostic, but it may still provide suggestive evidence for specific entities [eg, signs of aortic stenosis or idiopathic hypertrophic subaortic stenosis (IHSS)]. These clinical clues can be pursued with further testing to confirm or exclude particular entities as the causes of syncope. However, there remains a large group of patients in whom the initial clinical evaluation does not lead to a specific diagnosis and yields no suggestive findings about potential causes of syncope. Many cardiovascular tests are considered and often performed in these patients, but psychiatric illness also should be considered in the diagnostic work-up when correlates of psychiatric illnesses noted are present. Psychiatric illnesses should be particularly considered in patients who report multiple syncopal episodes with prodromal symptoms, and who describe nonspecific symptoms referable to several organ systems. These patients have the highest probability of having a psychiatric diagnoses. In younger male patients with unexplained syncope, alcohol/drug disorders should also be explored. In patients with clinical symptoms that are compatible with vasovagal syncope and those that are tilt positive, attention should be paid to stress and psychiatric illnesses, as they may be contributory factors. A detailed psychosocial history and screening instruments are recommended for use in these conditions. Disorder-specific screening instruments can be administered when the physician suspects a particular psychiatric illness and wishes to rule it in or out. For example, several well-validated instruments are available for mood disorder case-finding purposes.[18] When psychiatric illness in general is of concern but no specific DSM-IV disorder is suspected in relation to the syncope, the PRIME-MD[19] can be administered. This recently developed instrument consists of a patient self-report questionnaire covering somatoform, eating, depressive, and anxiety disorders, as well as alcohol abuse. When the patient acknowledges a minimal number of symptoms for a given disorder, the physician administers the appropriate module of the PRIME-MD's *Clinician Evaluation Guide* to ascertain whether the symptoms are sufficiently extensive and of sufficient duration to meet the DSM-IV criteria for the disorder.

References

1. Silverstein MD, Singer DE, Mulley A, et al. Patients with syncope admitted to medical intensive care units. *JAMA* 1982;248:1185–1189.
2. Day SC, Cook EF, Funkenstein H, Goldman L. Evaluation and outcome of emergency room patients with transient loss of consciousness. *Am J Med* 1982;73:15–23.
3. Kapoor W. Evaluation and outcome of patients with syncope. *Medicine* 1990; 69:160–175.
4. Kapoor WN, Fortunato M, Hanusa BH, Schulberg HC. Psychiatric illnesses in patients with syncope. *Am J Med* 1995:99;505–512.
5. Linzer M, Felder A, Hackel A, et al. Psychiatric Syncope: A new look at an old disease. *Psychosomatics* 1990;31:181–188.
6. *Diagnostic and Statistical Manual of Mental Disorders, 4th Edition.* Washington, DC: American Psychiatric Association; 1994.
7. Engel GL. Psychologic stress, vasodepressor (vasovagal) syncope, and sudden death. *Ann Intern Med* 1978;89:403–412.
8. Sledge WH. Antecedent psychological factors in the onset of vasovagal syncope. *Psychosom Med* 1978;40:568–579.
9. Carruthers M. Vagotonicity of violence: Biochemical and cardiac responses to violent films and television programs. *Br Med J* 1973;3:384.
10. Schmidt RT. Personality and fainting. *J Psychosom Res* 1975;19:21–25.
11. Steptoe A, Wardale J. Emotional fainting and the psychophysiologic response to blood and injury: Autonomic mechanisms and coping strategies. *Psychosom Med* 1988;50:402–417.
12. Small GW, Borus JF. Outbreak of illness in a school chorus. *N Engl J Med* 1983;308:632–635.
13. Levine RJ. Epidemic faintness and syncope in a school marching band. *JAMA* 1977;238:2373–2376.
14. Schulberg HC, Saul M, McClelland M, et al. Assessing depression in primary medical and psychiatric practices. *Arch Gen Psychiatry* 1985;42:1164–1170.

15. Lown B, DeSilva RA, Reich P, Murawski BJ. Psychophysiologic factors in sudden cardiac death. *Am J Psychiatry* 1980;137:1325–1335.
16. Koenig D, Linzer M, Pontinen M, Devine GW. Syncope in young adults: Evidence of a combined medical and psychiatric approach. *J Intern Med* 1992; 232;169–176.
17. Grubb BP, Gerard G, Wolfe DA, et al. Syncope and seizures of psychogenic origin: Identification with head-upright tilt table testing. *Clin Cardiol* 1992; 15:839–842.
18. Mulrow C, Williams J, Gerety M, et al. Case-finding instruments for depression in primary care settings. *Ann Intern Med* 1995;122:913–921.
19. Spitzer R, Williams J, Kroenke K, et al. Utility of a new procedure for diagnosing mental disorders in primary care: The PRIME-MD 1000 study. *JAMA* 1994; 272:1749–1756.

Neurally Mediated Hypotension and the Chronic Fatigue Syndrome

Hugh Calkins, MD and Peter C. Rowe, MD

Introduction

The chronic fatigue syndrome is a common medical disorder defined by profound fatigue lasting at least 6 months, often beginning abruptly after an acute viral infection, and not explained by known medical or psychiatric disorders.[1,2] The pathophysiological basis of chronic fatigue syndrome is uncertain, no pathognomonic signs or tests exist, and no consistently effective therapy has been identified.[3] Recent studies demonstrate a close association between the chronic fatigue syndrome and neurally mediated hypotension, a common abnormality of blood pressure regulation (also referred to as neurocardiogenic syncope or vasodepressor syncope).[4,5] Evidence to support this association includes an extensive overlap in symptoms and exacerbating features between these two conditions, a >90% prevalence of an abnormal response to upright tilt among patients with chronic fatigue syndrome, and an improvement in symptoms of chronic fatigue patients in response to therapy directed to neurally mediated hypotension.[5] The purpose of this chapter is to review the results of these initial studies and to review the current status of this rapidly evolving area of research.

Neurally Mediated Hypotension

Neurocardiogenic syncope, neurally mediated syncope, neurally mediated hypotension, vasodepressor syncope, vasovagal syncope, and "faint-

From Grubb BP, Olshansky B (eds.). *Syncope: Mechanisms and Management.* Armonk, NY: Futura Publishing Co., Inc.; © 1998.

ing" are different names for the common disorder of autonomic cardiovascular regulation.[6–11] Precipitating factors associated with the development of neurally mediated hypotension are those that either reduce ventricular filling or increase catecholamine secretion, such as prolonged standing, a warm environment or hot shower, exercise, and stressful situations. Under these types of situations, patients with this condition develop severe lightheadedness and/or syncope. It has been proposed that these clinical phenomena result from a paradoxical reflex that is initiated when ventricular preload is reduced by venous pooling. In response, susceptible individuals develop high concentrations of circulating catecholamines, which promote augmented inotropic activity and excessive stimulation of mechanoreceptors in the left ventricle as a result of vigorous contraction of a volume-depleted ventricle. Activation of these mechanoreceptors/nonmyelinated afferent C-fibers leads to a withdrawal of peripheral sympathetic tone and an increase in vagal tone, which in turn causes vasodilation and bradycardia. The ultimate clinical consequences are syncope or presyncope.[8–10]

Therapy for neurally mediated hypotension attempts to either prevent initiation of the abnormal reflex by increasing blood volume (through increased dietary sodium or fludrocortisone) and decreasing the inotropic effects of adrenergic stimulation (through β-adrenergic antagonists or disopyramide), or to alter the efferent limb of the response by minimizing the resultant bradycardia and vasodilation (through pacemaker therapy; α-adrenergic agonists such as midodrine or ephedrine; anticholinergic agents such as disopyramide; or serotonin reuptake inhibitors such as Zoloft, Prozac, or Serzone).[9,10,12-17] Neurally mediated syncope is more common in the young than in the elderly, more common in slender individuals, and more common in those with blood pressures in the lower part of the normal range.[8,9,11,18] A familial pattern has been reported.[19,20]

Chronic Fatigue Syndrome

The chronic fatigue syndrome is characterized clinically by profound fatigue, cognitive disturbances, and a variety of somatic symptoms including sore throat, headaches, myalgias, and postexertional fatigue.[21] An operational definition of CFS generated for research purposes was published by Holmes and colleagues[1] in 1988. The central feature of this and of the British and Australian CFS definitions is the presence of severe fatigue of new or definite onset for at least 6 months' duration that is sufficient to interfere in a substantial way with normal daily activities. In addition to this requirement, the recent 1994 CFS definition by Fukuda and colleagues[2] requires the concurrent occurrence of four of the following eight symptoms: cognitive disturbances (including difficulties with short-term memory and concentration), sore throat, tender cervical or axillary lymph nodes, muscle pain, multi-joint pain without joint swelling or redness, headaches, unrefreshing sleep, and postexertional malaise lasting more than 24 hours. The prevalence of CFS is difficult to measure with precision, but minimal estimates are available from several sources. Bates and colleagues[21] estimated that 3/1000 patients who attend a primary care practice in the United States have CFS, with the upper confidence limit of that estimate being 6/1000. This estimate is regarded as conservative, as data on the classification of fatigue were not available for 69% of patients reporting debilitating fatigue for at least 6 months. In a subtropical area of Australia, Lloyd and colleagues[22] estimated a prevalence of CFS of 37.1/100,000 (95% confidence interval 26.8–50.2), without unusual socioeconomic or racial distributions, and with a 1.3 to 1.0 female to male ratio. In this population, 43% of CFS patients were unable to attend school or work.

The etiology of CFS is unknown. Although the abrupt onset of symptoms in the setting of a flu-like illness suggests that infection is an important factor in the initiation of symptoms, no single pathogen has been identified as the predominant cause of the syndrome. The routine physical examination and routine laboratory tests are usually normal in those with CFS, although some investigators have reported chemical,[23] hormonal,[24] and immunologic abnormalities[25–27] of uncertain significance. Single-photon emission computed tomography (SPECT) scans of the brain demonstrate more regional perfusion defects in CFS patients than in healthy controls, a finding that has been interpreted to be consistent with chronic viral encephalitis,[28] but which could also be consistent with hypoperfusion of the cerebral circulation for other reasons.

No therapy has been found to be consistently effective for those with CFS. Trials of liver extract,[29] intravenous immunoglobulin,[30,31] acyclovir,[32] and essential fatty acids[33,34] have shown no reliable benefit. While a short-lived placebo effect has been observed in some of these studies, when measured carefully, the magnitude of that effect is usually small. In the study by Straus and colleagues[32] for example, the mean placebo effect was a 7.5 point improvement on a 100 point scale measuring general sense of well being.

Full recovery from CFS is uncommon. Wilson and colleagues[35] re-evaluated 103/139 (74%) of CFS patients originally enrolled in clinical trials. After a mean of 9.3 years of symptoms, only 6 had recovered completely. Recent estimates by Steele and colleagues[36] suggest that after 10 years, an estimated 70% remain ill.

Relationship Between Neurally Mediated Hypotension and Fatigue

In evaluating whether aspects of the clinical history could differentiate syncope caused by either ventricular tachycardia, heart block, or neurally mediated hypotension, Calkins and colleagues[11] noted that postsyncopal fatigue was strongly and uniquely associated with neurally mediated hypotension; it was reported by 94% of patients with neurally mediated hypotension as compared to 23% of patients with syncope resulting from ventricular tachycardia or heart block.[11] Furthermore, the presence of postsyncopal fatigue was identified as the single most powerful predictor of the cause of syncope. This observation expands on a relatively neglected observation by Sir Thomas Lewis[37] in his classic 1932 paper on vasovagal syncope. Lewis described a soldier who experienced vasovagal syncope followed by a 36-hour period of fatigue. Prolonged fatigue was thus observed to accompany neurally mediated hypotension over 60 years ago.

Subsequently, Rowe and colleagues[4] demonstrated that neurally mediated hypotension can be associated with chronic fatigue when they reported a consecutive series of seven adolescents with chronic fatigue but without syncope, each of whom had evidence of neurally mediated hypotension. The median duration of fatigue was 7 months (range 2 to 29 months); only one patient had fatigue for fewer than 6 months. In four, the fatigue and lightheadedness began suddenly in association with an episode of pharyngitis documented or suspected to be viral. These four patients satisfied the 1988 Centers for Disease Control criteria for the diagnosis of chronic fatigue syndrome. None of the subjects had a reduction in blood pressure >10 mm Hg within the first 5 minutes of being tilted upright; thus, no patient had orthostatic hypotension. However, as the procedure progressed, all seven developed clinically important hypotension; the median systolic blood pressure at the time the tilt test was stopped was 65 mm Hg (range, 37 to 75). In addition to triggering hypotension or bradycardia, tilt testing reproduced the clinical symptoms of lightheadedness and fatigue in all seven. Two became syncopal for the first time during the testing, and three others developed junctional bradycardia. After completion of the tilt test, all subjects were instructed to increase their salt intake, and all were treated with either a β-adrenergic antagonist or disopyramide. Four of seven experienced a substantial improvement in their symptoms within a week of beginning treatment with either atenolol 50 mg/day (n=2) or disopyramide 100 mg or 200 mg twice daily (n=2). Follow-up tilt testing was performed in two participants. One, whose symptoms had improved, had a normal follow-up tilt test, and the other, who had not improved on therapy, had a persistently abnormal response. In the four responders, symptoms of lightheadedness and postexertional fatigue have either resolved or are substantially better than before therapy, and improvements have been sustained for 12 months. These observations demonstrate an association between chronic fatigue and neurally mediated hypotension, even when syncope is not a clinical feature. The association is strengthened by the prompt and virtually complete response of four of the patients to treatment that is effective for neurally mediated hypotension.

The Relationship Between Neurally Mediated Hypotension and the Chronic Fatigue Syndrome

The observations outlined above, which linked neurally mediated hypotension to fatigue and chronic fatigue, led us to the hypothesis that a proportion of those with an established diagnosis of chronic fatigue syndrome actually may have treatable neurally mediated hypotension. Consistent with this hypothesis, the existing literature on the chronic fatigue syndrome suggests a substantial overlap in the clinical features of the chronic fatigue syndrome and neurally mediated hypotension. Comprehensive summaries based on data from a number of clinics and studies have identified lightheadedness in approximately 50% of those with the chronic fatigue syndrome.[38] Bell and colleagues[39] described syncope in 10% of adolescents with the chronic fatigue syndrome.

To test this hypothesis, Bou-Holaigah and colleagues[5] compared the clinical history and response to upright tilt testing in 23 patients with chronic fatigue syndrome and 14 controls. The 14 normal volunteers who participated in this study were eligible if they had never experienced syncope and if they were not fatigued. Patients were eligible for this study if they had an established diagnosis of chronic fatigue syndrome, were younger than 49 years of age, and were not taking medications that could interfere with tilt table responses. Each patient with the chronic fatigue syndrome completed a questionnaire that quantified the degree of functional impairment, identified medications used for fatigue, and solicited information about the type and severity of symptoms. In addition, these patients were asked to complete a questionnaire that rated their general sense of well being; their general health, using the 20-item Medical Outcome Study (MOS-20) short form survey[40]; their degree of cognitive dysfunction, using the Wood Mental Fatigue Inventory)[41]; and two measures designed for this study: a Symptom Change Score and an Activity Restriction Index. With the exception of the MOS-20, which asks about symptoms over 3-month intervals, the outcome assessments were repeated every 4 weeks following initiation of treatment.

Upright tilt testing was performed in a quiet room following a 4-hour fast. A three-stage, 70° upright tilt protocol was used. After 10 minutes in the supine position, the table was tilted to 70° for 45 minutes (stage 1). If an abnormal response was not observed, isoproterenol at a dose of 1 or 2 μg/min (titrated to achieve a 20% increase in heart rate) was infused for 10 minutes in the supine position and the upright tilt was repeated for 15 minutes (stage 2). If this stage was tolerated, the patient was returned to the supine position and the dose of isoproterenol was increased by 2 μg/min to 3 or 4 μg/min. After 10 minutes in the supine position, the upright tilt was repeated for 10 minutes (stage 3). An abnormal response required the development of syncope or severe presyncope with at least a 25 mm Hg decrease in systolic blood pressure and no associated increase in heart rate. Patients were instructed to increase their dietary salt intake, and were offered treatment with one or more medications commonly used in the management of patients with neurally mediated hypotension. Initial therapy was with fludrocortisone 0.1 mg daily. If fludrocortisone was ineffective, partially effective, or poorly tolerated, the dose was adjusted or it was supplemented or replaced by β-adrenergic antagonists (propranolol 10 to 40 mg/day, or atenolol 25 to 50 mg/day) or disopyramide (100 to 200 mg twice daily).

The clinical characteristics of chronic fatigue syndrome patients in this study are similar to those of prior reported populations. There were 18 women and five men with a mean age of 34 ± 12 years (range, 14–49 years). All 23 were Caucasian. Nineteen (83%) reported an abrupt onset of symptoms in association with an infectious illness that resembled influenza or mononucleosis. The median duration of illness was 5 years (range, 11 months to 36 years). Seventeen patients (74%) were unable to work or attend school regularly because of chronic fatigue syndrome. A median of two therapies directed at chronic fatigue syndrome had been ineffective. Symptoms compatible with neurally mediated hypotension and syncope among those with chronic fatigue syndrome were chronic lightheadedness (96%), nausea (96%), diaphoresis (83%), exacerbation of fatigue after physical exertion (100%), prolonged standing (78%), or hot shower (78%). Although 10 patients (43%) had experienced at least one episode of syncope, this symptom was not frequent, and had occurred more than 10 years prior to the development of chronic fatigue syndrome in eight patients, simultaneous with onset of chronic fatigue syndrome in one patient, and following onset of chronic fatigue syndrome in one patient. Sixty-one percent reported that they usually or always tried to avoid salt and salty foods. The median MOS-20 score was 50 (range 26–67); a score of 100 would indicate excellent health.

An abnormal response to upright tilt that was consistent with neurally mediated hypotension (a drop of at least 25 mm Hg in systolic blood pressure with no associated increase in heart rate) was observed in 22/23 patients with chronic fatigue syndrome (96%) versus 4/14 healthy controls (29%, $P=0.0001$). The stage of tilt during which an abnormal response was observed also differed (Table 1). During stage 1 of the upright tilt protocol in the absence of isoproterenol, an abnormal response to upright tilt was observed in 16 patients with chronic fatigue syndrome (70%) versus none of the controls ($P=0.0001$). Thirteen of 22 patients with an abnormal response became syncopal. The odds ratio for an abnormal response to upright tilt was 62 in those with chronic fatigue syndrome (lower 95% confidence interval, 5.4). During stage 1 of the upright tilt protocol, all patients with chronic fatigue syndrome complained of worse fatigue, and all but

_____ Table 1 _____

Response to Upright Tilt in Those With CFS and in Healthy Controls

| | Abnormal Response | | | |
	Stage 1	Stage 2	Stage 3	Normal
CFS	16	3	3	1
Controls	0	1	3	10

CFS = chronic fatigue syndrome.

one experienced symptoms commonly observed prior to neurally mediated hypotension and syncope including warmth (87%), lightheadedness (87%), and nausea (70%). All control patients remained asymptomatic during stage 1 of the upright tilt test ($P=0.0001$). Two patients elected not to begin treatment. Another patient was treated for less than 2 weeks. The remaining 20 have been treated with fludrocortisone (11), atenolol (1), midodrine (1), disopyramide (2), or a combination of fludrocortisone and atenolol. Of these 20, nine reported complete or near complete resolution of all symptoms (defined as a general sense of well being of ≥ 7, a Woods Mental Fatigue score of ≤ 8, and an Activity Restriction Index score of <2). Cognitive dysfunction, tender glands, myalgias, and sore throat improved as did the primary symptom of fatigue. Among the 20 patients treated for more than 2 weeks, each method of quantifying the patients' clinical status demonstrated a significant improvement in symptoms (Table 2).

The results of this study suggest that there is a close link between neurally mediated hypotension and the chronic fatigue syndrome, as evidenced by the extensive overlap in symptoms and exacerbating features between the two conditions, the almost uniform provocation of neurally mediated hypotension in chronic fatigue syndrome patients during upright tilt, and the exacerbation of chronic fatigue symptoms during upright tilt.

_____ Table 2 _____

Response to Treatment of Neurally Mediated Hypotension in CFS

Outcome Measure	Pretreatment*	On Treatment	P
Wood mental fatigue inventory	20.6 ± 8.1	6.9 ± 2.3	<0.0001
Activity restriction index	4.9 ± 1.0	3.0 ± 1.6	0.0001
General sense of well being	3.6 ± 1.5	6.9 ± 2.3	0.0001

CFS = chronic fatigue syndrome.
* All results are expressed as mean $\pm$ SD.

Furthermore, the results of this study also suggest that the symptoms of the chronic fatigue syndrome are potentially reversible with medications used for treatment of neurally mediated hypotension.

The findings of this study are also consistent with prior studies that have described the clinical features and treatment of a small series of patients who presented with fatigue and lightheadedness and were suspected of having autonomic dysfunction.[42,43] Streeten,[43] as well as Rosen and Cryer[44] had reported successful treatment of this condition with fludrocortisone and sodium loading. Fouad and colleagues[45] described a series of 11 patients with weakness and lightheadedness who had a tachycardic response to 10 minutes of upright tilt, and in whom symptoms resolved with salt and fludrocortisone. In 1992, Streeten and colleagues[43] documented a drop in blood pressure with prolonged standing in seven adults with fatigue, and hypothesized that chronic fatigue syndrome might be due to delayed orthostatic hypotension. We are not aware of any studies that followed from this speculation. Our observations are also consistent with a study by Schondorf and Low,[42] who described chronic fatigue and lightheadedness in 13/16 individuals with a related form of autonomic dysfunction, idiopathic postural orthostatic tachycardia syndrome (POTS). Whether these patients could be classified as having neurally mediated hypotension is unclear, as blood pressure was reported for only 2 to 3 minutes after upright tilt. Rosen and Cryer[44] had reported successful treatment of this condition with fludrocortisone and sodium loading. Similarly, Fouad and colleagues[45] described a series of 11 patients with weakness and lightheadedness who had a tachycardic response to 10 minutes of upright tilt, and in whom symptoms resolved with salt and fludrocortisone. More recently, Grubb and colleagues[46] reported the clinical characteristics, response to upright tilt testing, and response to treatment of a series of 28 patients with the postural orthostatic tachycardia syndrome. Patients were included in this series if they presented with at least a 6-month history of orthostatic intolerance manifested by weakness, lightheadedness, orthostatic tachycardia, fatigue, and near syncope. The diagnosis of postural orthostatic tachycardia syndrome was established by reproduction of the patients' clinical symptoms during upright tilt testing in conjunction with at least a 30-bpm increase in heart rate to a rate exceeding 110 bpm within 10 minutes of upright tilt. Twenty-one of 28 patients reported an improvement in symptoms with treatment with one or more pharmacological agents including fludrocortisone, atenolol, and erythropoietin.

The Pathophysiological Basis for the Chronic Fatigue Syndrome and its Relationship with Neurally Mediated Hypotension

Although the cause of the chronic fatigue syndrome has been the focus of intense research during the past 10 years, the pathophysiological basis for this disorder remains unclear.[1-3] Like the closely related (perhaps identical) condition neuromyasthenia, chronic fatigue syndrome often begins abruptly after an infectious illness. Initial studies proposed that the chronic fatigue syndrome resulted from a chronic Epstein-Barr virus infection, but more recent studies refute these findings.[47-50] Several causes of the chronic fatigue syndrome have been proposed, including: a Coxsackie or other enteroviral infection, an immune dysfunction, a psychiatric disorder, a hypothalamic-pituitary-adrenal insufficiency, or a disorder of serotonin metabolism.[3,25,26,47,51-55]

Although a number of these abnormalities might be more proximal causes of chronic fatigue syndrome, the results of the studies summarized above suggest that neurally mediated hypotension may be the final common pathway for symptoms in this disorder. This hypothesis provides a framework within which many of the clinical features of the syndrome can be understood. For example, patients with the chronic fatigue syndrome typically have great difficulty shopping, an activity that would be expected to trigger neurally mediated hypotension due to venous pooling.

The precise pathophysiological basis underlying the relationship between neurally mediated hypotension and the chronic fatigue syndrome remains uncertain. However, any mechanism that is proposed would have to account for the acuteness of onset and the high prevalence of preceding infectious processes. Within this framework, several potential mechanisms can be postulated. First, it is possible that this close relationship may reflect virally induced autonomic dysfunction[56,57] as had been suspected in neuromyasthenia.[58-60] This type of disorder may affect the ability of veno and/or arteriolar vasoconstriction, which may augment venous pooling on standing, thus increasing the susceptibility to neurally mediated hypotension. A second mechanism that may explain this close association is an abnormality of renal and/or adrenal function resulting in an inability to retain sodium. The elevation in serum angiotensin-converting enzyme reported in patients with chronic fatigue syndrome is also consistent with the hypothesis that these patients have abnormally low blood volume.[61] A third mechanism that can be postulated is that this relationship reflects an abnormality of serotonic metabolism, as serotonin reuptake inhibitors have been used in uncontrolled trials to treat both disorders.[3,15,46] Alternatively, patients with chronic fatigue syndrome may have a heightened sensitivity of mechanoreceptors. In this regard, it is notable that the response of pulmonary C-fiber mechanoreceptors can be increased dramatically with the activation of mast cells.[62] Whether the high prevalence of allergic disease in those with CFS contributes to mast cell activation and C-fiber stimulation remains to be determined.[63]

Although further speculation about other mechanisms is possible, the precise pathophysiological basis for the relationship between CFS and neurally mediated hypotension remains uncertain and awaits the results of future research efforts. Identification of a single abnormality or the classification of patients to appropriate subgroups, each linked by one of several pathophysiological conditions, may allow more rational approaches to therapy and possibly prevention of future cases of the chronic fatigue syndrome.

Current Approaches to Evaluation and Treatment

The improvement in symptoms typically associated with the chronic fatigue syndrome in response to treatment directed at neurally mediated hypotension reported recently by Bou-Holaigah and colleagues[5] must be interpreted with caution, as this study was performed in a small number of patients, had a short duration of follow-up, and was neither randomized, blinded, nor placebo-controlled.[5] We believe, however, that the magnitude and rapid time course of improvement in symptoms in response to treatment are difficult to attribute solely to a placebo effect. These findings must be considered unproven until the results of large prospective randomized trials are available. Despite these words of caution, many patients with the chronic fatigue syndrome are unwilling to delay potentially useful treatment. To this end, the approach to treatment of neurally mediated hypotension currently used by physicians at the Johns Hopkins Hospital is described in the following paragraphs.

The evaluation of a patient with chronic fatigue syndrome consists of an initial clinical evaluation during which history and prior laboratory tests are reviewed. Particular attention is focused on establishing whether the patient fulfills the diagnostic criteria for the chronic fatigue syndrome.[2] In this regard, it is important to recognize that patients with the chronic fatigue syndrome represent a small proportion of the approximately one fourth of the population who experience fatigue lasting at least 2 weeks in duration, and of the 24% of patients evaluated at general medical clinics who experience fatigue of at least 1 months' duration.[2,21] It is currently unknown whether neurally mediated hypotension is related to these more common fatiguing illnesses.

Attention is also focused on determining whether the patient's clinical history is compatible with neurally mediated hypotension. For example, patients frequently complain of lightheadedness with prolonged standing (eg, while on line at a grocery store). Other situations commonly associated with lightheadedness include hot showers or the moments immediately following exercise. Approximately one third of patients with the chronic fatigue syndrome will have experienced at least one episode of syncope, but for most this is a remote event. It is also helpful to determine whether the patient restricts his or her salt intake and whether the patient has a prior history of peripheral edema, hypertension, asthma, or other conditions that may alter the approach used to treat neurally mediated hypotension.

During the physical examination, particular attention should be focused on obtaining the patient's orthostatic vital signs. In normal adults, upright posture results in a slight fall in systolic blood pressure (5 to 10 mm Hg) and a similar and slight increase in the diastolic blood pressure (5 to 10 mm Hg). The heart rate normally increases by <20 bpm.[64] With typical orthostatic hypotension, the systolic and diastolic blood pressure fall with standing. Another pattern that may be observed is the presence of idiopathic postural orthostatic tachycardia. This type of response is characterized by an increase in heart rate by >30 bpm or to >110 bpm[43] with or without an associated decrease in systolic or diastolic blood pressure. Other potential causes of orthostatic hypotension such as autonomic neuropathy (amyloid, diabetes, familial), degenerative central nervous system disease (Parkinson's disease, pure autonomic failure, multiple system atrophy), prolonged bed rest, or spinal cord lesions must be excluded to classify the patient as having idiopathic postural orthostatic tachycardia syndrome. Patients with idiopathic postural orthostatic tachycardia syndrome frequently present with an abnormal red/blue color in their hands and feet with prolonged standing, suggesting the presence of some abnormality that results in marked venodilation.[46] The presence of postural orthostatic tachycardia syndrome does not preclude the presence of neurally mediated hypotension. In our experience, approximately 10% to 20% of patients with the chronic fatigue syndrome will demonstrate this type of response. The implications of this finding from a therapeutic standpoint remain uncertain.

Upright tilt table testing is a useful diagnostic test for patients with the chronic fatigue syndrome. Orthostatic intolerance as manifested by the provocation of symptoms is almost universal. An abnormal hemodynamic response to tilt table testing with reproduction of the patient's clinical symptoms is observed in approximately 90% of patients. Among the remaining patients, two subgroups can be identified: 1) those with a negative hemodynamic response without reproduction of clinical symptoms and 2) those with either a normal hemodynamic response or a hemodynamic response consistent with idiopathic postural orthostatic tachycardia syndrome in whom the clinical symptoms are reproduced. The efficacy of treatment in these two subgroups has not been studied in detail, but the consistent provocation of symptoms suggests that upright tilt testing may not capture the important pathophysiological abnormalities in these individuals.

The treatment of patients with chronic fatigue syndrome within the framework of neurally mediated hypotension consists of several components. Initially, it is recommended that the patient increase his or her intake of sodium and fluid and discontinue diuretics and other medications that act as either diuretics or vasodilators. An increase in daily sodium intake of at least 3000 mg can be readily accomplished by minor alterations in diet. If necessary, this can be supplemented with NaCl tablets. For most patients, changes in diet alone result in little or no improvement in symptoms, thus necessitating initiation of pharmacological therapy directed at neurally mediated hypotension. Fludrocortisone is a useful firstline agent (initial dose of 0.025 to 0.05 mg/day increasing to 0.1 to 0.2 mg/day). Administration of fludrocortisone in conjunction with K replacement (10 or 20 meq/day) improves clinical tolerance to fludrocortisone. If fludrocortisone is either ineffective or poorly tolerated, alternative pharmacological agents can be considered. These secondline therapeutic agents include β-blockers (ie, atenolol at doses of 0.5 to 1.0 mg/kg/day), disopyramide (Norpace CR 100 to 200 mg bid), or one of several serotonin reuptake inhibitors. If this is poorly tolerated or ineffective, less well-established approaches to therapy can be considered, including midodrine (an investigational α-agonist), ephedrine, methylphenidate, theophylline, or clonidine, which have been shown to be ineffective by others. For some, judicious use of combined therapy with fludrocortisone, a vasoconstrictor, and either a selective serotonin reuptake inhibitor (SSRI) or a negative inotropic agent has been associated with improvement in symptoms.

Future Directions

The results of the studies summarized in this chapter provide tantalizing evidence to suggest the presence of a relationship between fatigue, chronic fatigue, chronic fatigue syndrome, and neurally mediated hypotension, a common abnormality of blood pressure regulation. As with any new approach to a clinical problem, many very important questions remain unanswered. With focused research, the next 5 to 10 years should bring answers to these questions, as well as a rational approach to the evaluation and treatment of patients with the chronic fatigue syndrome and the related disorder fibromyalgia.

References

1. Holmes GP, Kaplan JE, Gantz NM, et al. Chronic fatigue syndrome: A working case definition. *Ann Intern Med* 1988;108:387–389.
2. Fukuda K, Straus SE, Hickie I, et al. The chronic fatigue syndrome: A comprehensive approach to its definition and study. *Ann Intern Med* 1994;121:953–959.
3. Lane RM. Aetiology, diagnosis and treatment of chronic fatigue syndrome. *J Serotonin Res* 1994;1:47–60.
4. Rowe PC, Bou-Holaigah I, Kan JS, et al. Is neurally mediated hypotension an unrecognized cause of chronic fatigue? *Lancet* 1995;345:623–624.
6. Engel, GL. *Fainting: Physiological and Psychological Considerations.* Springfield, IL: Charles C. Thomas; 1950.

7. Weissler AM, Warren JV. Vasodepressor syncope. *Am Heart J* 1959;57:786–794.
8. Van Lieshout JJ, Wieling W, Karemaker JM. The vasovagal response. *Clin Sci* 1991;81:575–586.
9. Kosinski DJ, Grubb BP. Neurally mediated syncope with an update on indications and usefulness of head-upright tilt table testing and pharmacologic therapy. *Curr Opin Cardiol* 1994;9:53–64.
10. Sra JS, Jazayeri MR, Dhala A, et al. Neurocardiogenic syncope: Diagnosis, mechanisms, and treatment. *Cardiol Clin* 1993;11:183–191.
11. Calkins H, Shyr Y, Frumin H, et al. The value of the clinical history in the differentiation of syncope due to ventricular tachycardia, atrioventricular block, and vasodepressor syncope. *Am J Med* 1995;98:365–373.
12. Sheldon R, Killam S. Methodology of isoproterenol-tilt table testing in patients with syncope. *J Am Coll Cardiol* 1992;19:773–779.
13. Sra J, Vishnubhakta SM, Jazayeri MR, et al. Use of intravenous esmolol to predict efficacy of oral beta-adrenergic blocker therapy in patients with neurocardiogenic syncope. *J Am Coll Cardiol* 1992;19:402–408.
14. Milstein S, Buetikofer J, Dunnigan A, et al. Usefulness of disopyramide for prevention of upright tilt-induced hypotension-bradycardia. *Am J Cardiol* 1990;65:1339–1344.
15. Grubb BP, Wolfe DA, Samoil D, et al. Usefulness of fluoxetine hydrochloride for prevention of resistant upright tilt induced syncope. *Pacing Clin Electrophysiol* 1993;16:458–464.
16. Calkins H, Seifert M, Morady F. Clinical presentation and long term follow-up of athletes with exercise induced vasodepressor syncope. *Am Heart J* 1995;159–164.
17. Grubb BP, Temesy-Armos PN, Samoil D, et al. Tilt table testing in the evaluation and management of athletes with recurrent exercise-induced syncope. *J Am Coll Sports Med* 1993;25:24–28.
18. Harrison MH, Kravik SE, Geelen G, et al. Blood pressure and plasma renin activity as predictors of orthostatic tolerance. *Aviat Space Environ Med* 1985;7:1059–1064.
19. Kleinknecht RA, Lenz J, Ford G, et al. Types and correlates of blood/injury level-related vasovagal syncope. *Behav Res Ther* 1990;28:289–295.
20. Camfield PR, Camfield CS. Syncope in childhood: A case control clinical study of the familial tendency to faint. *Can J Neurol Sci* 1990;17:306–308.
21. Bates DW, Schmitt W, Buchwald D, et al. Prevalence of fatigue and chronic fatigue syndrome in a primary care practice. *Arch Intern Med* 1993;153:2759–2765.
22. Lloyd AR, Hickie I, Boughton CR, et al. Prevalence of chronic fatigue syndrome in an Australian population. *Med J Aust* 1990;153:522–528.
23. Bates DW, Buchwald D, Lee J, et al. Clinical laboratory test findings in patients with chronic fatigue syndrome. *Arch Int Med* 1995;155:97–103.
24. Demitrack MA, Dale JK, Straus SE, et al. Evidence of impaired activation of the hypothalamic-pituitary-adrenal axis in patients with chronic fatigue syndrome. *J Clin Endocrinol Metab* 1991;73:1224–1234.
25. Landay AL, Jessop C, Lennette ET, et al. Chronic fatigue syndrome: Clinical condition associated with immune activation. *Lancet* 1991;338:707–712.
26. Klimas NG, Salvato FR, Morgan R, et al. Immunologic abnormalities in chronic fatigue syndrome. *Clin Microbiol* 1990;28:1403–1410.
27. Prieto J, Subira ML, Castilla A, et al. Naloxone-reversible monocyte dysfunction in patients with chronic fatigue syndrome. *Scand J Immunol* 1989;30:13–20.
28. Schwartz RB, Komaroff AL, Garada BM, et al. SPECT imaging of the brain: Comparison of findings in patients with chronic fatigue syndrome, AIDS dementia complex, and unipolar depression. *AJR* 1994;162:943–951.

29. Kaslow JE, Rucker L, Onishi R. Liver-extract-folic ácid-cyanocobalamin vs placebo for chronic fatigue syndrome. *Am J Med* 1990;89:554–560.
30. Peterson PK, Shepard J, Macres M, et al. A controlled trial of intravenous immunoglobulin G in chronic fatigue syndrome. *Am J Med* 1990;89:554–560.
31. Lloyd A, Hickie I, Wakefield D, et al. A double-blind, placebo-controlled trial of intravenous immunoglobulin therapy in patients with chronic fatigue syndrome. *Am J Med* 1990;89:561–568.
32. Straus SE, Dale JK, Tobi M, et al. Acyclovir treatment of the chronic fatigue syndrome: Lack of efficacy in a placebo-controlled trial. *N Engl J Med* 1988; 319:1692–1698.
33. Behan PO, Behan WMH, Horrobin D. Effect of high doses of essential fatty acids on the postviral fatigue syndrome. *Acta Neurol Scand* 1990;82:209–216.
34. Wilson A, Hickie I, Lloyd A, et al. The treatment of chronic fatigue syndrome: Science and speculation. *Am J Med* 1994;96:544–550.
35. Wilson A, Hickie I, Lloyd A, et al. Longitudinal study of outcome of chronic fatigue syndrome. *Br Med J* 1994;308:756–759.
36. Steele L, Reyes M, Dobbins JG, et al. Measuring the course and outcome of chronic fatigue syndrome: Results from longitudinal follow-up of 112 patients. Presented at: Development of Outcome Measures for Therapeutic Trials in Chronic Fatigue Syndrome, NIH, Bethesda, MD; April 11, 1995.
37. Lewis T. A lecture on vasovagal syncope and the carotid sinus mechanism. *Br Med J* 1932;1:873–876.
38. Komaroff AL, Buchwald D. Symptoms and signs of chronic fatigue syndrome. *Rev Infect Dis* 1991;13(suppl 1):S8–S11.
39. Bell KM, Cookfair D, Bell DS, et al. Risk factors associated with chronic fatigue syndrome in a cluster of pediatric cases. *Rev Inf Dis* 1991;13(suppl 1):S32–S38.
40. Stewart AL, Hays RD, Ware JE Jr. The MOS short-form general health survey: Reliability and validity in a general population. *Med Care* 1988;26:724–735.
41. Bentall RP, Wood GC, Marrinam T. A brief mental fatigue questionnaire. *Br J Clin Psychol* 1993;32:375–379.
42. Schondorf R, Low PA. Idiopathic postural orthostatic tachycardia syndrome: An attenuated form of acute pandysautonomia? *Neurology* 1993;43:132–137.
43. Streeten DHP, Anderson, GH. Delayed othostatic intolerance. *Arch Intern Med* 1992;152:1066–1072.
44. Rosen SG, Cryer PE. Postural tachycardia syndrome: Reversal of sympathetic hyperresponsiveness and clinical improvement during sodium loading. *Am J Med* 1982;72:847–850.
45. Fouad FM, Tadena-Thome L, Bravo EL, et al. Idiopathic hypovolemia. *Ann Intern Med* 1986;104:298–303.
46. Grubb BP, Kosinski DJ, Boehm K, et al. The postural orthostatic tachycardia syndrome: A neurocardiogenic variant identified during head up tilt table testing. *Pacing Clin Electrophysiol* 1997;20(8):2205–2213.
47. Manu P, Lane TH, Matthews DA. The pathophysiology of chronic fatigue syndrome: Confirmations, contradictions, and conjectures. *Int J Psych Med* 1992; 22:397–408.
48. Straus SE. Studies of herpes virus infection in chronic fatigue syndrome. *Ciba Found Symp* 1993;173:132–145.
49. Holmes GP, Kaplan JE, Stewart JA, et al. A cluster of patients with a chronic mononucleosis-like syndrome: Is Epstein-Barr virus the cause? *JAMA* 1987; 257:2297–2302.
50. Levine PH, Jacobson S, Pocinki AG, et al. Clinical, epidemiologic, and virologic studies in four clusters of the chronic fatigue syndrome. *Arch Intern Med* 1992;152:1611–1616.

51. Buchwald D, Cheney PR, Peterson DL, et al. A chronic illness characterized by fatigue, neurologic and immunologic disorders, and active human herpes virus type 6 infection. *Ann Intern Med* 1992;116:103–113.
52. Bond PA. A role for herpes simplex virus in the aetiology of chronic fatigue syndrome and related disorders. *Med Hypotheses* 1993;40:301–308.
53. DeFreitas E, Hilliard B, Cheney PR, et al. Retroviral sequences related to human T-lymphototropic virus type II in patients with chronic fatigue immune dysfunction syndrome. *Proc Natl Acad Sci U S A* 1991;88:2922–2926.
54. Hickie I, Lloyd A, Wakefield D, Parker G. The psychiatric status of patients with the chronic fatigue syndrome. *Br J Psychiatry* 1990;156:534–540.
55. Demitrack MA, Dale JK, Straus SE, et al. Evidence of impaired activation of the hypothalamic-pituitary-adrenal axis in patients with chronic fatigue syndrome. *J Clin Endocrinol Metab* 1991;73:1224–1234.
56. Fujii N, Tabira T, Shibasaki H, et al. Acute autonomic and sensory neuropathy associated with elevated Epstein-Barr virus antibody titre. *J Neurol Neurosurg Psych* 1982;45:656–661.
57. Neville BG, Sladen GE. Acute autonomic neuropathy following primary herpes simplex infection. *J Neurol Neurosurg Psychiatry* 1984;47:648–650.
58. Fog T. Vegetative (epidemic?) neuritis. *Ugeskr Laeger* 1953;115:1244–1250.
59. Henderson DA, Shelokov A. Epidemic neuromyasthenia — clinical syndrome? *N Engl J Med* 1959;260:757–764 and 814–818.
60. Henderson DA. Reflections on epidemic neuromyasthenia (chronic fatigue syndrome). *Clin Infect Dis* 1994;18(suppl 1):53–56.
61. Lieberman J, Bell DS. Serum angiotensin-converting enzyme as a marker for the chronic fatigue-immune dysfunction syndrome: A comparison to serum angiotensin-converting enzyme in sarcoidosis. *Am J Med* 1993;95:407–412.
62. Undem BJ, Riccio MM, Weinrich D, et al. Neurophysiology of mast cell-nerve interactions in the airways. *Int Arch Allergy Immunol* 1995;107:199–201.
63. Steinberg P, McNutt BE, Marshall P, et al. Immunodeficiency and other clinical immunology. *J Allergy Clin Immunol* 1996;97:119–126.
64. Robertson D, Robertson RM. Orthostatic hypotension: Diagnosis and therapy. *Mod Concepts Cardiovasc Dis* 1985;54(2):7–12.

Chapter 11

Carotid Sinus Hypersensitivity

Alan B. Wagshal, MD
and Shoei K. Stephen Huang, MD

Introduction

The fact that pressure on the carotid artery results in slowing of the heart rate and impairing of AV node conduction has been appreciated since before the turn of the century.[1,2] Although this effect was initially thought to result from stimulation of the vagus nerve,[3,4] in 1927 Hering[5] demonstrated that it was instead the result of stimulation of the carotid sinus. In 1961, Lown and Levine[6] showed that carotid sinus stimulation was a useful technique for analyzing many arrhythmias. Carotid sinus hypersensitivity has subsequently been recognized as one of the most common and best characterized of the neurally mediated syncopal syndromes (Figure 1).[7]

The first report of carotid sinus hypersensitivity as a cause of syncope was on a group of 15 patients in 1933 by Weiss and Baker.[8] These authors divided patients into the grouping used today, namely cardioinhibitory (bradycardia and/or prolonged asystole), vasodepressor type (abrupt hypotension without bradycardia), and the primary cerebral type (syncope or presyncope associated with neither hypotension or bradycardia). This third category is extremely rare and questions have been raised as to its existence,[8-10] attributing this finding instead to cerebrovascular disease aggravated by unilateral carotid artery occlusion. An additional category, the mixed cardioinhibitory and vasodepressor type, has also been defined.[11]

From Grubb BP, Olshansky B (eds.). *Syncope: Mechanisms and Management.* Armonk, NY: Futura Publishing Co., Inc.; © 1998.

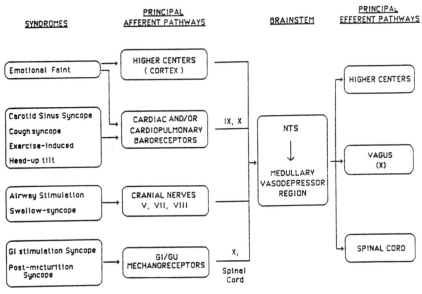

NTS = nucleus tractus solitarius

Figure 1. Diagrammatic representation of the relationship between various neurally mediated syncopal syndromes (far left), and their suspected afferent and efferent neural connections. Cranial nerves are indicated by conventional roman numeral designation. Reproduced with permission from Reference 7.

Anatomy and Physiology

The carotid sinus is a group of baroreceptors and nerve endings localized in an enlargement of the internal carotid artery at its origin from the common carotid artery.[12] The receptors are localized in the adventitia of the arterial wall. The afferent impulses are generated by localized stretch of the arterial wall and are transmitted through the sensory fibers of the carotid sinus nerve that travels with the glossopharyngeal nerve. The afferent pathways terminate in the nucleus tractus solitarius in the medulla, in close proximity to the dorsal and ambiguous nuclei, which control the vagus nerve (Figure 1). Although this disorder is classically considered an abnormal sensitivity of the carotid sinus itself, there is some evidence that at least in some patients the abnormality may reside in the brainstem itself.[13] The efferent pathways are transmitted widely through the cardiac branches of the vagus nerve and the sympathetic adrenergic nerves to both the heart and the peripheral vasculature. Sympathetic neural inhibition during carotid sinus massage was recently directly assessed using direct microneurographic recording of sympathetic nerve activity.[14] The result of carotid sinus stimulation is thus a combination of sinus node slowing, atrioventricular node block, and decreased cardiac output and vascular resistance. Physiologically, localized stretching of the carotid sinus receptors is produced by arterial hypertension, but this phenomenon can be duplicated by local external stimulation of the carotid sinus.

Technique

The patient should be supine with the neck slightly extended. The carotid pulsation should be palpated in the upper portion of the neck (just slightly below the angle of the jaw) where the carotid bifurcation is located. Pressure should be applied at this point in the direction of the vertebral column for 5 seconds. If no response is elicited with mild pressure, slightly increased degrees of pressure or massage can then be applied for successive 5-second intervals. Carotid sinus pressure should be limited to 5 seconds per attempt with a pause of at least 15 seconds between attempts.[15] Because the exact location of the carotid bifurcation, and thus the carotid sinus, is somewhat variable, several locations along the carotid artery should be tested. Both sides should be tested, but never simultaneously. For safety, the carotid artery should first be auscultated for bruits, and the presence of significant cerebrovascular disease should be excluded by history and examination. Because of the rare possibility of prolonged asystole or ventricular arrhythmias, a defibrillator and atropine and lidocaine should be available, as well as the ability for prolonged electrocardiographic recording. While there are several cases of ventricular tachycardia or ventricular fibrillation following carotid sinus massage reported in the literature,[16–24] most of these cases are in patients with serious underlying cardiac disease who are undergoing carotid sinus massage for help in the diagnosis or termination of supraventricular tachycardia or wide QRS-complex tachycardia.

The normal response to carotid sinus pressure is a transient decrease of the sinus rate and/or slowing of atrioventricular conduction, although the latter phenomenon is usually masked by the former. A sinus pause of up to 3 seconds is usually considered the upper limit of a normal response, and thus carotid sinus hypersensitivity is defined as a pause of at least 3 seconds in duration (Figure 2).[9,25] Some reports suggest that the right carotid sinus has a preferential effect on the sinus node, whereas the left carotid sinus has a preferential effect on the atrioventricular node,[16] but other studies do not show a clear-cut distinction.[6,26,27]

The vasodepressor form of carotid sinus hypersensitivity is defined as a fall of systolic blood pressure of 50 mm Hg or more (Figure 2), which is usually exaggerated in a sitting[9] or standing[28] position. Periodic cuff measurements of blood pressure are probably not adequate to diagnose this component in most patients; recently digital plethysmography has been shown to be a useful technique that allows accurate beat-to-beat measure-

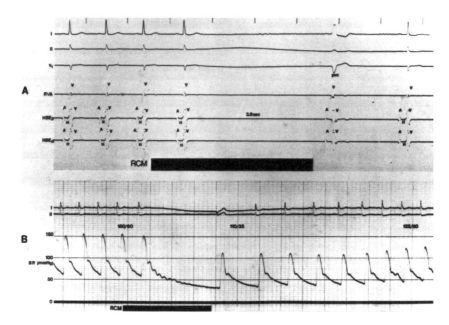

Figure 2. Typical mixed (cardioinhibitory and vasodepressor) response to carotid sinus massage in a patient with carotid sinus hypersensitivity. Panel A shows the surface electrocardiogram (leads I, II, and V₁) and intracardiac leads (right ventricular apex (RVA) and proximal and distal His bundle electrograms (HBE$_p$ and HBE$_d$) during right carotid sinus massage (RCM and black bar), which resulted in a 3.8-second pause. A ventricular escape beat or aberrantly conducted beat (labeled PVC) occurs simultaneously with resumption of atrial activity. Time line = 1 second; H = His bundle potential; A = atrial electrical activity; V = ventricular electrical activity. Panel B is a simultaneous recording of surface electrocardiograms leads I and II and femoral arterial blood pressure on a different strip-chart recorder during the same period of right carotid sinus massage shown in panel A. Note that systolic blood pressure declined from 160 mm Hg before the pause to 110 mm Hg after resumption of electrical activity and only gradually increased thereafter to 125 mm Hg by the end of the strip. Reproduced with permission from Reference 43.

ment of blood pressure.[29,30] At least one such unit is commercially available (Finapres, Ohmeda, Louisville, Colorado). In patients with a concomitant cardioinhibitory component, the diagnosis of a vasodepressor component requires either simultaneous administration of atropine or atrioventricular pacing, the latter being the preferred technique.

Various drugs such as propranolol[31,32] and methyldopa[33] have been shown to significantly exaggerate the bradycardic effects of carotid sinus pressure. This should be taken into account when interpreting the results of carotid sinus massage in patients taking one of these drugs.

While the finding of carotid sinus hypersensitivity in association with multiple episodes of syncope or near syncope is generally taken as cause-

and-effect evidence for a relationship, some authors insist on duplication of symptoms before ascribing the cause of syncope to carotid sinus hypersensitivity.[28] If such is the case, symptoms can be increased by performing carotid sinus massage during upright tilt table testing.[11,28,34,35]

Clinical Syndromes and Incidence of Carotid Sinus Hypersensitivity

Carotid sinus hypersensitivity is a fairly common cause of unexplained syncope, particularly in older patients. It is particularly common in older males with atherosclerosis.[27,36-38] Previous neck surgery, malignancy, and/ or radiation therapy to the neck have also been associated with carotid sinus hypersensitivity.[16,39,40]

Because of the predominant and dramatic sinus pause in the cardioinhibitory or mixed forms of the carotid sinus syndrome, syncope, when it occurs, is usually abrupt and indistinguishable from Stokes-Adams attacks. In this regard it differs from neurocardiogenic syncope in which syncope is more gradual and often precipitated by a prodrome of dizziness or lightheadedness (Figure 3).[30]

By use of either digital plethysmography or direct arterial blood pressure recordings, a majority of patients with carotid sinus hypersensitivity have been shown to have a vasodepressor component. For example, Gaggioli et al[29] showed that 57/68 (84%) patients with carotid sinus hypersensitivity had a vasodepressor component. A prominent vasodepressor component appears to be particularly common in older patients with carotid sinus hypersensitivity.[29,41]

The vasodepressor component of the carotid sinus reflex (either as an isolated finding or part of the mixed form) lasts longer than the cardioinhibitory portion.[27,41,42] In a study by Brown et al,[27] patients with the mixed form of carotid sinus hypersensitivity had hypotension that persisted for a mean of 27 seconds after cessation of carotid sinus massage, while patients with a pure vasodepressor response had even longer-lasting hypotension.

Huang et al[43] analyzed a group of 76 patients with unexplained syncope using carotid sinus massage and electrophysiological testing; a diagnosis of carotid sinus hypersensitivity was made in 21 (28%) patients. Most patients were treated with permanent pacemakers, and no patients who received a pacemaker had recurrent syncope, with a mean follow-up of 42±19 months. Morley et al[44] showed that approximately one third of patients requiring a permanent pacemaker for repeated syncopal spells had hypersensitive carotid sinus as the cause of syncope. However, the syndrome may be underdiagnosed if patients with recurrent syncope do not undergo carotid sinus massage before pacing is performed, and it is instead labeled idiopathic syncope or sick sinus syndrome.[30,45,46]

Carotid Sinus Syncope

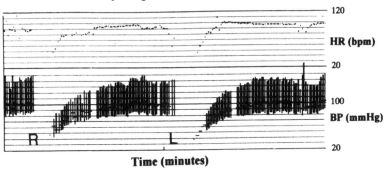

Vasovagal Syncope

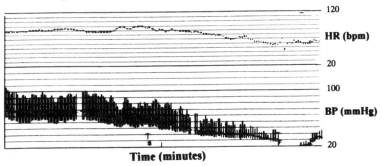

Figure 3. The typical differences between carotid sinus and vasovagal syncope. Both panels show 2 minutes of beat-to-beat heart rate and blood pressure recordings. The continuous blood pressure recordings were obtained noninvasively with digital plethysmography (Finapres). The top panel demonstrates positive right (R) and left (L) carotid sinus massage performed at 60° head-up tilt. Asystole develops suddenly and continues throughout the period of carotid sinus massage. The lower panel demonstrates vasovagal syncope developing after 18 minutes of 60° head-up tilt. The onset of the fall in blood pressure precedes that of the heart rate by about 15 seconds. Symptoms (S) occur relatively early, and are followed by a gradual fall in both blood pressure and heart rate that continues for about 1 minute before syncope intervenes (F), and the patient is returned supine. Reproduced with permission from Reference 30.

A particularly instructive study in this regard was performed by Brignole et al.[47] They analyzed 25 consecutive patients with syncope with documented asystolic pauses (either sinus or AV block) on prolonged Holter or telemetry monitoring that occurred during episodes of syncope. All patients underwent carotid sinus massage, head-up tilt table testing, and electrophysiological testing. Electrophysiological testing yielded a cause of syncope in 6 patients (5 patients with infra-Hisian block and 1 patient with sick sinus syndrome), whereas 17 of the 25 patients had an abnormal response to carotid sinus massage (n=14 patients) or tilt table testing (n=10 patients) or both (n=7 patients), which duplicated the findings seen on electrocardiographic monitoring. This suggests that in most patients with syncope, even with documented bradycardic events causing the syncope, a neurogenic rather than a cardiogenic cause is responsible. These findings correlate with and help to explain an earlier report that shows the poor yield of electrophysiological testing in patients with syncope even with documented bradycardia.[48]

The exact role that carotid sinus hypersensitivity plays in causing syncope, however, is difficult to determine because many patients without syncope exhibit abnormal responses to carotid sinus pressure. A prolonged sinus pause during carotid sinus pressure without a history of syncope or presyncope is particularly common among older males and patients with atherosclerosis; some studies show an incidence of up to 5% to 25% of this population.[9,11,38,42] Brown et al[27] performed carotid sinus massage in 55 consecutive patients who were being catheterized for coronary artery disease and found an incidence of carotid sinus hypersensitivity of 38%. Several studies have estimated that only 5% to 20% of patients exhibiting carotid sinus hypersensitivity actually have syncope of carotid sinus origin.[36,37,49] Whereas clinical syndromes such as syncope associated with wearing a tight collar or necktie, or with shaving or twisting of the neck, strongly suggest that carotid sinus hypersensitivity is the cause of syncope,[8] often the clinical precipitants are much less clear and thus it is harder to determine if the hypersensitive carotid sinus response induced by carotid sinus massage is indeed the cause of syncope.[6,34,35,50,51] Nelson et al[52] published a report on a series of patients with presumed carotid sinus hypersensitivity syncope who also had inducible sustained monomorphic ventricular tachycardia as a potential cause of syncope. An example of this problem is a 56-year-old male who recently presented to our hospital with the complaint of recurrent syncope after implantation of a permanent pacemaker for carotid sinus hypersensitivity. The original diagnosis of carotid sinus hypersensitivity had been made 3 months earlier after a syncopal spell that occurred while he was pheasant hunting and had just turned his neck to place his prey in a shoulder bag; complete invasive electrophysiological testing was negative except for a 4.5-second pause with right carotid pressure (Figure 4), which led to the pacemaker implantation. Further workup revealed evidence of temporal lobe epilepsy on electroencephalogram, with an actual seizure associated with syncope occurring while hooked up to the electroencephalogram. Pharmacological control of his seizure disorder also prevented further episodes of syncope. Since this syncopal spell was identical to his original presenting episode of syncope, the most likely situation was that the cause of both syncopal spells was temporal lobe sei-

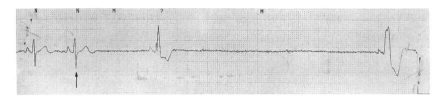

Figure 4. A telemetry strip showing a 4.5-second pause during right carotid sinus massage for 5 seconds (starting at arrow) in a 56-year-old male patient with recurrent syncope.

zures, and the abnormal response demonstrated by carotid sinus massage was an irrelevant finding (despite the story of syncope associated with head turning that would certainly have been compatible with carotid sinus hypersensitivity).

Associated Cardiovascular Diseases and Electrophysiological Abnormalities

In the series of 21 patients with carotid sinus hypersensitivity described by Huang et al,[43] all patients underwent comprehensive invasive electrophysiological testing as part of their initial diagnostic work-up for syncope. Abnormal sinus node function was found in 29% of the patients and abnormal AV node function was found in 33% of the patients. Similar incidences of sinus node and AV node dysfunction have been reported in other studies,[9,34,35,50,53-55] and suggest that although there is some overlap, the vast majority of patients with carotid sinus hypersensitivity have normal sinus node function, and thus in the vast majority of patients, sick sinus syndrome and carotid sinus hypersensitivity are separate entities.

While the classic presentation of syncope in the carotid sinus hypersensitivity syndrome is associated with some form of neck pressure or manipulation, many episodes of syncope in patients with documented hypersensitive carotid sinus syndrome are not related to neck manipulation, suggesting that there may be other triggers or receptors (such as, but not necessarily limited to, those described in the aortic arch, gastrointestinal tract, or genitourinary tract) (see Figure 1) for syncope in this condition.[15] In fact, patients with classic presentations of carotid sinus hypersensitivity have also had syncopal spells associated with other triggers such as coughing,[56] sneezing, straining at stool, or heavy lifting,[8,37,57] and micturition.[9]

Brignole et al[58,59] presented evidence suggesting an overlap between carotid sinus hypersensitivity and neurocardiogenic syncope; 40% of patients with carotid sinus hypersensitivity also had positive tilt table tests, and vice versa.[58,59] In a follow-up study,[60] the same investigators showed that patients with syncope from carotid sinus hypersensitivity who also had a positive tilt table study were more likely to have recurrence of syncope despite permanent DDD pacing (15/24 patients; 63%) than patients with a negative tilt table study (9/24 patients; 38%), whereas patients with no further episodes of syncope more frequently had a negative (90/145 patients; 62%) than a positive (55/145 patients; 38%) tilt table test. They concluded that in patients with carotid sinus syndrome, a positive response to head-up tilt testing suggests that a complex autonomic disease that involves multiple receptors and pathways is present. Furthermore, in any given patient, it is difficult to assess how much of the hypersensitivity resides in the afferent limb (ie, true hypersensitivity of the carotid sinus), and how much resides in the efferent limb (ie, an exaggerated vagal output in response to normal activity of the carotid sinus or an exaggerated sensitivity to normal vagal outputs). There is one study[13] that shows that there may be a neural defect underlying at least some cases of the carotid sinus syndrome. In this light, it is easy to see why there may be a significant overlap between carotid sinus hypersensitivity and other neurogenic causes of syncope.

Management of Patients with Carotid Sinus Hypersensitivity

Permanent pacing has been well established as the treatment of choice for patients with syncope that is proven or strongly suspected to be caused by a hypersensitive carotid sinus.[9,34,57,61] However, some patients with carotid sinus hypersensitivity may undergo spontaneous remission of symptoms.[34,43,62-64] Nevertheless, in a prospective study of pacing versus no pacing for carotid sinus syndrome, 57% of those patients randomized to the no-pacing limb experienced recurrent syncope over a mean follow-up of 36 months, compared with 9% in the paced group.

Formal guidelines for insertion of a permanent pacemaker in carotid sinus hypersensitivity were published by a joint task force from the American Heart Association and the American College of Cardiology in 1991 (Table 1).[65] It is of note that the wording is "recurrent syncope" as an indication for pacing—apparently to exclude patients with just a single episode of syncope. Clearly, however, most investigators would recommend a permanent pacemaker if the first episode of carotid sinus syncope resulted in significant injury to the patient. In a series of patients studied by Morley and Sutton,[15] 25% of the syncopal spells due to carotid sinus hypersensitivity were associated with significant injury, and thus pacing for all patients after a single syncopal spell was recommended. The finding of a high frequency of injury from syncope in these patients correlates with the usual abrupt onset of asystole and syncope seen in this disorder, as mentioned earlier in this chapter.

_____ Table 1 _____

Indications for Permanent Pacing in Hypersensitive Carotid Sinus and Neurovascular Syndromes

Class I. (Conditions for which there is general agreement that permanent pacemakers should be implanted)
  A. Recurrent syncope associated with clear, spontaneous events provoked by carotid sinus stimulation; minimal carotid sinus pressure induces asystole of >3 seconds' duration in the absence of any medication that depresses the sinus node or AV conduction.

Class II. (Conditions for which permanent pacemakers are frequently used, but there is divergence of opinion with respect to the necessity of their insertion)
  A. Recurrent syncope without clear, provocative events and with a hypersensitive cardioinhibitory response.

Class III. (Conditions for which there is general agreement that pacemakers are unnecessary)
  A. A hyperactive cardioinhibitory response to carotid sinus stimulation in the absence of symptoms.
  B. Vague symptoms such as dizziness or lightheadedness or both, with a hyperactive cardioinhibitory response to carotid sinus stimulation.
  C. Recurrent syncope, light-headedness or dizziness in the absence of a cardioinhibitory response.

AV = atrioventricular.
Reproduced with permission from Dreifus, L.S. et al: ACC/AHA task force report: Guidelines for implantation of cardiac pacemakers and antiarrhythmia devices. *J Am Coll Cardiol* 1991; 18:1–13.

The presence of an associated vasodepressor component makes treatment of carotid sinus hypersensitivity much more difficult, and is probably the major cause of recurrent syncope in patients treated with permanent pacemakers.[42] In several studies,[64,66] approximately 10% of patients with carotid sinus syndrome treated with a pacemaker had recurrent syncope. Atrioventricular sequential pacing is clearly preferred over ventricular pacing alone.[42,67] Morley et al[44] showed that atrioventricular sequential pacing alone was often enough to eliminate symptoms in patients with mixed cardioinhibitory and vasodepressor forms of the carotid sinus syndrome who continued to have symptoms with ventricular pacing alone. However, Almquist et al[42] showed that despite atrioventricular sequential pacing to maintain a constant heart rate of 80 bpm, the drop in systolic blood pressure in patients with a prominent vasodepressor component to carotid sinus pressure was little affected. A recent paper[68] suggests that use of dual-chamber pacing with automatic mode conversion that allows for automatic switching from AAI to DDD, plus atrial acceleration when AV block occurs, is more advantageous than DDD pacing alone. Surgical denervation of the carotid sinus is another potential treatment[69,70] that has proven effective in the treatment of the vasodepressor type or mixed form of carotid sinus syndrome when pacing therapy is inadequate to correct this disorder.[70]

Drugs that have been used to treat vasodepressive carotid sinus hypersensitivity include mineralocorticoids,[9] dihydroergotamine,[71] and ephedrine.[36,42] Ephedrine is probably the most effective of these drugs, but it is poorly tolerated, particularly in the elderly population, which comprises most patients with carotid sinus hypersensitivity, because of other sympathomimetic side effects.

Two patients who had prominent vasodepressor components to their carotid sinus syndrome and who had continued symptoms despite dual-chamber pacing were recently effectively treated with serotonin reuptake inhibitors (sertraline hydrochloride or fluoxetine hydrochloride), which both blocked the hypotensive component of carotid sinus massage and rendered the patients clinically free of symptoms.[72] This trial was motivated by earlier experiences of the same investigators, of a beneficial effect of fluoxetine hydrochloride on neurocardiogenic syncope.[73] Not only does this suggest a potential useful treatment for carotid sinus hypersensitivity that must be studied in larger numbers of patients, but it also adds to the speculation discussed earlier in this chapter that there is a close relationship between neurocardiogenic syncope and carotid sinus hypersensitivity.[30,58]

Conclusions

Carotid sinus hypersensitivity is an important cause of syncope that is probably under-recognized. It may be part of a more generalized syndrome of neurally mediated syncope that is becoming increasingly recognized as an important cause of syncope. While cardiac pacing is effective for the cardioinhibitory portion of the reflex, a coexisting vasodepressor component is frequently present, often unrecognized,[29] and a major cause of incomplete amelioration of symptoms with pacemaker therapy. Definitive therapy of the vasodepressor component is lacking and may require surgical denervation in some patients, although a possible association with other forms of neurocardiogenic syncope and some anecdotal reports of successful drug therapy in some patients suggest that more effective treatments for this aspect of the hypersensitive carotid sinus response may be forthcoming.

References

1. Parry CH. *An inquiry Into the Symptoms and Causes of the Syncope Anginosa.* Bath, England: R Cuttwell; 1799;102.
2. Cohn AE, Lewis T. The predominant influence of the left vagus nerve upon conduction between the auricles and ventricles in the dog. *J Exp Med* 1913; 18:739–744.

3. Burchell HB. A.V. Waller (1816-1870) and "vagus" pressure. *Pacing Clin Electrophysiol* 1988;11:1499–1501.
4. Waller AV. On the effects of compression of the vagus nerve in the cure and relief of various nervous affections. *Practitioner* 1870;4:193.
5. Hering HE. *Die Karotissinusreflexe auf Herz und Gefasse von Normal Physiologishen und Klinishen Standpunkt*. Dresden: Th. Steinkopff; 1927.
6. Lown B, Levine SA. The carotid sinus: Clinical value of its stimulation. *Circulation* 1961;23:766–789.
7. Benditt DG, Remole S, Bailin S, et al. Tilt table testing for evaluation of neurally-mediated (cardioneurogenic) syncope: Rationale and proposed protocols. *Pacing Clin Electrophysiol* 1991;14:1528–1537.
8. Weiss S, Baker JP. The carotid sinus reflex in health and disease: Its role in the causation of fainting and convulsions. *Medicine* 1933;12:297–345.
9. Walter PF, Crawley IS, Dorney ER. Carotid sinus hypersensitivity and syncope. *Am J Cardiol* 1978;42:396–403.
10. Gurjian ES, Webster JE, Hardy WC. Non-existence of the so-called cerebral form of carotid sinus syncope. *Neurology* 1958;8:818–826.
11. Stryjer D, Friedensohn A, Schlesinger Z. Carotid sinus hypersensitivity: Diagnosis of the vasodepressor type in the presence of the cardioinhibitory type. *Pacing Clin Electrophysiol* 1982;5:793–800.
12. Longhurst JC. Arterial baroreceptors in health and disease. *Cardiovascular Reviews & Reports* 1982;3:271–298.
13. Kenny RA, Lyon CC, Ingram AM, et al. Enhanced vagal activity and normal arginine vasopressin response in carotid sinus syndrome: Implications for a central abnormality in carotid sinus hypersensitivity. *Cardiovasc Res* 1987; 21:545–550.
14. Luck JC, Hoover R, Sutcliff G, et al. Measurement of sympathetic nerve activity in carotid sinus hypersensitivity. (Abstr) *Eur J Clin Pacing Electrophysiol* 1994; 4(suppl 4):25.
15. Morley CA, Sutton R. Carotid sinus syncope. *Int J Cardiol* 1984;6:287–293.
16. Schweitzer P, Teichholz LE. Carotid sinus massage: Its diagnostic and therapeutic value in arrhythmias. *Am J Med* 1985;78:645–654.
17. Meredith HC, Beckwith JR. Development of ventricular tachycardia following carotid sinus stimulation in paroxysmal supraventricular tachycardia. *Am Heart J* 1950;39:694–695.
18. Scherf D, Bernemann CA. Appearance of ventricular ectopic rhythm during carotid sinus pressure. *Chest* 1966;50:530–532.
19. Mathews CA. Ventricular tachycardia induced by carotid sinus stimulation. *J Maine Med Assoc* 1969;60:135–137.
20. Greenwood RJ, Dupler DA. Death following carotid sinus pressure. *JAMA* 1962;181:605–609.
21. Porus RI, Marcus FI. Ventricular fibrillation during carotid sinus stimulation. *N Engl J Med* 1963;268:1338–1342.
22. Alexander S, Ping WC. Fatal ventricular fibrillation during carotid sinus stimulation. *Am J Cardiol* 1966;18:289–291.
23. Hilal M, Massumi R. Fatal ventricular fibrillation after carotid sinus stimulation. *N Engl J Med* 1966;275:157–185.
24. Cohen MV. Ventricular fibrillation precipitated by carotid sinus pressure: Case report and review of the literature. *Am Heart J* 1972;84:681–686.
25. Fisher JD. Role of electrophysiologic testing in diagnosis and treatment of patients with known and suspected bradycardias and tachycardias. *Prog Cardiovasc Dis* 1981;24:25–90.

26. Sigler LH. The cardioinhibitory carotid sinus reflex: Its importance as a vago-cardiosensitivity test. *Am J Cardiol* 1963;12:175–183.
27. Brown KA, Maloney JD, Smith HC, et al. Carotid sinus reflex in patients undergoing coronary angiography: Relationship of degree and location of coronary artery disease to response to carotid sinus massage. *Circulation* 1980; 62:697–703.
28. Hammill SC, Holmes DR, Wood DL, et al. Electrophysiological testing in the upright position: Improved evaluation of patients with rhythm disturbances using a tilt table. *J Am Coll Cardiol* 1984;4:65–71.
29. Gaggioli G, Brignole M, Menozzi C, et al. Reappraisal of the vasodepressor reflex in carotid sinus syndrome. *Am J Cardiol* 1995;75:518–521.
30. Sutton R, Peterson MEV. The clinical spectrum of neurocardiogenic syncope. *J Cardiovasc Electrophysiol* 1995;6:569–576.
31. Reyes A. Propranolol and the hyperactive carotid sinus reflex syndrome. *Br Med J* 1973;2:662.
32. Berglund H, Rosenqvist M, Goukter S, et al. Responses to carotid sinus stimulation before and after propranolol. *Br Heart J* 1988;60:516–521.
33. Baurnfeind R, Hall C, Denes P, et al. Carotid sinus hypersensitivity with alpha methyldopa. *Ann Int Med* 1978;88:214–215.
34. Sugrue DD, Gersh BJ, Holmes DR, et al. Symptomatic "isolated" carotid sinus hypersensitivity: Natural history and results of treatment with anticholinergic drugs or pacemaker. *J Am Coll Cardiol* 1986;7:158–162.
35. Sugrue DD, Wood DL, McGoon MD. Carotid sinus hypersensitivity and syncope. *Mayo Clin Proc* 1984;59:637–640.
36. Thomas JE. Hyperactive carotid sinus reflex and carotid sinus syncope. *Mayo Clin Proc* 1969;44:127–139.
37. Nathanson MH. Hyperactive cardioinhibitory carotid sinus reflex. *Arch Int Med* 1946;77:491–502.
38. Hickler RB. Orthostatic hypotension and syncope. *N Engl J Med* 1977; 296:336–337.
39. Tulchinsky M, Krasnow SH. Carotid sinus syndrome associated with an occult primary nasopharyngeal carcinoma. *Arch Int Med* 1988;148:1217–1219.
40. Holmes FA, Glass PJ, Ewer MS, et al. Syncope and hypotension due to carcinoma of the breast metastatic to the carotid sinus. *Am J Med* 1987;82:1238–1242.
41. McIntosh S, Lawson J, Kenny RA. Clinical characteristics of vasodepressor, cardioinhibitory, and mixed carotid sinus syndrome in the elderly. *Am J Med* 1993;95:203–208.
42. Almquist A, Gornick C, Benson DW Jr, et al. Carotid sinus hypersensitivity: Evaluation of the vasodepressor component. *Circulation* 1985;71:927–936.
43. Huang SKS, Ezri MD, Hauser RG, et al. Carotid sinus hypersensitivity in patients with unexplained syncope: Clinical, electrophysiologic, and long-term follow-up observations. *Am Heart J* 1988;116:989-996.
44. Morley CA, Perrins EJ, Grant P, et al. Carotid sinus syncope treated by pacing: Analysis of persistent symptoms and role of atrioventricular sequential pacing. *Br Heart J* 1982;47:411–418.
45. Parsonnet V, Bernstein D. The 1989 World Survey of cardiac pacing. *Pacing Clin Electrophysiol* 1991;14:2073–2076.
46. Strasberg B, Pinchas A, Lewin RF, et al. Carotid sinus syndrome: An overlooked cause of syncope. *Isr J Med Sci* 1985;21:430–433.
47. Brignole M, Menozzi C, Bottoni N, et al. Mechanisms of syncope caused by transient bradycardia and the diagnostic value of electrophysiologic testing and cardiovascular reflexivity maneuvers. *Am J Cardiol* 1995;76:273–278.

48. Fujimura O, Yee R, Klein GJ, et al. The diagnostic sensitivity of electrophysiologic testing in patients with syncope caused by transient bradycardia. *N Engl J Med* 1989;321:1703–1707.

49. Strasberg B, Sagie A, Erdman S, et al. Carotid sinus hypersensitivity and the carotid sinus syndrome. *Prog Cardiovasc Dis* 1989;31:379–391.

50. Davies AB, Stephens MR, Davies AG. Carotid sinus hypersensitivity in patients presenting with syncope. *Br Heart J* 1979;42:583–586.

51. Heidorn GH, McNamara AP. Effect of carotid sinus stimulation on the electrocardiograms of clinically normal individuals. *Circulation* 1956;14:1104.

52. Nelson SP, Kou WH, de Buitleir M, et al. Value of programmed ventricular stimulation in presumed carotid sinus syndrome. *Am J Cardiol* 1987;60:1073–1077.

53. Hartzler GO, Maloney JD. Cardioinhibitory carotid sinus hypersensitivity. *Arch Int Med* 1977;137:727–731.

54. Morley CA, Hudson WM, Kwok HT, et al. Is there a difference between sick sinus syndrome and carotid sinus syndrome. *Br Heart J* 1983;49:620–621.

55. Gould L, Reddy CVR, Becker WH, et al. Usefulness of carotid sinus pressure in detecting sick sinus syndrome. *J Electrocardiol* 1978;11:261–268.

56. Wenger TL, Dohrmann ML, Strauss HC, et al. Hypersensitive carotid sinus syndrome manifested as cough syncope. *Pacing Clin Electrophysiol* 1980;3:332–339.

57. Peretz DI, Gerein AN, Miyagishima RT. Permanent demand pacing for hypersensitive carotid sinus syndrome. *Can Med Assoc J* 1973;108:1131–1134.

58. Brignole M, Menozzi C, Gianfranchi L, et al. Neurally mediated syncope detected by carotid sinus massage and head-up tilt test in sick sinus syndrome. *Am J Cardiol* 1991;68:1032–1036.

59. Brignole M, Menozzi C, Gianfranchi L, et al. Carotid sinus massage, eyeball compression, and head-up tilt test in patients with syncope of uncertain origin and in healthy control subjects. *Am Heart J* 1991;122:1644–1651.

60. Gaggioli G, Brignole M, Menozzi C, et al. A positive response to head-up tilt testing predicts syncopal recurrence in carotid sinus syndrome patients with permanent pacemakers. *Am J Cardiol* 1995;76:720–722.

61. Chughtai AL, Yans J, Kwatra M. Carotid sinus syncope: Report of two cases. *JAMA* 1977;237:2320–2321.

62. Holden W, McAnulty JH, Rahimtoola SH. Characterization of heart rate response to exercise in the sick sinus syndrome. *Br Heart J* 1978;40:923–930.

63. Brignole M, Menozzi L, Lolli G, et al. Natural and unnatural history of patients with severe carotid sinus hypersensitivity: A preliminary study. *Pacing Clin Electrophysiol* 1988;11:1628–1635.

64. Brignole M, Menozzi C, Lolli G, et al. Long termed outcome of paced and nonpaced patients with severe carotid sinus syndrome. *Am J Cardiol* 1992;69:1039–1043.

65. Dreifus LS, Fisch C, Griffin JC, et al. ACC/AHA Task Force Report: Guidelines for implantation of cardiac pacemakers and antiarrhythmia devices. *J Am Coll Cardiol* 1991;18:1–13.

66. Sutton R. Pacing in patients with carotid sinus and vasovagal syndromes. *Proc 4th Eur Symp Cardiac Pacing*, Stockholm. 1989;133–136.

67. Madigan MP, Flaker GC, Curtis JJ, et al. Carotid sinus hypersensitivity: Beneficial effects of dual-chamber pacing. *Am J Cardiol* 1984;53:1034–1040.

68. Blanc J-J, Cazeau S, Ritter P, et al. Carotid sinus syndrome: Acute hemodynamic evaluation of a dual chamber pacing mode. *Pacing Clin Electrophysiol* 1995;18:1902–1908.

69. Trout H, Brown L, Thompson J. Carotid sinus syndrome: Treatment by carotid sinus denervation. *Ann Surg* 1979;189:575–580.

70. Acquati F, Forgione FN, Caico SI, et al. Carotid sinus denervation in the treatment of carotid sinus syndrome. (Abstr) Circulation 1995;92:I–594.
71. Morley CA, Perrins EJ, Sutton R. Pharmacological intervention in the carotid sinus syndrome. (Abstr) *Pacing Clin Electrophysiol* 1983;6:A16.
72. Grubb BP, Samoil D, Kosinski D, et al. The use of serotonin reuptake inhibitors for the treatment of recurrent syncope due to carotid sinus hypersensitivity unresponsive to dual chamber cardiac pacing. *Pacing Clin Electrophysiol* 1994; 17:1434–1436.
73. Grubb BP, Wolfe DA, Samoil D, et al. Usefulness of fluoxetine hydrochloride for prevention of resistant upright tilt induced syncope. *Pacing Clin Electrophysiol* 1993;16:458–464.

Chapter 12

Miscellaneous Causes
of Syncope

Daniel J. Kosinski, MD

There are several unique etiologies of syncope that are not readily classified into the discussion in previous chapters. The purpose of this chapter is to review several of these etiologies of syncope.

Situational Syncope

Situational syncope is defined as syncope related to a particular circumstance (see Table 1). The various entities comprised in this condition have in common a mechanism that generally involves a combination of decreased preload, increased vagal activity, and/or decreased sympathetic activity. The afferent stimulus varies clinically, but the efferent response is varying degrees of cardioinhibitory and vasodepressor effects. In addition, some of these situations also involve a component of decreased cardiac filling.

Several of these situations deserve special mention, as the mechanisms involved are somewhat unusual. *Glossopharyngeal syncope* is generally precipitated by intense pain in the external auditory canal or posterior pharynx and is thought to occur due to vagal stimulation by way of afferent impulses originating in the glossopharyngeal nerve.[1] *Hot tub syncope* occurs generally upon abrupt exit from a hot tub or Jacuzzi. When an individual is immersed in such an environment, vasodilatation occurs as part of the normal compensation to heat. Abrupt standing to exit the tub leads to a normal displacement of volume with upright posture. However, this volume displace-

From Grubb BP, Olshansky B (eds.). *Syncope: Mechanisms and Management.* Armonk, NY: Futura Publishing Co., Inc.; © 1998.

_____ Table 1 _____

Causes of Situational Syncope

Micturition	Occulovagal
Glossopharyngeal	Instrumentation
Deglutition	Hot tub
Defecation	Postphlebotomy
Tussive	Sneeze
Postprandial	Trumpet/horn playing
Valsalva	(Valsalva mechanism)

ment in the face of vasodilatation can lead to excessive peripheral vascular pooling with a decrease in blood pressure that is sufficient to produce syncope.

Breath holding, particularly a problem in children, can lead to syncope via a vagal reflex.[2,3] These episodes may be mistaken for epilepsy.[4]*Airway stimulation* may also provoke syncope or cardiac arrest via a vagal mechanism.[5]

Syncopal episodes may also occur during or immediately following ingestion of a bolus of food. Patients who experience this type of syncope are often found to have an abnormality of the esophagus such as a diverticulum, stricture, or cancer. Thus, the patient with recurrent *swallow syncope* should be examined for these disorders. A similar situation is sometimes seen when a person who is quite hot takes a cold drink. In this situation it is thought that the cold liquid induces esophageal or gastric spasm (and pain) enough to produce a vagal reflex-mediated period of hypotension and bradycardia. Swallowing cold liquid while in an overheated state is reported to have resulted in death in otherwise healthy soldiers and athletes. A poem in *the Lancet* warns:

Full many a man, both young and old
Has gone to his sarcophagus
Through pouring water, ice cold, down
His too hot oesophagus.[6]

Syncope Due to Increased Intrathoracic Pressure

Increased intrathoracic pressure may lead to a decrease in venous return to the heart. The autonomic nervous system is generally able to compensate for this. However, in some instances compensatory mechanisms are overcome and syncope occurs. Such situations include but are not limited to trumpet playing, cough, or deliberate Valsalva maneuver.[6,7] *Cough syncope* is particularly interesting in that a single cough may cause only a brief increase in intrathoracic pressure. Severe paroxysms of cough, however, can severely elevate intrathoracic pressure. Syncope may occur as a consequence of decreased venous return or a vagal reaction triggered by a reflex overshoot of arterial pressure when coughing stops. *Sneeze syncope* is thought to be produced by a similar mechanism.[6]

Syncope Due to the Use of Therapeutic or Recreational Drugs

Many therapeutic agents have "prosyncopal" effects. The major culprit drugs are, in general, agents designed to lower heart rate or promote vasodilatation (primarily antihypertensive agents). These types of drugs may inhibit the body's ability to make proper adjustments for the maintenance of adequate cerebral perfusion.

Several other therapeutic agents can be responsible for syncope. Phenothiazine agents can cause syncope secondary to cardiac arrhythmia or sudden hypotension.[8] Tricyclic antidepressants can cause cardiac arrhythmias and can also cause hypotension through α-blockage.[9] Antiarrhythmic agents can cause syncope due to multiple effects including proarrhythmia phenomena, hypotension, and myocardial depression.

Several recreational drugs are also associated with syncope. Alcohol ingestion is associated with cardiac arrhythmia (the "holiday heart" syndrome), particularly atrial fibrillation. However, more serious arrhythmias may occur from alcohol ingestion.[10] Cocaine may cause syncope secondary to arrhythmia due to myocarditis, ischemia, sympathomimetic effects, or direct electrophysiological effects.[9]

Hair-Grooming Syncope Seizures

This is an unusual cause of syncope that is generally seen in young females. It involves convulsive syncope that occurs in relation to hair grooming.[11] The convulsive syncope is almost invariably preceded by a prodrome of presyncope, nausea, lightheadedness, diaphoresis, and visual disturbance. The reaction is thought to be a variant of vasovagal syncope that is triggered by hair pulling or scalp stimulation activating the trigeminal nerve.[11]

Syncope in Pacemaker Patients

When patients with pacemakers experience syncope, it is frequently assumed to represent either pacemaker dysfunction or pacemaker syndrome. However, Pavlovic et al[12] found that this is not necessarily so. They evaluated 46 patients who experienced syncope after pacemaker implantation. Extensive evaluation was performed on each patient. The etiology of syncope was found to be exit block in 4.3% of patients and failed sensing in 2.1%. The majority of the patients (36.9%) were found to have tilt table-induced syncope. In 30.4% of patients, no cause was assigned to syncope despite extensive evaluation. They concluded that pacemaker dysfunction is not a major cause of syncope in pacemaker patients, and that other causes, in particular neurally mediated syncope, should be considered.

Pulmonary Embolism

Although syncope is not recognized as a classic presentation of pulmonary embolism, as many as 13% of patients with pulmonary embolism present with syncope as the primary symptom.[13–17] The mechanism of this phenomenon is not completely clear, but it may be due to a fall in cardiac output and cerebral blood flow[18] or due to a reflex vagal reaction.[19]

Syncope During Sexual Activity

Sexual activity is quite naturally associated with sympathetic activation. Such activity can cause tachycardia, tachypnea, and transient hypertension. These changes return to baseline shortly after orgasm. In individuals without heart disease, the oxygen consumption of the heart is not substantially increased during sexual activity, and electrocardiographic abnormalities are not noted.[20] In patients with ischemic heart disease, the situation may be quite different and either symptomatic or silent ischemia may be generated. In such instances the combination of ischemia and sympathetic activation may lead to arrhythmia.[21]

In addition, in select patients without ischemic heart disease, sympathetic stimulation during sexual activity can lead to syncope. Such patients include those with long QT syndrome or neurocardiogenic syncope.

Syncope Due to Metabolic or Endocrine Abnormalities

Although certain metabolic abnormalities have been noted as etiologies of syncope, the proportion of episodes due to metabolic causes is likely low. In a study by Racco et al[22] only 5% of episodes of syncope could be identified as being of metabolic cause. In general, the most common metabolic causes of syncope are thought to be hypoglycemia, hypoxia, and forced or voluntary hyperventilation.[23]

Hypoglycemia is perhaps the most traditional metabolic abnormality associated with syncope. Accompanying symptoms are generally dizziness, diaphoresis, and altered behavior. To assign hypoglycemia as a cause of syncope, it is necessary to actually demonstrate hypoglycemia during the time of symptoms. This can be very difficult. Hypoglycemia may be spontaneous due to a number of endocrine abnormalities such as insulinoma or autoimmune hypoglycemia. Hypoglycemia, however, is often iatrogenic due to the use of insulin or oral hypoglycemic agent in diabetic patients. This is particularly a problem in elderly patients.

Hypoxemia has also been recognized as a cause of syncope. One study[22] identifies hypoxemia as a cause of syncope in 3% of the patients studied.

It has traditionally been viewed that hyperventilation can produce syncope through a reduction in cerebral blood flow. However, in a study of young subjects, forced hyperventilation alone could not induce syncope.[23] Therefore it is reasonable to hypothesize that syncope due to hyperventilation may have a psychological as well as a physical component.

One cause of syncope that deserves some mention is hypoadrenalism, which is a failure in the body's capacity to mount an adequate glucocorticoid response to stress. The disorder may either be primary in nature due to disordered adrenal gland function (Addison's disease) or may occur secondary to dysfunction of the anterior pituitary or due to failure of the hypothalmo-pituitary-adrenal axis (most frequently as a result of exogenous steroids).[24]

The clinical features of Addison's disease are somewhat nonspecific, consisting principally of extreme fatigue, nausea, and vomiting. Primary adrenal failure results in not only glucocorticoid loss, but mineral corticoid deficiency as well, giving rise to orthostatic hypotension and syncope. Syncope is the presenting complaint in up to 10% of patients with Addison's disease. Most often, the disease becomes evident when an apparently minor illness provokes a life-threatening sequence of abdominal pain, syncope, and death. One of the classic (and often forgotten) signs of Addison's disease is a pigmentation of nonexposed areas (for example the buccal mucosa) that occur due to the melanotrophic actions of elevations in corticotropin (ACTH). While reductions in serum sodium along with elevations in serum potassium are common, serum electrolytes are just as likely to be normal. The time of onset is usually in middle age, and it is often autoimmune in nature. The diagnosis is made through the measurement of cortisol levels as well as administration of the short tetracosactrin test.

There are numerous other metabolic or endocrine causes of syncope that are much less common. Such causes are listed in Table 2.

Summary

There are several unique and unusual causes of syncope. Their etiologies of may be commonly encountered in clinical practice. The diagnosis of these unique instances of syncope can often be established by a thorough history and limited noninvasive evaluation.

_____ Table 2 _____

Metabolic Causes of Syncope

Hypo/hyper kalemia	Hypoxia
Hypo/hyper calcemia	Hypoglycemia
Hypo/hyper magnesemia	Hyperventilation

Endocrine Disorders

Hypoadrenalism—may be due to hypopituitarism, Addison's disease, adrenal suppression.
Endocrine Disorders in which *vasoactive substances* are produced—carcinoid syndrome, pheocytochroma, mastocytosis.

References

1. Kong Y. Glossopharyngeal neuralgia associated with bradycardia, syncope, and seizure. *Circulation* 1964;3:109–113.
2. Bridge E, Livingston S, Tietze E. Breath holding spells. *J Pediatr* 1943;23:539–561.
3. Lombroso C, Lerman P. Breath holding spells. *Pediatrics* 1967;39:563–581.
4. Stephenson J. Reflex anoxic seizures while breath holding: Non-epileptic vagal attacks. *Arch Dis Child* 1978;53:193–200.
5. Johnson R, Lambie D, Spalding J. *Neurocardiology.* London: W.B. Saunders Co.; 1984;167–168.
6. Johnson R. Lambie D, Spalding J. *Neurocardiology.* London: W.B.Saunders Co.; 1984;174–176.
7. Faulkner M, Sharper-Schaefer E. Circulatory effects of trumpet playing. *Br Med J* 1959;1:685–686.
8. Leestma J, Koenig K. Sudden death and phenothiazines. *Arch Gen Psychiatry* 1988;18:137–148.
9. Hackel D, Reimer K. Role of recreational and therapeutic drugs in occurrence of sudden death. *Cardiovascular Reviews and Reports* 1994;7:321.
10. Ettinger P, Wu CF, De La Cruz L, et al. Arrhythmia and the "holiday heart": Alcohol-associated cardiac rhythm disorders. *Am Heart J* 1978;95:555–562.
11. Lewis P, Frank L. Hair grooming syncope seizures. *Pediatrics* 1993; 91(4):836–837.
12. Pavlovic S, Kocovic D, Djordjevic M, et al. The etiology of syncope in pacemaker patients. *Pacing Clin Electrophysiol* 1991;14(12):2086–2091.
13. Thames M, Alpert J, Dalen J. Syncope in patients with pulmonary embolism. *JAMA* 1977;238(23):2509–2511.
14. Edelson G, Reis N, Hettinger E. Syncope as a premonitory sign of fatal pulmonary embolism: Two case reports. *Acta Orthop Scand* 1988;59(1):71–73.
15. Bell WR, Simon T, Demets D. The clinical features of submassive and massive pulmonary emboli. *Am J Med* 1977;62(3):355–360.
16. Bush W, Renner U, Wirtfeld A, et al. Floating pulmonary embolism: Unusual cause of recurrent syncope. *Eur Heart J* 1984;5(7):602–605.

17. Wilk J, Nardone A, Jennings C, et al. Unexplained syncope: When to suspect pulmonary embolism. *Geriatrics* 1995;50(10):46–50.
18. Fred H, Willerson J, Alexander J. Neurological manifestations of pulmonary thromboembolism. *Arch Int Med* 1967;120:33–37.
19. Simpson R, Pedolak R, Mangano C, et al. Vagal syncope during recurrent pulmonary embolism. *JAMA* 1983;249(3):390–393.
20. Hellerstein H, Friedman E. Sexual activity and the post coronary patient. *Arch Int Med* 1970;125:987–999.
21. Opie L, Coetzge W. Metabolic components of ischemia and fibrillation. In: Zipes, Jalife J (eds): *Cardiac Electrophysiology From Cell to Bedside.* Philadelphia: W.B. Saunders Co.; 456–462 and 90.
22. Racco F, Sconocchini C, Reginelli R. La sincope in una popolazone generale: Diagnosi ezilogoca e follow-up. *Minerva Med* 1993;84:249–261.
23. Wayne H. Clinical differentiation between hypoxia and hyperventilation. *J Aviation Med* 1958;29:307–315.
24. Robertson D, Taylor R. Metabolic and endocrine causes of syncope. In: Kenny (ed): *Syncope in the Older Patient.* London: Chapman and Hall Medical; 1995;249.

Chapter 13

Syncope in the Child and Adolescent

Bertrand Ross, MD and Blair P. Grubb, MD

Syncope is a relatively common complaint among both children and adolescents. Derived from the Greek work *synkoptein,* meaning "to cut short," it refers to a transient loss of consciousness and postural tone with spontaneous recovery. Both a sign and a syndrome, it may result from a number of different causes, some of which may ultimately culminate in death. It has been estimated that one in five children will have a syncopal episode by the time he or she reaches adulthood. The frequency of the problem is compounded by the fact that syncope produces a tremendous amount of anxiety among parents and athletic and school officials. Indeed the social repercussions of recurrent syncope may have a more dramatic impact on a child than the syncope itself. As children differ from adults, so too do the causes of syncope. In this chapter some of the common causes of syncope in children are discussed. When these causes are covered in detail elsewhere, the differences between the pediatric and the adult patient are emphasized.

Classification and Approach

The causes of syncope in children and adolescents may be classified in a variety of different ways. A simple yet useful way of organizing the various potential etiologies is found in Table 1.

As with the adult patient, the history and physical examination is key. When available, descriptions of the episode by bystanders are particularly

From Grubb BP, Olshansky B (eds.). *Syncope: Mechanisms and Management.* Armonk, NY: Futura Publishing Co., Inc.; © 1998.

_____ Table 1 _____

Causes of Syncope in Children

I. Neurally Mediated Syncopes
   A. Neurocardiogenic (vasovagal)
   B. Dysautonomic (orthostatic)
   C. Cerebral (vasoconstrictive) syncope
II. Cardiovascular Syncope
   A. Cardiac
      1. Primary cause
         a. Hypercyanotic spells
         b. Low cardiac output
         c. Myocardial infarction
      2. Arrhythmic
         a. Supraventricular tachycardia
         b. Ventricular tachycardia
         c. SA and AV nodal dysfunction
   B. Other Vascular Causes
      1. Cerebrovascular accident
      2. Subclavian steal syndrome
III. Noncardiovascular Syncope
   A. Psychogenic (hysteric)
   B. Epilepsy

See text for details.
SA = sinoatrial; AV = atrioventricular.

helpful, as the child may have difficulty remembering and may be frightened by the questioning process. It is important to find out if there is any history of unexplained sudden death among family members, and to learn the circumstances surrounding these deaths. One should endeavor to determine the frequency of episodes, the conditions under which the episodes occurred, whether there was a prodrome, the duration of loss of consciousness, and whether injury resulted from the fall. Was there tonic-clonic activity? Incontinence? A postictal state?

As in adults, one of the principal determinations to be made in children and adolescents is whether the heart is structurally normal. Aspects of the history may provide a clue to the potential for cardiac etiologies. For example, occurrence of syncope in the supine position suggests a cardiac source. In addition, the absence of any prodrome prior to loss of consciousness is more common in cardiac syncope.

Neurally Mediated Syncopes

Over the last few years a large body of research has demonstrated that transient alterations in the autonomic nervous system's control of heart rate and blood pressure may lead to hypotension and loss of consciousness. This type of syncope is quite common in pediatric patients, particularly in adolescents. Rather than a single entity, this type of syncope represents a group of different disorders, each of which occurs due to a disturbance in autonomic control. Although it is dealt with in more detail in other chapters, a brief description of each of these entities with regard to the pediatric population is provided.

Neurocardiogenic Syncope (see Chapter 3)

Also referred to as the common faint or vasovagal syncope, this disturbance in neuroregulatory control of vascular tone is by far the most common cause of syncope in otherwise healthy children and adolescents.[1–6] The episodes themselves are characterized by a sudden fall in blood pressure that is associated with lightheadedness, dizziness, and loss of consciousness, frequently accompanied by signs of autonomic nervous system hyperactivity such as diaphoresis, nausea, pallor, hyperventilation, and tachycardia followed by bradycardia. The pathophysiological aspects of this disorder are dealt with in detail elsewhere in this text, however a brief description is appropriate. Current thought holds that a sudden increase in peripheral vascular pooling results in a sudden reduction in venous return to the heart, allowing for over-vigorous ventricular contractions.[7] These hyperdynamic beats activate myocardial C-fibers (which usually only respond to stretching of the myocardial wall during periods of increased blood pressure), sending a sudden surge in neural traffic to the brain stem, thus conveying the false impression that the patient is hypertensive. The brain stem then responds with an apparent "paradoxic" lowering of blood pressure by sympathetic withdrawal, leading to vasodilation and bradycardia. Thus, these patients demonstrate a sudden profound drop in blood pressure followed by a fall in heart rate. As opposed to adults, we have found that children often panic at the onset of prodromal signs, and begin to hyperventilate due to anxiety, an act which may further reduce cerebral perfusion by producing systemic hypocapnia.

The clinical presentation may take a variety of forms in the pediatric patient. Classically, these episodes are often provoked by environmental stimuli such as anxiety, blood drawing (or just the sight of a needle), pain, or even the sight of blood.[8] However, it is just as common to hear that the patient had been engaged in normal activities (such as playing, shopping, or walking outside), when he or she suddenly turned pale, appeared sweaty, and then lost consciousness.[9] Interestingly, in 33% of children with tilt-confirmed neurocardiogenic syncope, there is a family history of syncope. In adolescents there is often a history of a period of rapid growth that precedes the onset of symptoms. In young women there is a trend for episodes to be more frequent at the time just preceding menses. We have also noted an increased frequency of episodes among adolescents who lose a large amount of weight quickly during crash dieting.

Tilt table testing is used to confirm the diagnosis (a detailed discussion of this is found in Chapter 3.)[1-6] It should be kept in mind that classic tilt table testing, which produces an orthostatic stress on the autonomic nervous system's ability to maintain blood pressure, may not be an adequate stress for smaller children, given their shorter stature and smaller body surface area. A more prolonged upright time or other increase in orthostatic stress (such as the use of provocative agents such as isoproterenol) may be necessary.[8]

Heart rate variability studies using power spectral analysis have shown abnormal responses to orthostatic stress in children with recurrent syncope.[10] Interestingly, these abnormal findings occurred while the mean heart rate and blood pressure were still normal and the patient was asymptomatic. These findings preceded the eventual syncopal event by 5 or more minutes.

Therapeutic options for pediatric and adolescent patients are discussed in detail elsewhere in this text, and tend to be somewhat different from those for adults. Treatment of this condition with fludrocortisone has been an option for a number of years. Adult patients, however, have had problems with side effects, most notably hypertension. This may be much less of a problem for pediatric or adolescent patients. We have used fludrocortisone as our first treatment option, and in over 10 years we have had only two episodes of hypertension that required discontinuation of the medication. In one of those two patients, after continued treatment failures with other medical regimens, the medication was restarted at the family's request, and with reinstitution there was no recurrence of hypertension.

Permanent pacing has been used as a treatment for this condition, especially in those children with prolonged asystole associated with a positive tilt table test. Although the most effective and appropriate treatment is unclear, it has been our experience that almost all of our pediatric-aged patients have opted for treatment medically without the need for permanent pacing. We have had several patients who have had asystole for 20 to 30 seconds during testing and were treated medically (with various agents) without pacing. These patients are now asymptomatic and are off all therapy up to 5 years later.

We generally treat children and adolescents medically until they have been without symptoms for 12 months. Based on our experience over the last 11 years, we have found that the majority require only 12 months of therapy, while a small number need therapy for up to several years. Similarly, a significant majority of patients, as they mature, have no or few further episodes, although a minority (usually those most severely affected) continue to have symptoms but at differing frequencies.

Dysautonomic Syncope (see Chapter 4)

Upon assumption of an upright posture, there is usually a gravity-mediated downward displacement of up to 500 cc of blood to the more dependent areas of the body. This is compensated for by a reflex-mediated increase in both heart rate and force of contraction and peripheral vasoconstriction. In dysautonomic syncope one or more of the compensatory mechanisms for orthostatic stress fails, with a resultant fall in blood pressure and cerebral perfusion that leads to syncope. In contrast to classic neurocardiogenic syncope, there is less of a prodrome and an absence of bradycardia or diaphoresis. Often there are other signs and symptoms of autonomic failure present.

Cerebral syncope is a recently recognized (although rare) condition in which inappropriate degrees of cerebral vasoconstriction alone may result in syncope despite a normal systemic blood pressure.[11]

Cardiovascular Syncope

Cardiac syncope may occur as a result of primary hemodynamic events, or it may be secondary to disturbances in cardiac rhythm.

One of the more important primary cardiac causes of syncope is the hypercyanotic spell. These spells may be seen in a variety of different conditions including tetralogy of Fallot, transposition of the great arteries with left ventricular outflow tract obstruction (subpulmonary or pulmonary stenosis), tricuspid atresia, and Eisenmenger's syndrome.[12,13] Severe hypercyanotic episodes are also referred to as "tetralogy spells." The spell often begins with crying, and then progresses to deep rapid breathing. Crying results in the prolonged forced expiration of air, leading to an increase in intrathoracic pressure, which in turn leads to a reduction in pulmonary blood flow and a greater degree of right-to-left shunting. The resultant decrease in oxygen saturation and pH of blood leading to the heart produces more cyanosis and results in a compensatory increase in respirations and/or crying, causing the cycle to repeat itself. When the hypoxia is severe enough, loss of consciousness ensues. The episode may be ended in a variety of fashions, the most frequent of which occurs by calming the child and bringing the knees to the chest (often by squatting). This augments systemic vascular resistance thereby increasing blood flow to the pulmonary vasculature.

Syncope may also result from conditions that reduce cardiac output due to an obstruction to blood flow. These conditions include any form of stenosis of the aortic valve as well as subvalvular or supravalvular aortic stenosis. In children and adolescents as in adults, syncope associated with congenital or acquired aortic stenosis is a marker of severe obstruction, and may indicate the need for valve replacement or repair. Patients who reach adulthood with a history of severe aortic stenosis that had been treated with moderate success in childhood may, over time, develop subendocardial fibrosis, which may lead to ventricular dysrhythmias secondary to ischemia.

Children who suffer from hypertrophic cardiomyopathy may have syncope due either to hemodynamic or dysrhythmic causes.[14] Unfortunately, both signs and symptoms may be much more subtle in the pediatric age group, and death is often the presenting sign of the illness. In many patients the first indication of a problem may be syncope, and a single episode can be the only warning of impending sudden death. It is important to determine if any other family members are affected with the disorder.

Syncope may also be seen with severe pulmonic stenosis or in pulmonary hypertension. Syncope in the setting of increased pulmonary vascular resistance may occur from the hypercyanotic spells discussed previously or from a significant and abrupt increase in pulmonary vascular resistance that causes a rapid reduction in cardiac output and precipitates acute right ventricular failure.[12] It is thought that the cessation of blood flow that occurs from the sudden increase in pulmonary resistance leads to sudden death in patients with Eisenmenger's syndrome.[13] There is generally no effective cure for the increase in pulmonary vascular resistance (PVR) that produces varying degrees of decreased cardiac output. Palliative therapies such as phlebotomy with fluid administration to lower the hematocrit, or atrial septostomy to increase right-to-left atrial level shunt and thereby increase cardiac output may be of some benefit.[15,16] However, each carries a risk. If the intra-atrial communication is made too large, patients may shunt right-to-left to such a degree that effective pulmonary blood flow is reduced, and the patient may expire from low cardiac output. Similarly, if the systemic vascular resistance decreases too much relative to the pulmonary vascular resistance during phlebotomy for polycythemia, cardiac output may decrease precipitously, and a death spiral may be started.

The practitioner should be aware that there may be patients who have had repair of a ventricular septal defect in childhood to prevent pulmonary vascular obstructive disease, yet still develop pulmonary hypertension from end-stage pulmonary vascular obstructive disease. As patients are being operated on in infancy, this is much less likely to occur in the future.

A somewhat uncommon, but nonetheless important, cause of syncope in children may be myocardial infarction. The most frequent cause in pediatric patients is anomalous coronary arteries, most often when the left coronary artery arises from the pulmonary artery. Alternatively, the left coronary artery may take an anomalous course between the trunks of the aorta and pulmonary arteries, leaving it vulnerable to compression during exercise. Myocardial infarction may also be seen as a sequela of coronary narrowing due to Kawasaki's disease.[12]

Dysrhythmias: Normal Heart

Disturbances of the heart rhythm that are severe enough to result in syncope are relatively rare in the patient with a structurally normal heart. These disturbances are essentially similar to those problems seen in older patients that are discussed in more detail elsewhere in this text.

As with their adult counterparts, children rarely experience syncope caused by supraventricular tachycardia. The two most common forms of supraventricular tachycardia in children, atrioventricular reentry via an accessory atrioventricular connection and atrioventricular nodal reentry, are essentially the same in children as in adults, and the interested reader is directed to the chapters of this text that deal with supraventricular tachycardia.

Syncope associated with exercise or emotion in a patient with a structurally normal heart should raise suspicion of the long QT syndrome.[17] The syncope that occurs in the long QT syndrome is due to the hemodynamic compromise caused by a polymorphic "torsade de pointes" ventricular tachycardia. Episodes of sudden loss of consciousness have been associated with fright or being awakened by a loud noise. Most patients first exhibit symptoms sometime in the first 2 decades of life, and there may be several tragic sudden deaths among members of the same family. This disorder may be misdiagnosed as seizures. Mortality in the syndrome can be high (approximately 71%) in untreated patients. Mortality rates fall to 7% if patients are treated with β-blocking agents (with implantable defibrillators or ganglionectomy reserved for refractory cases).

Arrhythmogenic right ventricular dysplasia (ARVD) may result in ventricular tachycardia and syncope.[18,19] The disorder seems more common in parts of Europe than in North America. ARVD should be suspected in any patient with exercise-induced ventricular tachycardia with a left bundle branch pattern. The ventricular tachycardia occurs secondary to a patchy right ventricular cardiomyopathy. As definite structural changes do not become manifest until the third to fourth decade of life, it is not surprising that the signs and symptoms may be difficult to detect in children.

Dysrhythmias: Repaired or Palliated Structural Disease

In the pediatric population, congenital heart disease is the single most common cause of arrhythmias that lead to syncope. More often than not, these patients have undergone a prior correction or palliation of a congenital cardiac defect, with the arrhythmia presenting at a later time. The type and anatomic location of the arrhythmia are usually related to the site of the surgical intervention.

Some atrial repairs, for example, will produce sick sinus syndrome, which if severe enough may lead to syncope or even death. Although there are a number of definitions of what constitutes sick sinus syndrome, the most common is that of sinus bradycardia or arrest either with or without supraventricular tachycardia. Interestingly, there is evidence to suggest that the tachycardias are the more important cause of syncope, as patients continue to experience syncope after pacemaker implantation. The actual syncopal episode is of sudden onset and usually of a brief duration. Treatment for these problems often involve antiarrhythmic therapy combined with permanent pacemaker implantation.

In a similar manner, those patients who have undergone atrial surgery are more prone to both atrial flutter and atrial fibrillation. These disorders seem particularly common in those patients who have undergone atrial baffling repairs such as the Senning and Mustard operations, which were the standard repairs for transposition of the great arteries for over 20 years.[20] These patients often have atrial flutter with a rapid ventricular response combined with sinus node dysfunction, which may produce hemodynamic compromise and syncope.[21] These problems may also be seen in atrial septal defect repairs, mitral valve annuloplasties or replacements, tricuspid valve annuloplasty for Ebstein's anomaly, and atrioventricular canal repairs. Syncope in these patients must be taken quite seriously, as it may foretell impending sudden death.

Atrioventricular block in the pediatric population may either be congenital or acquired (usually following cardiac surgery).[22] Congenital complete heart block (often associated with maternal lupus) in the presence of a normal heart frequently does not require pacing. One study found that syncope in this group was associated with a heart rate during exercise of <50 bpm.[12,22] Thus, pacing should be considered in congenital heart block patients with rates lower than 50 bpm who have experienced syncope or heart failure. L-transposition of the great vessels (or "anatomically corrected" transposition) has a more superiorly and superficially placed atrioventricular (AV) node and is associated with an increased risk for the development of AV block.[12]

Ventricular tachycardia and ventricular fibrillation are seen in either children with damaged ventricles or in those whose repairs produce large amounts of ventricular scarring.[18] A classic example of the latter is seen following repair of tetralogy of Fallot.[20,23] This condition is the most common single cause of death in children between 1 and 16 years of age (although deaths due to firearms may soon surpass it). The ventricular arrhythmias can originate from any area in the ventricle that is associated with a large amount of scarring. Patients with significant residual obstruction or poor ventricular function appear to be at increased risk, as are those who undergo the repair later in life. Arrhythmias may make their appearance years after surgery.

Myocarditis and dilated cardiomyopathy may both present with syncope secondary to ventricular arrhythmias. In infants, ventricular tumors (such as Purkinje cell tumors) are an important cause of ventricular tachycardia.

Noncardiovascular Syncope

One of the important causes of syncope in pediatrics (especially in adolescents) is psychogenic (or hysteric) syncope (see Chapter 9). Patients who suffer from psychogenic causes of syncope are often distinguished by the extreme frequency of the episodes (sometimes 2 to 3 per day) and the fact that episodes are usually not associated with injury.[24] In those individuals the loss of consciousness may be quite prolonged (occasionally as long as an hour), during which time heart rate and blood pressure are normal, and assumption of a recumbent position does not terminate the event. These patients may seem to display a remarkable indifference to their syncope. During tilt table testing these patients may suddenly faint without observable changes in heart rate, blood pressure, transcranial Doppler blood flow, or electroencephalographic recording.[25] After detailed psychiatric evaluations, many of these individuals are found to be suffering from conversion reactions, most frequently due to sexual abuse. It is important to realize that patients who experience conversion reactions are not consciously aware of their actions.[26] Indeed, these events may be the only way an abused child or adolescent will be able to "cry for help."

We have also seen parents who claim that their child has experienced multiple syncopal episodes, and in order to hide evidence of physical abuse, claim that the child injured himself during the falls associated with these events. A close history will often reveal inconsistences, and a physical exam will reveal wounds of such a nature and location that they are unlikely to have occurred during a fall. Any such suspicions must be reported to the proper authorities. In addition, we have seen cases of Munchausen's by proxy, where a parent will secretly administer a diuretic or vasodilator to a child so as to produce hypotension and syncope. One such case was uncovered only after a toxicology screen was obtained in the emergency department after the mother brought the child following a syncopal event. Only later was it discovered that the mother was deeply emotionally disturbed.

Another group of patients who seem to display a high degree of indifference (as well as open hostility to the physician) is the group of patients whose syncope may result from illicit drug use. Unfortunately, substance abuse is occurring in increasingly younger age groups. Toxicology screens will often provide important clues to the diagnosis, as patients will rarely volunteer this information (particularly when their parents are present). The presence of needle marks ("tracks") may be revealing, as may evidence of nasal septal damage.

Seizures are an uncommon cause of syncope.[27] Episodes are usually associated with tonic-clonic movements, incontinence, and prolonged loss of consciousness. An akinetic seizure (also called atonic seizure) is manifested by a sudden fall to the ground. The episode may be so dramatic that onlookers describe the patient as "having been thrown to the ground," an event which may be accompanied by head or facial trauma. This type of seizure occurs most often between the ages of 2 and 8 years, and rarely in adolescence. The electroencephalogram is often quite abnormal, demonstrating generalized or multifocal epileptiform discharges. These seizures are often quite challenging to treat, with the highest success rates seen with valproic acid or clonazepam. Some patients have responded to use of the medium chain triglyceride (MCT) variant of the ketogenic diet.

Occasionally, patients may suffer from hyperventilation syndrome. Often associated with panic attacks, hyperventilation syndrome is manifested by rapid and frequently deep breathing, tightness in the chest, palpitations, and a feeling of dyspnea.[12] If it is sufficient to produce hypocapnia, hyperventilation will be associated with circumoral hand numbness and tingling. Episodes may last up to half an hour, and the patient will be able to reproduce his or her symptoms by hyperventilation. It should be kept in mind however that some children may begin to hyperventilate due to the anxiety provoked during an episode of neurocardiogenic syncope. We have found that biofeedback training may be helpful in hyperventilation.

Summary

Recurrent syncope in the pediatric patient can be an important symptom of a variety of disorders that range from a simple faint to potentially lethal ventricular arrhythmias. Episodes must be taken seriously, with the history and physical examination serving as the basis for subsequent laboratory investigations. Syncope in patients with congenital heart disease should be cause for particular concern.

References

1. Ross BA, Hughes A, Anderson E, et al. Orthostatic versus electrophysiologic testing in unexplained syncope in children and adolescents. *J Cardiovasc Electrophysiol* 1992;3:418–422.
2. Samoil D, Grubb BP, Kip K, Kosinski D. Head upright tilt table testing in children with unexplained syncope. *Pediatrics* 1993;92:426–430.
3. Thilenius OG, Quinones JA, Husayni TS, Novak J. Tilt table test for diagnosis of unexplained syncope in pediatric patients. *Pediatrics* 1991;87:334–338.
4. Hannon D, Ross BA. Head up tilt testing in children who faint. *J Pediatrics* 1991;118:731–732.
5. Lerman-Sagie T, Rechavia E, Strasberg B, et al. Head up tilt for the evaluation of syncope of unknown origin in children. *J Pediatrics* 1991;118:676–679.

6. Grubb BP, Temesy-Armos P, Moore J, et al. The use of head upright tilt table testing in the evaluation and management of syncope in children and adolescents. *Pacing Clin Electrophysiol* 1992;15:742–748.
7. Kosinski D, Grubb BP. Pathophysiological aspects of neurocardiogenic syncope. *Pacing Clin Electrophysiol* 1995;18:716–721.
8. Grubb BP, Kosinski D. Current trends in the etiology, diagnosis and management of neurocardiogenic syncope. *Curr Opin Cardiol* 1996;11:32–41.
9. Thilenius OG, Ryd KJ, Husanyi J. Variations in expression and treatment of transient neurocardiogenic instability. *Am J Cardiol* 1992;69:1193–1195.
10. Ross BA, Aknan AA, Schneider DS, et al. Abnormal heart rate variability responses to standing in children and adolescents with recurrent unexplained syncope. *Circulation* 1993;88 (suppl):4841–4851.
11. Grubb BP, Samoil D, Kosinski D, et al. Cerebral syncope, loss of consciousness associated with cerebral vasoconstriction in the absence of systemic hypotension. *Pacing Clin Electrophysiol* (in press).
12. O'Laughlin MP. Syncope. In: Gillette P, Garson A (eds): *Pediatric Arrhythmias: Electrophysiology and Pacing.* Philadelphia: W.B. Saunders Co.; 1990;600–615.
13. Brammell HL, Vogel JHK, Pryor R, et al. The Eisenmenger syndrome: A clinical and physiologic reappraisal. *Am J Cardiol* 1971;28:679–692.
14. Canedo MI, Frank MJ, Abdulla AM. Rhythm disturbances in hypertrophic cardiomyopathy: Prevalence, relation to symptoms and management. *Am J Cardiol* 1980;45:848–855.
15. Rich S, Lam W. Atrial septostomy as palliative therapy for refractory primary pulmonary hypertension. *Am J Cardiol* 1983;51:1560–1561.
16. Austen WG, Morrow AG, Berry WB. Experimental studies of the surgical treatment of primary pulmonary hypertension. *J Thoracic Cardiovasc Surg* 1964; 48:448–455.
17. Schwartz PJ, Moss AJ. Prolonged Q-T interval: What does it mean? *J Cardiovasc Med* 1982;7:1317.
18. Rocchini AP, Chun PO, Dick M. Ventricular tachycardia in children. *Am J Cardiol* 1981;47:1091–1097.
19. Thiene G, Nava A, Corrado D, et al. Right ventricular cardiomyopathy and sudden death in young people. *N Engl J Med* 1988;318:129–133.
20. Vaksmann G, Fournier A, Davignon A, et al. Frequency and prognosis of arrhythmias after operative "correction" of tetralogy of Fallot. *Am J Cardiol* 1990;66:346–349.
21. Trusler GA, Castaneda AR, Rosenthal A, et al. Current results of management in transposition of the great arteries, with special emphasis on patients with associated ventricular septal defect. *J Am Coll Cardiol* 1987;10:1061–1071.
22. Ross BA, Trippel DL. Atrioventricular block. In: Garson A, Bricker JT, Fisher DJ, Neish SR (eds): *The Science and Practice of Pediatric Cardiology.* Baltimore: Williams and Wilkins; 1995.
23. Walsh EP, Rockenmacher S, Keane JF, et al. Late results in patients with tetralogy of Fallot repaired in infancy. *Circulation* 1988;77:1062–1067.
24. Linzer M, Varia I, Pontinem M, et al. Medically unexplained syncope: Relationship to psychiatric illness. *Am J Med* 1992;92:185–245.
25. Grubb BP, Gerard G, Wolfe D, et al. Syncope and seizures of psychogenic origin: Identification with upright tilt table testing. *Clin Cardiol* 1992;15:839–842.
26. Shihabuddin L, Shehadeh A, Agla D. Syncope as a conversion mechanism. *Psychosomatics* 1994;35:496–498.
27. Wiederholt WG. Seizure Disorders. In: Wiederholt (ed): *Neurology for Nonneurologists.* Philadelphia: W.B. Saunders Co.;1995;211–231.

Chapter 14

Syncope in the Athlete

Daniel J. Kosinski, MD

Due in part to the recent unfortunate deaths of several high-profile athletes,[1,2] there exists a renewed concern over the evaluation of athletes who suffer syncope. These syncopal episodes range in clinical presentation from syncope occurring during vigorous activity to syncope occurring during modest exertion or at rest. In addition, the patient population involved ranges from the elite professional athlete to the purely recreational participant. The differential diagnosis will therefore be quite broad, and it will be affected by numerous variables. Despite such complexity, it is reasonable to attempt to construct a framework in which to evaluate patients with syncope that is related to athletic activity.

Why is evaluation necessary? In part, because many causes of syncope are treatable, and thus morbidity may be decreased. In addition, it is paramount to identify individuals in whom a serious or potentially lethal condition exists. Maron et al[3] report that 17% of young athletes with sudden death had a history of syncope or presyncope. A publication by Driscoll and Edwards[4] reports that in children and adolescents the figure is 23%. In a report by Kramer et al,[5] 86% of young soldiers who experienced exercise-related sudden death had a history of syncope. Given these data, it is clear that with proper evaluation, an impact can be made in terms of potential mortality reduction.

As with any cardiovascular condition, the evaluation of syncope should begin with a detailed history and physical examination. Prior work by Calkins et al[6] shows that the clinical history itself may be of value in narrowing the differential diagnosis of syncope. Therefore, a thorough description of the syncopal episode(s) should be obtained. Other relevant points in the

From Grubb BP, Olshansky B (eds.). *Syncope: Mechanisms and Management.* Armonk, NY: Futura Publishing Co., Inc.; © 1998.

history include a review of any current or prior cardiac conditions, family history, concurrent illness, and a review of current medications including the use of nonprescription medications. The clinician must also explore the possibility of recreational drug use. It is very necessary to make these inquiries, as syncope or even sudden death may occur due to the role of therapeutic or recreational drugs.[7]

It is also necessary to attempt to define as best as possible the "type of athlete" the patient is. Although the definition of a "competitive athlete" has been outlined,[8] lesser degrees of athletic activity are difficult to quantify. In addition, a recent publication by Mitchell et al[9] provides insight into the concept that different types of athletic activity command different degrees of cardiovascular compensation. Dynamic exercise (such as swimming) generally involves an increase in heart rate and stroke volume with a decrease in end-systolic volume. Static exercise (such as weight lifting) involves minimal changes in heart rate and ventricular volumes. Arterial pressure and ventricular contractility, however, are increased. In general, most athletic activity requires a combination of static and dynamic activity. And although there are no data to suggest that either type of exercise presents a greater risk of syncope, it is helpful to make such an assessment in regard to the interpretation of noninvasive testing.[10–12]

In addition to the learning the types of athletic activity the patient is engaged in, the clinician must also ascertain the degree to which the individual participates in such activities. These data are important not only for developing a differential diagnosis but also for interpreting the results of noninvasive testing such as echocardiography and electrocardiography.[11–15]

Physical Examination

The physical examination should include a thorough ausculatory examination as well as testing for orthostatic hypotension.

At the conclusion of the history and physical examination, it is sometimes possible to define a reasonable etiology for the syncopal event(s). Further evaluation should then be directed toward that etiology. However, if the history and physical examination are nondiagnostic, further data should be pursued.

Electrocardiography

The initiation of noninvasive evaluation should begin with the scalar electrocardiogram. As with the evaluation of any individual with syncope, attention should be directed toward identifying a potential etiology for syncope. The electrocardiogram should be evaluated for evidence of preexcitation, long QT syndrome, right ventricular dysplasia, and ventricular hypertrophy (see Figures 1 and 2). In addition, any evidence for coronary

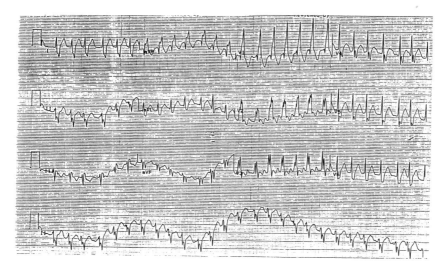

Figure 1. Wide complex tachycardia seen in a 17-year-old male with syncope accompanied by palpitations. The patient was a competitive athlete.

artery disease (pathological Q waves, bundle branch block) should be noted. The presence or absence of conduction disease should also be identified. The presence of an abnormality does not constitute a diagnosis of the etiology of syncope, but it may certainly provide information that is

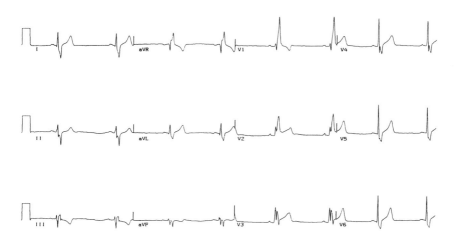

Figure 2. Electrocardiogram in sinus rhythm showing right bundle branch block in the 17-year-old male shown in Figure 1. Further evaluation including cardiac magnetic resonance imaging and right ventriculography lead to the diagnosis of right ventricular dysplasia.

useful for directing further evaluation. In addition, the absence of any such pathology is also helpful.

When evaluating patients with syncope that is related to athletic activity, it is important to understand that certain electrocardiographic features are or may be common in athletes. The electrocardiogram may show resting bradycardia with high voltage in the left chest leads.[10] In fact, voltage criteria for left ventricular hypertrophy may be met.[16] In addition, intraventricular conduction defects[10] and repolarization abnormalities[10,14] may be seen in these patients.

In addition to resting bradycardia, other resting bradyarrhythmias that may not be pathological may be seen. These bradyarrhythmias may include junctional rhythm, prolonged atrioventricular (AV) conduction, or Wenckebach phenomena.[17–19] And although unusual, Mobitz type II block and even complete atrioventricular block have been reported.[20] A common feature of resting AV block in athletes, however, is that these abnormalities disappear with exercise.[10,21]

The ST segment may be elevated or depressed and the T wave may be biphasic or even inverted on these patients' electrocardiograms.[10]

Therefore, changes in the electrocardiogram that appear pathological may or may not be. These issues are often difficult to resolve without further noninvasive evaluation.

Echocardiography

It is our opinion, as well as the opinion of others, that in evaluating syncope related to athletic activity, it is imperative to evaluate for structural heart disease.[22,23] This includes potentially lethal conditions such as hypertrophic cardiomyopathy, right ventricular dysplasia, anomalous coronary arteries, valvular heart disease, myocarditis, congenital heart disease, and coronary artery disease. Although the absolute yield of echocardiography in this subgroup of patients with syncope is unknown, it is likely to be low. However, multiple potentially lethal disorders that are readily identifiable by echocardiography may present initially as syncope.[24] To this end, echocardiography may be highly valuable. Furthermore, echocardiography is safe and in most instances readily available.

When interpreting echocardiography in athletic individuals, one must be cognizant of changes that may be seen. The "athlete's heart" as a physiological phenomenon has been recognized for many years.[25] However, only recently has this phenomenon been to a large extent clarified.[25,26] Suffice it to say that highly trained athletes have a larger calculated left ventricular mass than sedentary persons. This observed increase in mass is mainly due to the presence of a larger left ventricular cavity size.[27] Left ventricular wall thickness may, however, also be increased, and the differentiation of this phenomenon from hypertrophic cardiomyopathy is of concern. Pellicia[26] reported that in 98% of athletes the maximal wall thickness is ≤12 mm. Wall thickness ≥13 mm is seen in only 1.7% of athletes.[25] The greatest maximal diameter is 16 mm. In addition, although the septum is usually thickened to a greater degree than other segments, the disproportionality to other segments is minor.[26] Therefore, a thickness of ≥13 mm is uncommon in athletes, with the exception of those involved in rowing sports, and should raise concern about hypertrophic cardiomyopathy. This is particularly of concern if the maximal thickness is ≥16 mm.[25,26]

If maximal thickness appears to be in the 13 mm to 16 mm range, other factors are helpful. As previously mentioned, in physiological hypertrophy cavitary enlargement should be seen.[25,26,28] In addition, tissue reflectivity between hypertrophied and normal segments should not vary.[26] In the athlete's heart syndrome, however, Doppler studies may be the most helpful feature for differentiating normal from abnormal hypertrophy. Patients with physiological hypertrophy show consistently normal or augmented diastolic function, in contrast to patients with hypertrophic cardiomyopathy in whom impaired diastolic function is usually present.[25,26,29,30]

It is of interest that the athlete's heart syndrome appears to be a male phenomenon.[25-31] Pellicia et al[25] noted that of 209 elite female athletes, none had a maximal ventricular wall thickness ≥11 mm. Nakata et al[30] noted the effects of 2 years of endurance training in left ventricular dimensions and function in three female athletes. As in the athletes studied by Pellicia, no significant hypertrophy occurred. Therefore, it is uncertain whether lesser degrees of hypertrophy (≥11 mm) may be of significance in female athletes.

Finally, it should be understand that in trained athletes with physiological hypertrophy, a period of deconditioning should produce regression of wall thickness.[32,33]

In addition to assessing for hypertrophy, echocardiographic evaluation should include evaluation for disorders such as congenital heart disease, ischemic heart disease, valvular heart disease, right ventricular dysplasia, and myocarditis. In addition, an attempt should be made to visualize for coronary artery ostia. A recent publication[34] demonstrated that in athletes, echocardiography in assessment for coronary artery anomalies was reliable in a high percentage of patients.

If significant echocardiographic abnormality is noted, further investigation should of course be directed appropriately. If both the electrocardiographic data and the echocardiographic data are benign, either exercise stress testing, head-upright tilt testing, or both should be performed next.

Exercise Stress Testing

If the individual episode(s) of syncope are exclusively or frequently related to exertion, we proceed with exercise stress testing. Exercise testing can be of value for providing information as to the etiology of syncope in a variety of patients (see Figures 3 and 4, Figures 5 and 6).

Obviously, syncope during exertion can be due to ischemic-induced arrhythmia. This can be secondary to a permanent substrate such as a healed myocardial infarction site, but it may also be due to a transient ischemic-induced substrate in patients without prior infarction.[35] Ischemic-induced arrhythmia is more common in older patients, however it may also occur in younger patients. In a study of sports-related sudden death by Burke et al,[36] 26% of sudden deaths were due to severe atherosclerosis. The mean age of the individuals was 32 years old and only one patient had a history of prior infarction. In addition, younger patients may experience a transient ischemic phenomenon from abnormal coronary ostia,[37,38,39] hypoplastic coronary arteries,[40] or tunnel coronary arteries.[37]

In the absence of structural heart disease or occult coronary disease, stress testing may still be of considerable value. Patients, particularly young patients, may have exercise-induced or exercise-aggravated tachyarrhythmias.[35,41-45] Syncope is not an uncommon manifestation of such disorders and the patients may not have inducible tachycardia on electrophysiological study.[40,41] (See Figures 7,8, and 9)

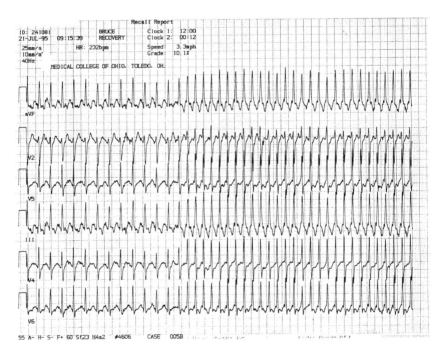

Figure 3. Narrow complex tachycardia initiated during exercise testing in a 34-year-old male. The tachycardia spontaneously terminated with an episode of nonsustained polymorphous ventricular tachyardia.

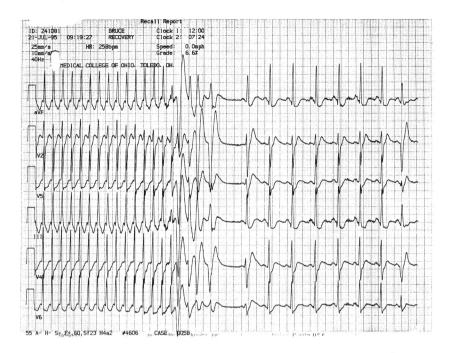

Figure 4. Narrow complex tachycardia initiated during exercise testing in the 34-year-old male shown in Figure 3. The tachycardia spontaneously terminated with an episode of nonsustained polymorphous ventricular tachyardia.

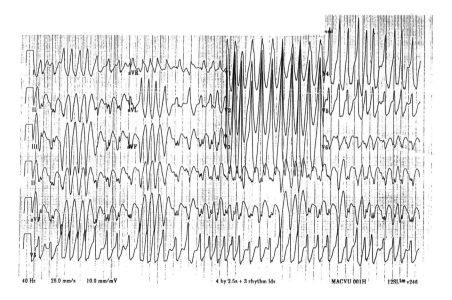

Figure 5. Wide complex tachycardia in a 23-year-old male who presented with severe presyncope that occurred during a bowling tournament. Atrial fibrillation with a rate of >200 bpm is seen in bundle branch aberrance.

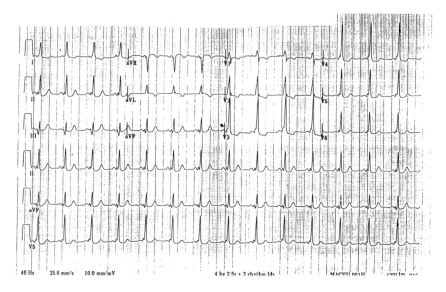

Figure 6. Electrocardiogram taken after cardioversion in the 23-year-old male shown in Figure 5. Preexcitation is manifest. The episode shown is the patient's first symptomatic episode.

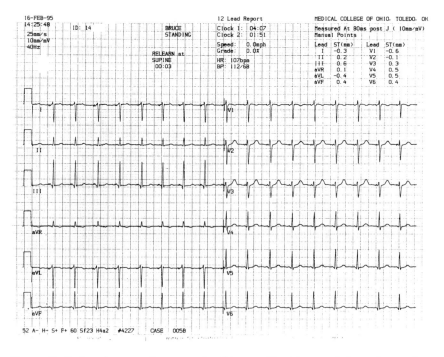

Figure 7. Scalar elecrocardiogram of a 24-year-old with complaints of exercise-induced palpitations associated with dizziness.

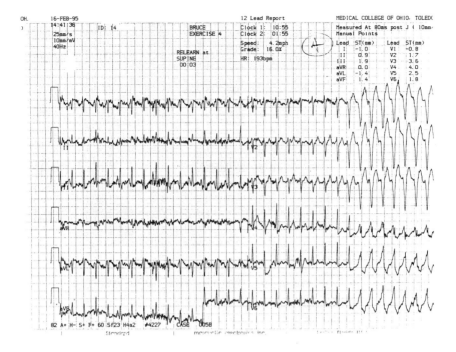

Figure 8. Shown at peak exercise, the initiation of a wide-complex tachycardia in the patient shown in Figure 7.

In addition, a syndrome of exercise-induced polymorphic ventricular tachycardia has been described in adults with normal QT intervals and no structural heart disease.[46] Electrophysiological study was negative in these patients, however, isoproterenol produced polymorphic ventricular tachycardia in 75% of the patients studied. The majority of these patients presented with syncope or presyncope. These patients responded well to treatment with β-blockers.

Nonarrhythmic exercised-induced syncope also occurs in patients with normal hearts. A syndrome of symptomatic sinus arrest provoked by deep inspiration has been described in three athletes.[47] In addition, postexercise asystole has also been described in patients presenting with exercise-related syncope.[48–50] This phenomenon is believed to be due to a neurally mediated mechanism.[50] It has been suggested that this may be an etiology of some cases of exercise-related death.[50]

Postexercise asystole is different from the phenomenon of postexercise postural hypotension. This disorder is defined as a postexercise orthostatic decrease of 20 mm Hg or more in systolic blood pressure. This phenomenon was first described by Gordon[51] near the turn of the century. Subsequent to that, Eichna et al[52] found the phenomenon to be present after vigorous exercise in as many as 50% of healthy individuals. In addition, syncopal spells were noted in some individuals. The authors believed the mechanism to be venous pooling and vasodilatation.

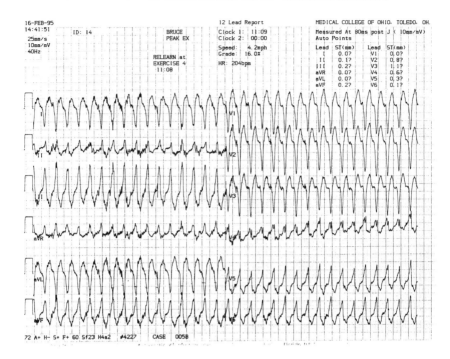

Figure 9. A ventricular tachycardia with a left bundle branch block configuration. On electrophysiological study, no tachycardia could be initiated despite aggressive stimulation and the use of isoproterenol (see Figures 7 and 8).

Most recently Holtzhausen and Noakes[53] investigated the prevalence of this phenomenon in marathon runners. They also evaluated the runners for changes in body weight, plasma volume, and degree of dehydration after an 80 km foot race. They found an average weight loss of 3.5 kg and an average decrease in plasma volume of 12.8%. The average level of dehydration was 4.6%. Postexercise postural hypotension was found in 21 of 38 runners (68%). No runners experienced postural syncope. However, 7 (23%) had blood pressures of <90 mm Hg in the erect position. Symptoms of dizziness and nausea were present in all of these subjects. The authors found it conceivable that if these individuals had been allowed to remain erect, syncope may have occurred.

Exercise Testing and Head-Upright Tilt Test to Evaluate for Exercise-Induced Neurocardiogenic Syncope

In 1978, Rasmussen et al[54] described syncope due to excessive vagal tone in three young athletes. However, the concept that vagally mediated or neurocardiogenic syncope could occur during exercise was not well substantiated. In addition, some felt that the data that existed to suggest the specificity of tilt testing in athletes was highly nonspecific.[55] Other authors have demonstrated that although the tilt test in runners, particularly distance runners, was nonspecific it may have been of value.[56] Data from our institution indicate that the specificity of tilt testing in athletic individuals is acceptable and similar to the specificity seen in the general population.[57,59] In addition, recent publications have clearly documented the phenomenon of exercise-induced neurally mediated syncope.

Sakaguchi et al[22] conducted a restrospective 8-year review of patients referred to the University of Minnesota Hospitals for syncope associated with exercise. Tilt-induced syncope was the leading cause of syncope in these patients. The diagnosis was established by head-upright tilt testing. It is of note that the patients were without structural heart disease. Calkins et al[23] had similar results when evaluating 17 patients referred for syncope that occured during or immediately after exercise. However, the most compelling evidence of this phenomenon came in reports by Sneddon et al,[59] Kosinski et al,[60] and Tse et al.[50] These three publications describe patients with exercise-induced syncope in whom symptomatic hypotension could be demonstrated in both exercise testing and head-upright tilt. Furthermore, it was possible with medical treatment to render patients tilt table and/or stress test negative and symptom free.

Electrophysiological Testing

If exercise stress testing and head-upright tilt testing are negative, electrophysiological study may be considered. Recent American College of Cardiology/American Heart Association (ACC/AHA) guidelines[61] provide a Class II indication to electrophysiological study in patients with unexplained syncope in whom no structural heart disease is present and in whom head-up tilt testing is negative. However, the yield on this group of patients is uncertain (see Figure 10).

Data on electrophysiological studies in the evaluation of syncope and in general are difficult to evaluate. Factors that affect the analysis are the heterogeneity of patients included, the ability to establish a cause-and-effect relationship, and the presence of nonspecific findings on study.[62] In addition, the majority of data involving electrophysiological testing in the diagnosis of syncope involve a wide range of patients, and do not address the role of electrophysiological study in syncope related to athletic activity.[22,62-73]

Sakaguchi et al[22] performed electrophysiological testing in 9 of 12 patients referred for syncope associated with exercise. Seven of these patients were without structural heart disease, and a basis for syncope was identified in two patients. It is of note that they also performed electrophysiological testing in 30 patients with syncope not associated with exer-

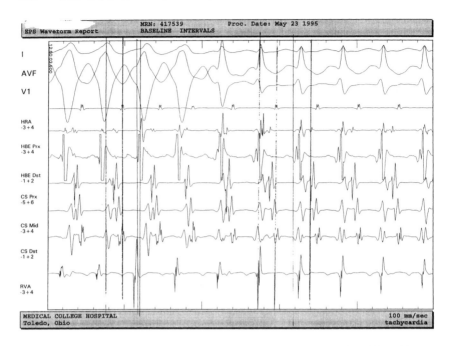

Figure 10. Electrophysiological study tracing of a tachycardia induced in a 16-year-old male with episodes of severe presyncope during athletic activity. The event recorded during one episode revealed a wide complex tachycardia. At electrophysiological testing a tachycardia was induced during isoproterenol stimulation. The first several beats are in a left bundle branch block configuration, and thereafter, in a right bundle branch block configuration. The R-P and P-R intervals are virtually identical, and earliest retrograde activation is at the proximal coronary sinus. The V-A interval remained constant throughout. A premature ventricular extrastimulus during His bundle refractoriness could not preexcite the atria, and the administration of adenosine during sinus rhythm eliminated retrograde conduction. The tachycardia was eliminated by anatomic radio frequency application in AV nodal "slow" pathway area.

cise, and they identified a basis for syncope in only one patient. Calkins et al[23] performed electrophysiological testing in 4 of 17 patients without structural heart disease who were referred for evaluation of exercise-induced syncope. A basis for syncope was not established in any of these patients. In our own experience with electrophysiological study in patients who experience exercise-associated syncope but have no form of structural heart disease or primary conduction abnormality, the yield has been low. However, in select patients such as those with recurrent syncopal episodes, those wishing to participate in vigorous competitive sports, contact sports, or sports with a high risk of injury, professional athletes, or those with a family history of syncope or sudden death, electrophysiological testing should be more seriously considered.

Coronary Angiography and Myocardial Biopsy

The principal role of coronary angiography in the evaluation of syncope of unknown etiology is to evaluate for coronary disease. This disease is often apparent in, or suspected by, the history and/or noninvasive testing, and coronary angiography in these cases is not an issue. The issue is the role angiography plays in the assessment of athletic-associated syncope when the history, physical exam, and noninvasive testing do not provide sufficient support for coronary artery disease. Another question to consider is: what is the role of angiography in the assessment of anomalous coronary artery disease?

There are no substantial data to assess the utility of coronary angiography in the evaluation of syncope related to exercise in younger individuals. Therefore, any recommendations are to be viewed in that light. However, other data can be considered. In reviewing data on the cause of sudden death in competitive athletes 35 years old, Maron et al[71] found that coronary heart disease was responsible for 10% of deaths, and coronary artery anomalies was responsible for 14% of deaths. However, the majority of affected individuals did not experience syncope prior to their fatal event. Burke et al[37] found that in exercise-associated sudden death in patients under the age of 30, coronary artery anomalies were the second leading cause of death. Furthermore, exercise-induced syncope was frequently present. Other authors have also reported exertional syncope in patients with coronary artery anomalies prior to the fatal event.[75]

The congenital coronary anomaly that is most commonly associated with sudden death is origin of the left main coronary artery from the right (anterior) sinus of Valsalva.[37] In 1974, Cheitlin et al[76] recognized the potential for sudden death with this variant. Burke et al,[37] in a review, found this anomaly to be associated with a 46% incidence of sudden death.[37] Most deaths (81%) occurred during or after exercise and occurred at a young age. Although sudden death was frequently unheralded, a surprising proportion of individuals were reported to have experienced prodromal symptoms such as exertional syncope or chest pain.

Other potentially lethal anomalies of the coronary arteries include the right coronary artery arising anomalously from the left coronary sinus and coursing between the aorta and pulmonary trunk, either coronary artery arising from the posterior sinus, or a single coronary ostium giving of all three major arteries.[37,77] In addition, both hypoplastic coronary arteries[37] and "tunnel coronary arteries"[37,78] due to myocardial bridging have been described as a cause of exercise-related sudden death. With this in mind, recommendation can be made, however, clinical judgment should be given wide latitude in this area. Given that anomalous coronary arteries can be reliably screened for with ultrasound,[34] and that other anomalies (including tunnel coronary arteries and hypoplastic arteries) are thought to cause sudden death on the basis of arrhythmia generated by transient ischemia,[78] stress testing (with a radionuclide agent if necessary) would seem to be a reasonable screening tool. Prinzmetal (vasospastic) angina[79-82] has also been reported as a cause of syncope, including exercise-induced syncope.[82] The diagnosis of this disorder is generally made by coronary angiography and pharmacological challenge. However, these publications involve only a small number of patients, therefore data on this entity are extremely limited. Consequently, our recommendations for coronary angiography in the evaluation of syncope in young athletes (≤35 years old) or related to exercise in young patients would be indicated if 1) coronary artery disease is known or suspected on history, physical exam, or noninvasive evaluation; 2) anomalous coronary artery distribution is suspected from ultrasound examination; 3) syncope occurred or occurs during exercise, ultrasound examination is nondiagnostic for coronary artery origin, and no other reasonable cause for syncope is found; 4) syncope occurred or occurs during exercise, noninvasive evaluation failed to provide an etiology of syncope, and the clinical suspicion is sufficient to suspect a transient ischemic-mediated event; 5) by clinical history and/or noninvasive evaluation, syncope due to vasospastic angina is suspected.

We realize that these guidelines are somewhat broad and vague, however, due to a lack of data in this area, sufficient latitude must be afforded the clinician.

In patients ≥35 years old, coronary artery disease is much more prevalent as a cause for sudden death[37,74] in athletes (as high as 80%), and therefore angiography should be strongly considered when evaluating for syncope in this age group. However, we feel that unless evidence for coronary artery disease is found by history, physical exam, electrocardiography or echocardiography, stress testing (with a radionuclide agent if necessary) should be used as a screening tool.

Myocardial biopsy in the evaluation of syncope in athletes or syncope related to exercise is limited to diagnosing those patients with suspected myocarditis or intrinsic myocardial disease such as sarcoid or amyloid. These causes are, in general, quite rare,[37,74] and biopsy should be almost exclusively reserved for individuals in whom history, physical exam, and noninvasive testing provide evidence for the possibility of such a condition. A possible exception is sarcoid. A review by Roberts et al[83] includes data on six patients with sarcoid in whom death occurred during exertion and in whom death was the initial manifestation of sarcoidosis. In individuals with a benign history and physical exam and a normal noninvasive evaluation (including echocardiogram, electrocardiogram, and stress testing), data cannot be marshalled to support a recommendation to biopsy as a routine diagnostic tool.

Summary

The evaluation of syncope in athletes or of syncope associated with exercise is challenging. Diagnosis is necessary to prevent further episodes and also to identify individuals in whom a potentially serious or life-threatening condition may exist. The crux of the issue is to separate the individual with a normal heart from the individual with either structural heart disease (including coronary anomalies) or primary electrical abnormalities. This can generally be done by history, physical exam, and a thorough noninvasive examination. If such conditions are discovered, aggressive evaluation is warranted (see Figure 11). If a potentially serious condition is not identified during noninvasive evaluation, aggressive evaluation is only necessary in select individuals. However, due to a lack of

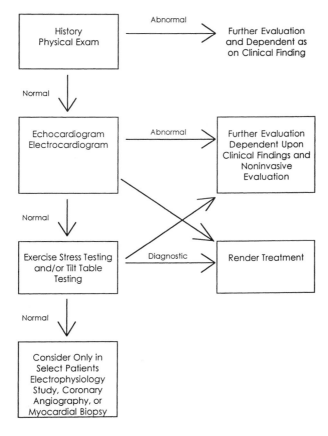

Figure 11. An algorithm for the evaluation of syncope in an athlete or syncope related to athletic activity.

reliable prospective data in many of these areas, clinical judgment should be given sufficient latitude in pursuing evaluation.

References

1. Maron B. Sudden death in young athletes: Lessons from the Hank Guthers affair. *N Engl J Med* 1993;329(1):55–57.
2. Swift EM. A city in mourning. *Sports Illustrated* 1993;79(Aug9):20–27.
3. Maron BJ, Roberts WC, McCallister WA, et al. Sudden death in young athletes. *Circulation* 1980;62:218–229.
4. Driscoll DJ, Edwards WD. Sudden unexpected death in children and adolescents. *J Am Coll Cardiol* 1985;5:118–121.
5. Kramer MR, Dvori Y, Leu B. Sudden death in young soldiers: High incidence of syncope prior to death. *Chest* 1988;93(2):345–347.
6. Calkins H, Shyr Y, Frumin H, et al. The value of the clinical history in the differentiation of syncope due to ventricular tachycardia, atrioventricular block, and neurocardiogenic syncope. *Am J Med* 1995;98:365–373.
7. Hackel D, Reimer K. Sudden death: Cardiac and other causes: Role of recreational and therapeutic drugs in occurrence of sudden death. *Cardiovascular Reviews and Reports* 1994;15(4):16–32.
8. Maron B, Mitchell J. Revised eligibility recommendations for competitive athletes with cardiovascular abnormalities. *J Am Coll Cardiol* 1994;24(4):848–850.
9. Mitchell J, Haskell W, Raven P. Classification of sports. *J Am Coll Cardiol* 1994;24(4)864–866.
10. Oakley C. The electrocardiogram in the highly trained athlete. *Cardiol Clin* 1992;10(2):295–302.
11. Pellicia A. Outer limits of physiologic hypertrophy and the relevance to the diagnosis of primary cardiac disease. *Cardiol Clin* 1992;12(2):267–277.
12. Fagard R. Impact of different sports and training on cardiac structure and function. *Cardiol Clin* 1992;10(2):241–256.
13. McFarlane N, Northridge DG, Wright AR, et al. A comparative study of left ventricular structure and function in elite athletes. *Br J Sports Med* 1991;25(1):45–48.
14. Bjornstad H, Storstein L, Meen HD, Hals O. Electrocardiographic findings of repolarization in athletic students and control subjects. *Cardiology* 1994;84(1):51–60.
15. Pellicia A, Maron B, Spataro A, et al. The upper limit of physiologic cardiac hypertrophy in highly trained elite athletes. *N Engl J Med* 1991;324:295–301.
16. Moore NE, Goineau JP, Patterson DG. Incomplete right bundle branch block: An electrocardiographic enigma and possible misnomer. *Circulation* 1975;45:678–687.
17. Cullen KJ, Colin R. Daily running causes Wenckebach heart block. *Lancet* 1964;2:729–730.
18. Grimby G, Saltin S. Daily running causing Wenckebach heart block. *Lancet* 1964;2:962–963.
19. Sargin O, Alp C, Tansi C. Wenckebach phenomenon with nodal and ventricular escape in marathon runners. *Chest* 1970;57:102–105.
20. Shamroth L, Kohl E. Marked sinus and A-V nodal bradycardia with interference dissociation in an athlete. *J Sports Med Phys Fitness* 1969;9:128–129.
21. Oakley D, Oakley CM. Significance of abnormal electrocardiograms in highly trained athletes. *Am J Cardiol* 1982;30:985–989.

22. Sakaguchi S, Shultz J, Renole S, et al. Syncope associated with exercise, a manifestation of neurally-mediated syncope. *Am J Cardiol* 1995;75:476–481.
23. Calkins H, Seifert M, Morady F. Clinical preservation and long-term followup of athletes with exercise-induced vasodepression syncope. *Am Heart J* 1995; 129:1159–1164.
24. Maron BJ, Roberts WC, McCallister HA, et al. Sudden death in young athletes. *Circulation* 1980;62:218–229.
25. Pellicia A, Maron B, Spataro A, et al. The upper limit of physiologic cardiac hypertrophy in highly trained athletes. *N Eng J Med* 1991;324:295–301.
26. Pellicia A. Outer limits of physiologic hypertrophy and relevance to the diagnosis of primary cardiac disease. *Cardiol Clin* 1992;10(2):267–277.
27. Maron BJ. Structural features of the athlete's heart: As defined by echocardiography. *J Am Coll Cardiol* 1986;7:190–203.
28. Lo YS, Chin MK. Echocardiographic left ventricular hypertrophy in Chinese endurance athletes. *Br J Sports Med* 1990;24(11):274–276.
29. MacFarlane N, Northridge DB, Weight AR, et al. A comparative study of left ventricular stucture and function in elite athletes. *Br J Sports Med* 1991;25(1):45–48.
30. Lewis JA, Spirito P, Pellicia A. Usefulness of Doppler echocardiographic assessment of diastolic filling in distinguishing "athlete's heart" from hypertrophic cardiomyopathy. *Br Heart J* 1992;68:296–300.
31. Nakata H, Mimura K, Sakuyama K, et al. Effects of long-term endurance training on left ventricular dimensions and function in female distance runners. *Ann Phys Anthropol* 1994;13(1):1–8.
32. Maron B. Hypertrophic cardiomyopathy. *Curr Probl Cardiol* 1993;10(11)637–704.
33. Maron BJ, Pellicia A, Spataro A. Reduction in left ventricular wall thickness after deconditioning in highly trained olympic athletes. *Br Heart J* 1993;69:125–128.
34. Pelliccia A, Spataro A, Maron B. Prospective echocardiographic screening for coronary artery anomalies in 1,360 elite competitive athletes. *Am J Cardiol* 1993;72:978–979.
35. Coumel P, Leenhardt A, Haddad G. Exercise ECG: Prognostic implications of exercise-induced arrhythmias. *Pacing Clin Electrophysiol* 1994;17:417–427.
36. Burke A, Farb A, Virmani R, et al. Sports-related and nonsports-related sudden cardiac death in young adults. *Am Heart J* 1991;121(2):568–575.
37. Burke A, Farb A, Virmani R. Causes of sudden death in athletes. *Cardiol Clin* 1992;10(2):303–315.
38. Scully R. Case records of the Massachusetts General Hospital. *N Eng J Med* 1990;320(22):1475–1483.
39. Liberthson RR, Zaman L, Wegman A, et al. Aberrant origin of the left coronary artery from the proximal right coronary artery: Diagnostic features and pre-post operative course. *Clin Cardiol* 1982;5:377–381.
40. McClellan JT, Jokl E. Congenital anomalies of coronary arteries as a cause of sudden death associated with physical exertion. *Medicine and Sport* 1971;5:91.
41. Gilman J, Naccarelli G. Sudden cardiac death. *Curr Probl Cardiol* 1992;17(11):719.
42. Palileo EJ, Ashley WW, Sriryn S. Exercise provocative right ventricular outflow tachycardia. *Am Heart J* 1982;104:185–193.
43. Woelfel A, Foster JR, Simpson RJ. Reproducibility and treatment of exercise-induced ventricular tachycardia. *Am J Cardiol* 1984;53:751–756.
44. Wu D, Kou HC, Hung JS. Exercise-triggered paroxysmal ventricular tachycardia: A repetitive rhythmic activity possibly related to after depolarization. *Ann Intern Med* 1981;95:410–414.
45. Levy M, Villain E, Philippe F, Kachaner J. Catecholamine-induced ventricular tachycardia: A cause of severe syncope during adolescence. *De Diatrie* 1993; 48(7–8):533–535.

46. Eisenberg S, Scheinman M, Oullet N, et al. Sudden cardiac death and polymorphic ventricular tachycardia in patients with normal QT intervals and normal cardiac systolic function. *Am J Cardiol* 1995;75:687–692.
47. Buja G, Folino AF, Bittante M, et al. Asystole with syncope secondary to hyperventilation in three young athletes. *Pacing Clin Electrophysiol* 1989;12(3):406–412.
48. Osswald S, Brooks R, O'Nunain S, et al. Asystole after exercise in healthy persons. *Ann Intern Med* 1994;120:1008–1011.
49. Fleg JL, Asante AV. Asystole following treadmill exercise in man without organic heart disease. *Arch Int Med* 1983;143:1821–1822.
50. Tse H, Lau C. Exercise-associated cardiac asystole in persons without structural heart disease. *Chest* 1995;107(2):572–576.
51. Gordon G. Observations on the effect of prolonged sense exertion on the blood pressure of healthy athletes. *Edinburgh Med J* 1907;22:53–56.
52. Eichna L, Horvath S, Bean W. Post-exertional orthostatic hypotension. *Am J Med Sci* 1947;213:641–654.
53. Holtzhausen LM, Noakes T. The prevalence and significance of post exercise (postural) hypotension in ultra marathon runners. *Med Sci Sports Exerc* 1995;27(12):1595–1601.
54. Rasmussen V, Haunso S, Skagen K. Cerebral attacks due to excessive vagal tone in heavily trained persons. *Acta Med Scand* 1978;204:401–405.
55. Ebert T, Denattan T. Hemodynamic responses of high fit runners during head up tilt testing to syncope. (Abstr) *1993 Proc Am Autonomic Society Annual Scientific Sessions* p. 11.
56. Ferrario G, Peci P, Tiberio N, et al. Long distance runner's heart: Is it a condition at risk for malignant vasovagal syndrome? (Abstr) *Pacing Clin Electrophysiol* 1993;16:936.
57. Grubb BP, Temesy-Armos P, Samoil D, et al. Tilt table testing in the evaluation and management of athletes with recurrent exercise-induced syncope. *Med Sci Sports Exerc* 1993;25:24–28.
58. Frederick S, Kosinski D, Grubb BP, et al. Comparison of aerobic capacity, parasympathetic modulation and orthostatic tolerance. *Clin Auton Res* 1995;6(5):334.
59. Sneddon J, Scalia G, Ward D, et al. Exercise-induced vasodepressor syncope. *Br Heart J* 1994;71:554–557.
60. Kosinski D, Grubb BP, Kip K, Hahn H. Exercise-induced neurocardiogenic syncope: A case report. *Am Heart J* (in press).
61. Zipes D, DiMarco J, Gillette P, et al. Guidelines for clinical intracardiac electrophysiologic and catheter ablation procedures. *J Am Coll Cardiol* 1995;26(2):555–573.
62. Kapoor W. Diagnostic evaluation of syncope. *Am J Med* 1991;90:91–106.
63. Morillo C, Zandri S, Klein G. Usefulness of signal-average ECG/head up tilt test and electrophysiologic studies in patients with unexplained syncope. (Abstr) *J Am Coll Cardiol* 1995?b Special Issue:92A.
64. Bass EB, Elson JJ, Fogoros RN, et al. Long-term prognosis of patients undergoing electrophysiologic studies for syncope of unknown origin. *Am J Cardiol* 1988;62:1186–1191.
65. DeMarco JP, Garan H, Harthorue JW, Ruskin J. Intracardiac electrophysiologic techniques in recurrent syncope of unknown cause. *Ann Intern Med* 1981;95:542–548.
66. Akhtar M, Shenasa M, Denker S, et al. Role of cardiac electrophysiologic studies in patients with unexplained recurrent syncope. *Pacing Clin Electrophysiol* 1983;6:192–201.
67. Sugrue D, Holmes D, Hammill J. Intracardiac electrophysiologic studies in patients with unexplained syncope. (Abstr) *Chest* 1985;88(suppl):645.

68. Olshansky B, Mazuz M, Martins JB. Significance of inducible tachycardia in patients with syncope of unknown origin: A long-term followup. *J Am Coll Cardiol* 1985;5:216–233.
69. Denes P, Ezri M. Role of electrophysiologic study in the management of patients with unexplained syncope. *Pacing Clin Electrophysiol* 1985;424–435.
70. Eichman SL, Felder SD, Matos JA, et al. The value of electrophysiologic studies in syncope of unknown origin: Report of 150 cases. *Am Heart J* 1985;110:469–479.
71. Doherty JU, Pembrook-Rogers D, Grogan EW. Electrophysiologic evaluation and followup characteristics of patients with recurrent unexplained syncope and pre-syncope. *Am J Cardiol* 1985;55:703–708.
72. Hess DS, Morady F, Scheiman M. Electrophysiologic testing in the evaluation of patients with syncope of unknown origin. *Am J Cardiol* 1982;50:1309–1315.
73. Gulamhusein S, Naccarelli GV, Ko PT. Value and limitations of clinical electrophysiologic study in assessment of patients with unexplained syncope. *Am J Med* 1982;73:700–705.
74. Maron B, Epstein S, Roberts W. Causes of sudden death in competitive athletes. *J Am Coll Cardiol* 1986;7:204–214.
75. Pedoe I, Teufel M. Sudden cardic death in childhood due to an abnormal coronary artery origin. *Deutsche Melizinische Woch en Schrift* 1993;118(23):861–866.
76. Cheitlin M, DeCastro C, McAllister H. Sudden death as a complication of anomalies left coronary origin from the anterior sinus of Valsalva. *Circulation* 1974;50:780–787.
77. Virmani R, Rogan K, Cheitlin M. Congenital coronary anomalies: Pathologic aspects. In: Virmani R, Forman MB (eds): *Nonatherosclerotic Ischemic Heart Disease.* New York: Raven Press; 1984.
78. Morales AR, Romanelli R. The mural left anterior descending artery, strenuous exertion and sudden death. *Circulation* 1980;62:230–237.
79. Tanabe Y, Yamazoe M, Igaroshi Y, et al. Importance of coronary artery spasm in alcohol-related unexplained syncope. *Jpn Heart J* 1992;33(2):135–144.
80. Watanaba K, Inomata T, Miyakita Y, et al. Electrophysiology study and ergonovine provocation of coronary spasm in unexplain syncope. *Jpn Heart J* 1993;34(2):171–182.
81. Tomcsanyi J, Karlocai K, Tarjan Z, et al. Prinzmetal angina as syncope. *Orv Hetil* 1991;132(51):2861–2862.
82. Havranek EP, Dunbar D. Exertional syncope caused by left main coronary artery spasm. *Am Heart J* 1992;123(3):792–794.
83. Roberts WC, McAllister HA, Ferrans VJ. Sarcoidosis of the heart: A clinicopathologic study of 35 necropsy patients (group I) and review of 78 previously described necropsy patients (group II). *Am J Med* 1977;63:86–103.

Chapter 15

Syncope in the Elderly

Gohar Azhar, MBBS and Lewis A. Lipsitz, MD

Introduction

Syncope is a common and potentially life threatening syndrome that increases in prevalence with age[1] and is associated with high morbidity secondary to fall-related injuries.[2] Syncope accounts for approximately 3% of emergency room visits and 2% to 3% of hospital admissions, 80% of which are in individuals over 65 years of age.[3–5] However, in only approximately 50% of patients is an etiologic diagnosis reached after an extensive evaluation.

In the institutionalized elderly the incidence of syncope is 6% annually with a high recurrence rate of 30%.[6] Each syncopal recurrence portends further decline and increasing functional dependence for this frail group of people. Due to alterations in cardiovascular control of the circulation, the accumulation of multiple illnesses, and the use of numerous medications, older people are particularly vulnerable to the development of hypotension and syncope.

Age-Related Physiological Changes Predisposing to Syncope

Cerebral Circulation

The final common pathway leading to syncope is a sudden reduction in the supply of oxygen and/or metabolic substrates delivered to the brain.

Supported by the Hebrew Rehabilitation Center for Aged, the Brockton/West Roxbury VA Medical Center, and Grants AG04390, AG08812, and AG09538 from the National Institute on Aging, Bethesda, Maryland.

From Grubb BP, Olshansky B (eds.). *Syncope: Mechanisms and Management*. Armonk, NY: Futura Publishing Co., Inc.; © 1998.

Normally, autoregulation of cerebral blood flow maintains an optimal supply of oxygen and glucose to the brain. Autoregulation is operative over a wide range of mean arterial blood pressures, normally between 60 mm Hg and 150 mm Hg.[7,8] Limited research has been done on cerebral blood flow changes with aging, but resting blood flow appears to be preserved.[9] Hypertension increases the threshold of cerebral autoregulation to a higher blood pressure level, thus increasing the susceptibility of hypertensive elderly patients to syncope during reductions in blood pressure to levels that would be considered normal in normotensive individuals.

Abnormal vascular reactivity has been well documented in the cerebral vessels in aging animals.[10] In human beings, paradoxical vasoconstriction of the cerebral arteries has been shown during head-up tilt induced syncope.[11] One of the underlying mechanisms could be abnormal endothelial dysfunction, which occurs with aging.[12] A recent transcranial Doppler study of elderly subjects demonstrated increased cerebral arteriolar vascular resistance despite reductions in blood pressure following a meal, a finding that could explain the increased propensity of elderly individuals for postprandial syncope.[13]

Sympathetic Nervous System

The sympathetic nervous system undergoes several age-related changes. There is an increase in plasma norepinephrine levels with age, due to greater spillover from sympathetic nerve terminals and a reduced clearance rate.[14-16] Despite increased circulating norepinephrine levels[17] the β-adrenergic mediated cardioacceleratory response to sympathetic activation is diminished. Alpha-adrenergic-mediated vasoconstrictor[18] and β-adrenergic vasodilatory[19] vascular responses are also impaired. These changes may be due in part to downregulation of adrenergic receptors in response to high plasma norepinephrine levels. The density of β-receptors on cardiomyocytes and lymphocytes is unchanged with age. However there appears to be a defect in the G-protein receptor[20] complex and reduced activity of adenyl cyclase in the aging heart.[21-23] The reduced β- adrenergic vasodilatory response may contribute to an increased peripheral vascular resistance with aging.

Parasympathetic Nervous System

Aging is also associated with a reduction in cardiac vagal tone, although the exact underlying mechanisms have not been delineated. A number of studies of heart rate variability show a reduction in vagal control of heart rate in response to respiration,[24-27] cough,[28,29] and the Valsalva maneuver.[30] Reduced heart rate variability with advancing age suggests a diminution in vagal control of heart rate which may afford some protection from the development of vasovagal syncope. Elderly patients with syncope have been shown to have reduced heart rate variability in response to deep breathing, compared to age-matched subjects without syncope.[28]

Baroreflex Sensitivity

Reflex changes in heart rate in response to alterations in blood pressure are mediated by the baroreflex, which loses its sensitivity with age.[29,31] The impairment in baroreflex control is manifested as diminished cardioacceleration in response to hypotension.[32,33] This may be due to a defect in β-adrenergic responsiveness, as described above. Most elderly people can compensate for this with increased vasoconstriction[34] unless challenged by vasodilator medications or hypovolemia. Therefore, elderly individuals are particularly vulnerable to syncope during vasodilator therapy or in response to volume contraction.

Heart Rate

Autonomic control of heart rate is altered in the elderly by impairments in both sympathetic and parasympathetic branches of the nervous system, as discussed above. The relative contributions of each component of the autonomic nervous system has been assessed by frequency domain analysis of heart rate variability.[35] Low-frequency heart rate oscillations (0.06 Hz to 0.15 Hz) are thought to represent baroreflex-mediated sympathetic and parasympathetic influences on heart rate variability, while high-frequency (0.15 Hz to 0.5 Hz) oscillations generally represent the vagally mediated respiratory sinus arrhythmia. Healthy aging is associated with a reduction in both frequencies, but with a relatively greater loss of the vagally mediated higher- frequency oscillations.[36–38]

There is also an age-associated loss of pacemaker cells in the sinus node, and an increase in elastic and collagenous tissue in the cardiac conduction system. By age 75, there are less than 10% of the sinoatrial cells that were present at maturity.

With age, the atrioventricular (AV) valves undergo some calcification that may extend into the AV node and into parts of the conduction system. These changes contribute to a higher incidence of conduction block, bradyarrhythmias, and sick sinus syndrome in the elderly, predisposing them to the development of syncope.

Cardiac Relaxation

Cardiac hypertrophy probably occurs with aging in response to increased stiffness of the vasculature, and as a result, cardiac contractile function at rest is maintained. However, during diastole, removal of calcium from the contractile proteins to the sarcoplasmic reticulum is impaired in aging hearts, resulting in slower isometric relaxation.[39–41] Diastolic dysfunction occurs with aging even in the absence of left ventricular hypertrophy. The reduced compliance of the ventricle in diastole restricts early diastolic filling, making the heart more dependent on preload and atrial contraction during diastole to fill adequately.[42,43] Consequently, any condition that produces volume contraction and reduces cardiac preload will decrease stroke volume, threaten blood pressure, and increase the risk of cerebral ischemia. Furthermore, any condition that impairs atrial contraction and late diastolic filling can reduce cardiac output and lead to the development of hypotension and syncope.

Vascular Tone

Due to diminished baroreflex control of heart rate, systemic vasoconstriction plays a major role in defending the circulation from hypotensive stress.[34] Although there is marked variability in forearm vascular response to the hypotensive stress of posture change with age,[44] most elderly individuals can increase peripheral resistance sufficiently to maintain blood pressure in response to upright posture.[34,45] A blunted α-adrenergic response may not account for all the variability of peripheral vasoconstriction with age, and deficient responses to other vasoconstrictors such as endothelin may be present.

One study shows that endothelin concentrations rise with age.[46] A few other studies[47,48] demonstrate an elevation in plasma endothelin concentrations in response to tilt, suggesting a role for this peptide in maintaining vascular tone during posture change. Since endothelin is a powerful vasoconstrictor, an age-related increase in this peptide may offset impairments in adrenergic control of peripheral vascular resistance.

Other humoral mediators that influence vascular tone are the vasoconstrictors angiotensin and vasopressin, and vasodilators atrial natriuretic peptide (ANP), prostacyclin, and nitric oxide. There is considerable interaction between these mediators and the catecholamines in blood pressure regulation. ANP, which is both a potent vasodilator and promoter of natriuresis, rises in the plasma with age.[49] In severe hypertension and congestive heart failure, ANP levels are even higher and may exert a beneficial effect by promoting natriuresis. High ANP levels may also exert deleterious effects by causing salt loss in the elderly in the presence of reduced fluid intake or increased insensible losses. This may lead to dehydration and syncope.

In contrast to ANP, renin and aldosterone levels fall with age, reducing sodium reabsorption. The cumulative effect of the changes in ANP, renin, and aldosterone is to shift the balance in favor of greater salt and water excretion by the kidneys.[50] Elderly individuals also have an impaired thirst-sensing mechanism[51] and do not compensate for hyperosmolality by drinking more fluid.

Hence, special attention must be given to the fluid requirements of a sick geriatric patient in order to prevent dehydration and syncope.

Effect of Hypertension

Approximately 30% of elderly people over the age of 75 have systolic hypertension.[52] Systolic hypertension has been identified in several studies as a significant risk factor for orthostatic[53-55] and postprandial hypotension.[56] The elderly patients who are at greatest risk for the development of *hypotension* are those with resting supine systolic *hypertension.* Other changes associated with hypertension include myocardial hypertrophy, reduced ventricular compliance, and shifting of cerebral autoregulation to a higher threshold.[7,9,57] All of these factors enhance the vulnerability of the aging individual to the development of hypotension and syncope.

Common Causes of Syncope in the Elderly

Hypotensive Syndromes

As previously discussed, many age-related physiological and pathological changes increase the vulnerability of elderly people to syncope. The superimposed stresses of acute illnesses, prolonged bed rest, dehydration, or antihypertensive medications can cause hypotension and syncope. Potent arteriolar and venous vasodilators such as α-blockers and nitrates are especially liable to cause sudden acute reductions in blood pressure that can overwhelm the baroreflex responses and cerebral autoregulation, and result in syncope.

Two hypotensive syndromes that are particularly prevalent and are common causes of syncope in elderly people are orthostatic hypotension and postprandial hypotension.

Orthostatic Hypotension

Orthostatic hypotension is defined as a decline in systolic blood pressure of 20 mm Hg, or a decline in diastolic blood pressure of 10 mm Hg on the assumption of an upright posture. Approximately 30% of community-dwelling elderly over the age of 75 have orthostatic hypotension,[58] and the prevalence rises with age and with the level of blood pressure.[59] Two previous epidemiological studies have demonstrated that a reduction of systolic blood pressure of >20 mm Hg within 3 minutes of standing is a significant risk factor for falls[60] and for syncope.[61] However, a recent study by Liu et al[62] did not find a relationship between orthostatic hypotension and falls. This may be due to the fact that orthostatic hypotension is common in elderly subjects, with and without falls and syncope, thereby making it unlikely to emerge as a significant risk factor in multivariate analysis. Also, many elderly people have large intraindividual variability in postural blood pressure throughout the day,[63] but remain asymptomatic. Syncope may occur only when the right combination of circumstances impedes optimal cerebral blood flow to maintain consciousness. The higher prevalence of orthostatic hypotension with increased age is due in part to age-associated changes in baroreflex sensitivity and vasoconstriction, as discussed previously. Orthostatic hypotension may also be due to diseases of autonomic function, which are common in old age (see below), or the medications used to treat these and other conditions.

Postprandial Hypotension

A number of studies during the past decade identify postprandial hypotension as an important cause of syncope in elderly patients[64,65] and in those with autonomic insufficiency.[66,67] Postprandial hypotension also appears to be more common than orthostatic hypotension in the elderly, although both may coexist in the same individual.[68] Previous studies of nursing home residents show that between 24% and 30% of residents have decreases in systolic blood pressure of >20 mm Hg within 75 minutes of eating a meal.[65,69] In most cases, postprandial hypotension is asymptomatic. However, in elderly institutionalized patients with syncope, 8% were found to have postprandial hypotension as the probable cause.[61] The exact pathophysiology of postprandial hypotension is still not fully understood, although studies show that there is a failure to maintain systemic vascular resistance after a meal during the phase of splanchnic blood pooling. Elderly patients without postprandial hypotension have similar splanchnic pooling of blood, but they are able to increase their systemic vascular resistance appropriately. Furthermore, elderly subjects with a postprandial decline in blood pressure have no change in their forearm vascular resistance in response to a meal, suggesting a defect in peripheral vasoconstriction as one of the underlying mechanisms.[70] This hypothesis is further supported by the ability of somatostatin to ameliorate postprandial reductions in blood pressure by decreasing splanchnic blood flow and increasing forearm vascular resistance.[71-73]

Many vasoactive gastrointestinal peptides have been studied for their possible role in the pathogenesis of postprandial hypotension, but none have shown a clear association. Postprandial hypotension is often unrecognized because clinical symptoms may be subtle, consisting of only dizziness or weakness. However, falls, syncope, coronary insufficiency, and strokes can occur if there is a large meal-related fall in blood pressure. All of these symptoms can occur up to 75 minutes after a meal. An increased awareness of this syndrome is essential in the overall assessment of a geriatric patient with syncope.

Cardiovascular Syncope

Syncope in the elderly is precipitated by a cardiac cause in 21% to 34% of cases.[74] Amongst all causes of syncope, various cardiac arrhythmias comprise 16%; sick sinus syndrome, 3% to 6%; aortic stenosis, 4% to 5%; myocardial infarction, 2% to 6%; and heart block, 1% to 3%.[61,74] Aortic stenosis is by far the most common structural lesion associated with syncope in the elderly. The prevalence of aortic stenosis increases with age; 75% of community-dwelling elderly people over the age of 85 have mild calcification of the aortic valve on echocardiography, and 6% have critical aortic stenosis.[75] Syncope affects approximately 25% of patients with symptomatic aortic stenosis. The patients who experience syncope have an increased incidence of sudden cardiac death.[76,77] Typically, syncope in a patient with aortic stenosis occurs with exercise, but it can also occur in response to directly acting vasodilators or even vasodilatation induced by a hot bath.

Another underrecognized cause of cardiovascular syncope in the elderly is hypertrophic cardiomyopathy. Approximately 5% to 25% of patients with hypertrophic cardiomyopathy experience syncope at rest or on exercise.[78] Although there are no current demographic data on the incidence of hypertrophic cardiomyopathy in community-dwelling elderly, one study[79] shows that 83% of patients were over 50 years of age at the time of diagnosis.

An important cause of postoperative syncope in the elderly is pulmonary embolism. Pulmonary embolism should be included in the differential diagnosis of syncope in all patients, as it is common and often overlooked. In one recent study,[80] 18% of elderly patients who were admitted to an acute geriatric ward had pulmonary embolism. Other less common cardiovascular causes of syncope include cardiac tamponade, aortic dissection, obstructive cardiac tumors, and thrombotic occlusion of a prosthetic cardiac valve.

Asymptomatic arrhythmias are common in healthy elderly individuals, and it is difficult to determine if an arrhythmia is responsible for syncope unless there is electrocardiographic confirmation during the episode. Since syncopal episodes are unpredictable and infrequent, even prolonged ECG monitoring may yield a low diagnostic rate. Bass et al[81] performed Holter monitoring in 95 patients with unknown syncope and discovered major ECG abnormalities in 15% of patients within the first 24 hours. Of the remaining patients, 11% showed ECG abnormalities when monitored for another 24 hours. Beyond 48 hours, the yield of Holter monitoring was poor. However, in this study as in a number of previous studies, there was no significant correlation between ECG abnormalities and symptoms of syncope.

An advancement in technique is the use of patient-activated loop recorders, which can retroactively record up to 4 minutes of ECG prior to the syncopal episode. These are useful in patients with frequent episodes of syncope and in those individuals who have sufficient understanding to be able to activate them at the time of an episode.

Neurological Diseases

Autonomic Dysfunction

The prevalence of autonomic dysfunction and associated orthostatic and postprandial syncope rises with age. Autonomic insufficiency, commonly seen in the elderly, occurs in association with central nervous system diseases such as Parkinson's disease and chronic strokes. Other less common central causes include multiple system atrophy (Shy-Drager syndrome), Huntington's disease, and Guillian Barre syndrome.

Pure autonomic failure (Bradbury-Eggleston syndrome) is a disease of peripheral sympathetic nerve terminals characterized by significant postural hypotension with low basal norepinephrine levels, reduced norepinephrine response to tyramine, and noradrenergic supersensitivity.

Other diseases that interrupt either afferent or efferent pathways of the peripheral autonomic nervous system include diabetes mellitus, tabes dorsalis, amyloidosis, porphyria, alcoholism, and various spinal cord problems and peripheral neuropathies.

Clinical features of autonomic dysfunction depend on the underlying disease plus the balance of sympathetic and parasympathetic losses. In general, however, symptoms of postural hypotension and syncope are accompanied by fatigue, reduced sweating, constipation, urinary incontinence or retention, visual disturbances, and erectile dysfunction and impotence in men.

Cerebrovascular Disease

Syncope, by definition, is a transient ischemic attack, but this is rarely due to cerebrovascular disease unless there are accompanying focal neurological deficits. Occasionally transient posterior circulation ischemia can result in loss of consciousness, but other brain stem abnormalities are usually present. Large cortical or subcortical strokes or ischemic events that result in loss of consciousness usually cause prolonged unresponsiveness or coma, and rarely result in full recovery characteristic of syncope.

Reflex Mechanisms

Carotid Sinus Hypersensitity

The prevalence of carotid hypersensitivity is approximately 10% in the elderly population, although only 5% to 20% of these patients develop spontaneous carotid sinus syncope.[82]

There are three subtypes of carotid hypersensitivity, with vasodepressor being the most common (37%), followed by cardioinhibitory (29%), and mixed (34%). The term "hypersensitivity" itself is probably a misnomer, as in most patients the cardioinhibitory component is produced by vigorous carotid compression and not by trivial stimuli such as shaving or tight collars.[83] Carotid sinus syncope has also been seen in patients with surgical denervation of the carotid sinus.[84] Although the exact pathophysiology of carotid hypersensitivity is unclear, a recent hypothesis suggests that carotid hypersensitivity is a marker of generalized atherosclerotic disease with reduced carotid sinus compliance. This, in turn, may reduce the afferent baroreflex traffic, producing an upregulation of brain stem postsynaptic α_2-adrenoreceptors, which mediate the reflex vasodilatation and cardioinhibition produced by carotid sinus baroreceptor stimulation.

Carotid hypersensitivity occurs with greater frequency in male patients with hypertension, coronary heart disease, and with use of digitalis, methyldopa, and β-blockers.[85-90] It is associated with considerable morbidity from fall-related injuries and fractures. Therefore, testing for this syndrome should be part of the routine work-up of syncope in patients without contraindications (see below).

Micturition/Defecation/Cough Syncope

Syncope may occur in any condition that produces a Valsalva maneuver, thus reducing venous return to the heart. These conditions include micturition, defecation, coughing, lifting heavy weights, and other physiological stresses. Micturition syncope is often seen in males with prostatic hypertrophy who strain to void while standing up. Also, rapid emptying of the bladder when blood is pooling in the lower extremities can cause reflex vasodilatation and hypotension.

Neurally Mediated/Neurocardiogenic/ Vasovagal Syncope

The above labels all refer to syncope in response to excessive vagal outflow, which produces hypotension, usually in association with bradycardia.

The exact mechanisms of neurally mediated syncope have not been elucidated, but this phenomenon is most commonly observed during intense sympathetic stimulation of the heart,[91] when venous return is reduced by upright posture or hypovolemia. In susceptible individuals, sympathetic activation is thought to generate an exaggerated ionotropic response[92] around a relatively empty ventricular chamber, thus activating cardiac mechanoreceptor C-fibers, which stimulate reflex vagal outflow from the medulla. The efferent response is vasodilatation and bradycardia, which results in hypotension and syncope. It is also possible that the cardiac mechanoreceptors are activated by chemical bonding with various neuropeptides (epinephrine, serotonin, vasopressin),[93,94] because vasovagal syncope has been seen in patients with transplanted and denervated hearts.[95]

Neurally mediated syncope may be less common in the elderly than in the young, especially in the oldest old (over 80) who have reduced β-adrenergic cardiac responsiveness and reduced cardiac vagal tone.[45] Nevertheless, vasovagal syncope does occur in the elderly and may be precipitated by inferior wall cardiac ischemia.

Endocrine Diseases

Diabetes mellitus, its complications, and its treatment can produce syncope via different mechanisms. Diabetic autonomic neuropathy can produce orthostatic hypotension and syncope, as discussed above. Hypoglycemia may occur in any illness in which the patient is not eating well. One should be aware of interactions between sulphonylureas and high dose salicylates, phenylbutazone, sulphonamides, chloramphenicoi, and dicoumarol, all of which reduce clearance of sulphonylureas and enhance their hypoglycemic effects. Reduced creatinine clearance due to renal impairment will also enhance susceptibility to hypoglycemic effects of insulin and oral hypoglycemics. Uncontrolled diabetes mellitus can cause an osmotic diuresis and dehydration, resulting in syncope.

Other endocrine causes of hypotension and syncope include Addison's disease, chronic adrenal suppression from steroid use, and hypopituitarism, all of which can produce hypoglycemia and hypovolumia. Conditions that are associated specifically with fluid loss are diabetes insipidus and salt-losing nephropathies. Other rarer entities, such as systemic mastocytosis, carcinoid, and pheochromocytoma, produce syncope via release of vasoactive substances such as histamine, epinephrine, and serotonin, respectively.

Evaluation and Management of Syncope in the Elderly

History

Among cases of syncope for which an explanation can be found, approximately 70% to 80% can be diagnosed by a good history and physical examination. It is important to get a detailed account of the situation in which syncope occurred, since many common everyday activities can impose significant stress on an elderly individual and produce hypotension (see above). Antihypertensives, especially the directly acting vasodilators, and psychoactive medications can produce orthostatic hypotension and syncope. Although a recent study of nursing home residents suggests that long-term use of cardiovascular medications has no significant effect on orthostatic or postprandial blood pressure,[68] caution must still be exercised in selected elderly patients who may be more susceptible to adverse drug effects because of autonomic dysfunction or impairments in renal or hepatic clearance of hypotensive medications. Many over-the-counter cold or antimotility bowel medications have anticholinergic side effects that can induce tachyarrhythmias and syncope. Ophthalmic β-blockers have been implicated in bradyarrhythmias and cardiac conduction blocks. Medications therefore need to be reviewed diligently in the elderly patient with syncope.

Syncope associated with exercise is usually secondary to left or right ventricular outflow tract obstruction from aortic stenosis, hypertrophic cardiomyopathy, pulmonary hypertension, or pulmonary embolus. Patients who experience prodromal nausea, dizziness, or diaphoresis may have vasovagal syncope. Sudden onset of syncope without warning is usually associated with arrhythmias or conduction blocks. Strokes and seizure activity usually have accompanying neurological signs and symptoms. Since approximately 6% of myocardial infarctions present as syncope, the history should also elicit risk factors and symptoms of coronary artery disease.

Physical Examination

A detailed physical examination should include blood pressure and pulse measurements in the supine position, then after 1 minute of standing, and after 3 minutes of standing. Postural hypotension is frequently asymptomatic in the elderly, but a drop in systolic blood pressure of more than 20 mm Hg should be regarded as a potentially dangerous finding that may predispose to syncope. If postprandial hypotension is suspected, blood pressure and pulse should be measured before a meal as well as 30 minutes and 60 minutes after the meal. The cardiovascular examination should include auscultation of the heart for murmurs of aortic stenosis, hypertrophic cardiomyopathy, mitral stenosis, and regurgitation.

There are differences in the examination of the geriatric patient that are helpful to remember. The carotid upstroke may not be reduced in aortic stenosis because of stiffening of the vessel wall and consequent rapid rate of rise of the upstroke. The murmur of aortic stenosis may be displaced and better heard at the apex rather than the base of the heart. As the aortic valve becomes calcified, the intensity of the aortic component of the second heart sound diminishes. The gap between the aortic and the pulmonary component of the second heart sound shortens with increasing severity of aortic stenosis until A2 may follow P2; this is called paradoxical splitting. The systolic murmur of hypertrophic cardiomyopathy may be difficult to differentiate from that of aortic stenosis or mitral regurgitation. Therefore, to adequately evaluate a murmur, echocardiography may be required. The salient features that distinguish hypertrophic obstructive cardiomyopathy from other causes of systolic murmurs are a decrease in the intensity of the murmur with squatting and an increase in the murmur with standing and the performance of the Valsalva maneuver. The intensity of the murmur is directly proportional to the gradient of the blood flow from the left ventricle to the subaortic region.

Autonomic dysfunction can be assessed by simple tests of heart rate responses to deep breathing and Valsalva.[28] Deep breathing is done with simultaneous recording of the ECG. The patient is asked to take slow deep breaths with 5 seconds for inspiration and 5 seconds for expiration, for a total of 3 minutes. The ratio of the R-R interval during expiration to the R-R interval during inspiration in the elderly should be >1.15.[28] This test provides an estimate of the integrity of the efferent vagal neural pathway to the heart.

The Valsalva maneuver tests heart rate responses to the changes in blood pressure that occur with straining maneuvers. The patient is asked to strain as if moving their bowels without holding their breath for 10 seconds. Another method is to blow into a tube attached to a mercury sphygmomanometer to maintain a pressure of 30 mm Hg for 10 seconds. The ratio of the longest R-R interval after the release of the Valsalva to the shortest R-R interval during the procedure should be >1.2.[26] This ratio indicates normal vagal withdrawal in response to a decrease in cardiac output during straining, and vagal activation due to the blood pressure overshoot following release of the Valsalva.

Carotid sinus massage should be done under ECG monitoring in patients who have no evidence of cerebrovascular disease, carotid bruits, cardiac conduction disease, or a recent myocardial infarction. One carotid sinus is massaged for 5 seconds, and the blood pressure is measured immediately before and after the procedure. If there is no response, massage should be repeated on the other side. Three types of responses may be produced: a reduction in heart rate, a drop in blood pressure, or both. Carotid sinus syndrome is diagnosed if there is a sinus pause of more than 3 seconds, a drop in systolic blood pressure of more than 50 mm Hg (or 30 mm Hg in the presence of symptoms), or occurrence of both responses simultaneously.

Tilt testing is occasionally helpful[96–98] to detect neurocardiogenic syncope and orthostatic hypotension, and it can also be used to evaluate the effectiveness of treatment for these conditions. Although there is no standard protocol for tilt, an angle of 60° for 45 minutes has been found to be useful for eliciting symptoms. Shorter duration of tilt may give false-negative results. If the tilt test is negative, isoproterenol is sometimes used to provoke neurally mediated syncope by mimicking the intense sympathetic response that precedes loss of consciousness. This is generally avoided in the elderly because it may produce myocardial ischemia.

Some studies show that vasovagal syncope and presyncope in response to tilt is less common in old age.[45] However, a number of recent studies suggest that neurocardiogenic syncope is underrecognized in elderly individuals,[99] and therefore recommend tilt table testing for diagnosis. However, 10% to 30% of healthy subjects without a history of syncope can have a positive test. Hence, a positive test does not necessarily mean that a vasovagal reaction was the cause of the patient's syncopal event.

Echocardiographic evaluation and Holter monitoring are recommended in patients with suspected cardiac causes of syncope. It is important for heart rate to be monitored during activities similar to those that were associated with syncope, and not only during bed rest in the hospital. Loop recorders may be used in patients with frequent episodes of syncope, but they require activation at the time of symptoms, which might not be possible for elderly patients with impaired cognition. Finally, as discussed above, electrophysiological studies may be used in the diagnosis of unexplained syncope in the elderly. Kapoor et al[74] studied 400 patients with syncope who underwent electrophysiological studies; electrophysiological testing was diagnostic in 1% of younger patients and in 2% of elderly patients. The role of electrophysiological studies for the diagnosis and management of syncope in the elderly is controversial. Wagshal et al[100] performed electrophysiological studies on 45 octogenarians, 53% of whom had syncopal episodes; in this group, electrophysiological studies were negative in 75% of patients, however 8% of the patients had induced ventricular tachycardia and 17% had conduction abnormalities that required pacemaker implantation. The overall incidence of complications was between 2% and 3%, and not significantly different from other age groups.

Electrophysiological studies are of low yield in patients without organic heart disease. Patients with coronary or structural heart disease with an ejection fraction <40%, an abnormal resting ECG, and a history of injury caused by syncope have more than a 95% chance of significant electrophysiological abnormalities.[101] However, unless symptoms of near syncope or syncope are reproduced, it is difficult to determine if the abnormalities on electrophysiological testing are the cause of syncope. The greatest value of electrophysiological testing lies in the management of ventricular tachycardia and fibrillation, in determining the efficacy of antiarrhythmic therapy, and in the placement of pacemakers. In very elderly patients where mortality is not an issue, electrophysiological testing may not be necessary for the work-up of syncope. Detailed discussion of the role of electrophysiological studies in syncope is covered in other chapters. A suggested algorithm for the evaluation of the syncopal elderly patient is shown in Figure 1.

Treatment

The management of elderly patients with syncope requires an understanding of their vulnerability to hypotension due to age- and disease-

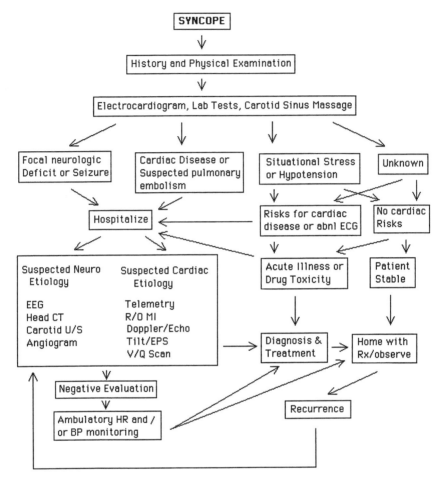

Figure 1. A suggested algotrithm for the evaluation of syncope in the elderly patient.

related physiological changes that impair compensation for hypotensive stress. Patients should be educated about preventive measures. For example, elderly patients should be advised to avoid dehydration, prolonged inactivity, or bed rest after an illness. Waist-high support stockings can be worn, or low-dose fludrocortisone (0.1 mg to 1 mg) can be prescribed for hypotensive syndromes, provided there is careful monitoring for hypertension, congestive heart failure, and hypokalemia. Patients with postprandial hypotension should take a brief walk or rest in the supine position after a meal. Large carbohydrate meals and alcoholic drinks should be avoided. Antihypertensives should not be given to coincide with meals, as they may exacerbate postprandial hypotension. As a general rule, the number of

_____ Table 1 _____

General Principals of Treatment for the Elderly Patient With Syncope

1. *Nonpharmacological Treatment*

   Avoid hypotensive stresses

   a. prolonged standing or sitting; particularly after meals
   b. nitrates and vasodilators
   c. diuretics during acute illnesses
   d. excessive heat
   e. large meals with alcohol

   Maximize venous returns

   a. exercise
   b. support hose
   c. volume—if no history of hypertension or congestive heart failure
   d. avoid sudden assumption of upright position, straining maneuvers (eg, at defecation)

   Driving precautions

   Advise not to drive if frequent syncopal episodes. Driving-free period postsyncope until evaluation of syncope is completed and appropriate treatment/precautions prescribed.

2. *Pharmacological Treatment*

   Adjust medication doses for altered pharmacokinetics

   a. decreased hepatic oxidation, eg, quinidine, procainamide, lidocaine amiodarone
   b. decreased renal clearance, eg, digoxin, procainamide

   Altered pharmacodynamics

   a. increased β-blocker effect
   b. increased confusion in response to drugs

   Monitor drug interactions

   a. exacerbation of hypoglycemia, enhanced effect of sulfonylurea in combination with alcohol, high dose salicylates, phenylbutazone, sulphonamides, warfarin
   b. exacerbation of orthostatic hypotension
      1. β-blockers with negative chronotropic drugs such as digoxin, diltiazem, verapamil, and negative ionotropes as nifedipine, which can cause congestive heart failure
      2. nitrates with directly acting vasodilators as prazosin and other potent antihypertensives
      3. tricyclics and trazodone with antihypertensives cause hypotension

Medications Useful for Autonomic Failure

1. Mineralocorticoid, eg, florinef (0.1–1.0 mg/day)
   Increased salt and water retention
   Useful in orthostatic hypotension

continues

_____ Table 1   Continued _____

General Principals of Treatment for the Elderly Patient With Syncope

2. β-Blockers/calcium channel blockers (propanolol, atenolol, disopyramide)
   Counteract sympathetic stimulation—useful in vasovagal syncope
   β-Blockers also prevent vasodilation in orthostasis
3. Prostaglandin synthetase inhibitors, eg, indomethacin—counteract vasodilation
   Caution in elderly subjects—GI and renal side-effects
4. Serotonin reuptake inhibitors
   —Fluoxetine
   downregulation of postsynaptic serontonin receptors used in vasovagal/
   neurocardiogenic
5. Gut peptide release inhibitor
   Octreotide (50 mg SQ 30 minutes before each meal) vasoconstrictor
   In severe orthostatic/postprandial hypotension
   Caution—diarrhea
6. Adenosine receptor blocker
   —Caffeine
   2 cups of coffee (250 mg) before a meal
7. Alpha agonists
   eg, midodrine (2.5–10 mg TID po), phenylephrine (60 mg BID, QID) in severe
   orthostatic hypotension
8. Dopamine agonist
   eg, DOPS—dihydroxphenylserine 25 mg po TID titrated to blood pressure
   In isolated dopamine β—orthostatic hypotension deficiency with orthostasis
9. Erythropoietin 25–75 U/kg three times a week SQ/IV
   Increases hematocrit and blood pressure
   Useful in autonomic failure with anemia

TID = three times a day; BID = twice daily; QID = four times a day; po = by mouth (*per os*);
SQ/IV = subcutaneous/intravenous.

medications should be minimized to avoid additive side effects. Venodilators such as nitrates should be avoided if possible in patients with diastolic dysfunction and cardiac outflow tract obstruction, as they can precipitate syncope.

Structural heart disease is generally amenable to surgical treatment, even in the very elderly. Syncope associated with aortic stenosis may be the harbinger of sudden death, and it requires urgent attention. The operative mortality of aortic valve surgery in elderly patients over the age of 80 has been shown to be <6% in one series.[102] However mortality is much higher (24% to 35%) if coronary artery bypass graft (CABG) or mitral valve surgery is performed.[102] Percutaneous balloon dilatation of the aortic valve has a high restenosis rate, but it may significantly improve the quality of life in patients who are at high risk for major operative procedures.[103]

Age is not a contraindication to pacemaker therapy. VVI pacing should generally be reserved for chronic atrial fibrillation; in every other case in which the atria are functioning, an A-V sequential or DDD mode is preferable in order to preserve the atrial contrution to cardiac output. VVI pacing in the elderly can cause retrograde conduction through the AV node. This can produce atrial contraction during ventricular systole, resulting in presyncope or syncope. The constellation of signs and symptoms associated with asynchronous atrioventricular contraction with VVI pacing is termed the "pacemaker syndrome." It may vary from simple fatigue to facial edema, dyspnea, chest pain, palpitations, and syncope. There may be associated cannon "A" waves in the neck and retrograde P waves on ECG. Treatment of the pacemaker syndrome involves conversion to a more physiological mode of pacing.

The elderly have a narrower margin for drug toxicity than do younger individuals, primarily because of their reduced renal and hepatic clearance of drugs. Drugs such as lidocaine, procainamide, quinidine, and digoxin may accumulate to toxic levels at usual doses. As with all medications in the elderly, the axiom should be "start low and go slow," and the first dose of any vasodilator should be given in the supine position with blood pressure monitoring, if possible.

A detailed account of treatment for specific causes of syncope is covered in other chapters. General and specific modalities for treatment of syncope in the elderly are described in Table 1.

References

1. Savage DD, Corwin L, McGee DL, et al. Epidemiological features of isolated syncope: The Framingham Study. *Stroke* 1985;16(4):626–629.
2. Kapoor WN. Evaluation of syncope in the elderly. *J Am Geriatr Soc* 1987;35:826–828.
3. Day SC, Cook EF, Funkenstein H, et al. Evaluation and outcome of emergency room patients with transient loss of consciousness. *Am J Med* 1982;73:15–23.
4. Doherty JU, Pembrook-Rogers D, Grogan EW, et al. Electrophysiologic evaluation and follow-up characteristics of patients with recurrent unexplained syncope and pre-syncope. *Am J Cardiol* 1985;55:703–708.
5. Lipsitz LA. Syncope in the elderly patient. *Hosp Pract* 1986;21:33–44.
6. Lipsitz L, Wei JY, Rowe JW. Syncope in an elderly, institutionalized population: Prevalence, incidence, and associated risk. *Q J Med* 1985;55:45–54.
7. Strandgraard S. Autoregulation of cerebral flow in hypertensive patients: The modifying influence of prolonged antihypertensive treatment on the tolerance to acute, drug induced hypotension. *Circulation* 1976;53:720–727.
8. Strandgraard S, Olesen J, Skinhoj E, et al. Autoregulation of brain circulation in severe arterial hypertension. *Br Med J* 1973;1:507–510.
9. Wollner L, McCarthy ST, Soper NDW, et al. Failure of cerebral autoregulation as a cause of brain dysfunction in the elderly. *Br Med J* 1979;1:1117–1118.
10. Mayhan WG, Faraci FM, Baumbach GL, et al. Effects of aging on responses of cerebral arterioles. *Am J Physiol* 1990;27:H1138–H1143.
11. Grubb BP, Gerard G. Cerebral vasoconstriction during head-upright tilt-induced vasovagal syncope. *Circulation* 1991;84:1157–1164.

12. Taddei S, Virdia A, Mattei P, et al. Aging and endothelial function in normotensive subjects and patients with essential hypertension. *Circulation* 1995;91:1981–1987.

13. Krajewski A, Freeman R, Ruthazer R, et al. Transcranial Doppler assessment of the cerebral circulation during postprandial hypotension in the elderly. *J Am Geriatr Soc* 1993;141:19–24.

14. Linares OA, Halter JB. Sympathochromaffin system activity in the elderly. *J Am Geriatr Soc* 1987;35:448–453.

15. Morrow LA, Linares OA, Hill TJ, et al. Age differences in plasma clearance mechanisms for epinephrine and norepinephrine in humans. *J Clin Endocrinol Metab* 1987;65:508–511.

16. Supiano MA, Linares OA, Smith MJ, et al. Age related difference in norepinephrine kinetics: Effect of posture and sodium-restricted diet. *Am J Physiol* 1990;259:E422–E431.

17. Rowe JW, Troen BR. Sympathetic nervous system and aging in man. *Endocr Rev* 1980;1:167–179.

18. Hogikyan RV, Supiano MA. Arterial a-adrenergic responsiveness is decreased and SNS activity is increased in older humans. *Am J Physiol* 1994;266:E717–E724.

19. Pan HYM, Blaschke TF. Decline in beta-adrenergic receptor-mediated vascular relaxation with aging in man. *J Pharm Exptl Therap* 1986;239:802–807.

20. Brodde OE, Zerkowski HR, Schranz D, et al. Age-dependent changes in the beta-adrenoceptor G-protein adenyl cyclase system in human right atrium. *J Cardiovasc Pharmacol* 1995;26(1):20–26.

21. Ford GA, Hoffman BB, Vestal RE, et al. Age related changes in adenosine and beta-adrenoceptor responsiveness of vascular smooth muscle in man. *Br J Clin Pharmacol* 1992;33:83–87.

22. Abrass IB, Davis JL, Scarpace PJ, et al. Isoproterenol responsiveness and myocardioal β-adrenergic receptors in young and old rats. *J Gerontol* 1982;37:156–160.

23. Abrass IB, Scarpace PJ. Human lymphocte beta-adrenergic receptors are unaltered with age. *J Gerontol* 1981;36:298–301.

24. Waddington JL, MacCullough MJ, Sambrooks JE, et al. Resting heart rate variability in man declines with age. *Experientia* 1979;35:1197–1198.

25. Jennings JR, Mack ME. Does aging differentially reduce heart rate variability related to respiration? *Exp Aging Res* 1984;10:19–23.

26. Gautschy B, Weidmann P. Autonomic function tests as related to age and gender in normal man. *Klin Wochenschr* 1986;64:499–505.

27. O'Brien IAD, O'Hare P, Corrall RJM, et al. Heart rate variability in healthy subjects: Effects of age and derivation of normal ranges for tests of autonomic function. *Br Heart J* 1986;55:348-354.

28. Maddens ME, Lipsitz LA, Wei JY, et al. Impaired heart rate responses to cough and deep breathing in elderly patients with unexplained syncope. *Am J Cardiol* 1987;60:1368–1372.

29. Wei JY, Rowe JW, Kestenbaum AD, et al. Post-cough heart rate response: Influence of age, sex, and basal blood pressure. *Am J Physiol* 1983;245:R18–R24.

30. Shimada K, Kitazumi T, Ogura H, et al. Differences in age-independent effects on blood pressure on baroreflex sensitivity between normal and hypertensive subjects. *Clin Sci* 1986;70:489-494.

31. Gribbin B, Pickering TG, Sleight P, et al. Effect of age and high blood pressure on baroreflex sensitivity in man. *Circ Res* 1971;29:424–431.

32. Smith JJ, Hughes CV, Ptacin MJ, et al. The effect of age on hemodynamic response to graded postural stress in normal men. *J Gerontol* 1987;42:406–411.

33. Minaker KL, Menielly GS, Young JB, et al. Blood pressure, pulse, and neuro-humoral responses to nitroprusside-induced hypotension in normative aging in men. *J Gerontol Med Sci* 1991;46:M151–M154.

34. Taylor JA, Hand GA. Sympathoadrenalcirculatory regulation of arterial pressure during orthostatic stress in young and older men. *Am J Physiol* 1992; 263:R1147–R1155.

35. Pomeranz B, Macaulay RJB, Caudill MA, et al. Assessment of autonomic function in humans by heart rate spectral analaysis. *Am J Physiol* 1985;248:H151–H153.

36. Billman GE, Dujardin JP. Dynamic changes in cardiac vagal tone as measured by time-series analysis. *Am J Physiol* 1990;258:H869–H902.

37. Simpson DM, Wicks R. Spectral analysis of heart rate indicates reduced baroreceptor mediated heart rate variability in elderly persons. *J Gerontol* 1988; 43(1):M21–M24.

38. Lipsitz LA, Mietus J, Moody GB, et al. Spectral characteristics of heart rate variability before and during postural tilt: Relations to aging and risk of syncope. *Circulation* 1990;81(6):1803–1818.

39. Froehlich JP, Lakatta EG, Beard E, et al. Studies of sarcoplasmic reticulum function and contraction duration in young and aged rat myocardium. *J Mol Cell Cardiol* 1978;10:427–438.

40. Orchard CH, Lakatta EG. Intracellular calcium transients and developed tensions in rat heart muscle: A mechanism for the negative interval-strength relationship. *J Gen Physiol* 1985;86:637–651.

41. Wei JY, Spurgeon HA, Lakatta EG, et al. Exitation-contraction in rat myocardium: Alterations in adult aging. *Am J Physiol* 1984;246:H784–H791.

42. Bryg RJ, Williams GA, Labovitz AJ. Effect of aging on left ventricular diastolic filling in normal subjects. *Am J Cardiol* 1987;59:971–974.

43. Miyatake K, Okamoto M, Kinoshita N, et al. Augmentation of atrial contribution to left ventricular inflow with aging as assessed by intracardiac doppler flowmetry. *Am J Cardiol* 1984;53:586–589.

44. Lipsitz LA, Bui M, Stiebeling M, et al. Forearm blood flow response to posture change in the very old: Non-invasive measurement by venous occlusin plethysmography. *J Am Geriatr Soc* 1991;39:53–59.

45. Lipsitz LA, Marks ER, Koestner JS, et al. Reduced susceptibility to syncope during postural tilt in old age: Is beta-blockade protective? *Arch Intern Med* 1989;149:2709–2712.

46. Miyauchi T, Yanagisawa M, Iida K, et al. Age - and sex-related variation of plasma endothelin-1 in normal and hypertensive subjects. *Am Heart J* 1992; 123:1092–1094.

47. Kaufman H, Oribe E, Oliver JA. Plasma endothelin during upright tilt: Relevance for orthostatic hypotension? *Lancet* 1991;338:1542–1545.

48. Stewart DJ, Cernacek P, Costello KB, et al. Elevated endothelin-1 in heart failure and loss of normal response to postural change. *Circulation* 1992; 85:510–517.

49. Haller BG, Zust H, Shaw S, et al. Effects of posture and ageing on circulating atrial natriuretic peptide levels in man. *J Hypertens* 1987;5:551–556.

50. Epstein M, Hollenberg NK. Age as a determinant of renal sodium conservation in normal man. *J Lab Clin Med* 1976;87:411–417.

51. Phillips PA, Phil D, Rolls BJ, et al. Reduced thirst after water deprivation in healthy elderly men. *N Engl J Med* 1984;311(12):753-759.

52. Kannel WE. Hypertension and aging. In: Finch CE, Schneider EL (ed)s: *Handbook of the Biology of Aging*. New York: Van Nostrand Reinhold; 1985;859–863.

53. Harris T, Lipsitz LA, Kleinman JC, et al. Postural change in blood pressure associated with age and systolic blood pressure: The national health and nutrition examination survey II. *J Gerontol* 1991;46:M159–M163.
54. Applegate WB, David BR, Black HR, et al. Prevalence of postural hypotension at baseline in the systolic hypertension in the elderly program (SHEP) cohort. *J Am Geriatr Soc* 1991;39:1057–1064.
55. Valvanne J, Sorva A, Erkinjuntti T, et al. The occurrence of postural hypotension in age cohorts of 75, 80, and 85 years: A population study. *Arch Gerontol Geriatr* 1991;2:421–424.
56. Lipsitz LA, Ryan SM, Parker JA, et al. Hemodynamic and autonomic nervous system responses to mixed meal ingestion in healthy young and old subjects, and dysautonomic patients with postprandial hypotension. *Circulation* 1993;87:391–400.
57. Barry DI. Cerebral blood flow in hypertension. *J Cardiovasc Pharmacol* 1985; 7:594–598.
58. Caird FL, Andrews GR, Kennedy RD, et al. Effect of posture on blood pressure in the elderly. *Br Heart J* 1973;35:527–530.
59. Harris T, Kleinman J, Lipsitz LA, et al. Is age or level of systolic blood pressure related to positional blood pressure change? *Gerontologist* 1986;26:59A.
60. Tinetti ME, Williams TF, Mayewski R. Fall risk index for elderly patients based on number of chronic disabilities. *Am J Med* 1986;80:429–434.
61. Lipsitz LA, Pluchino FC, Wei JY, et al. Syncope in institutionalized elderly: The impact of multiple pathological conditions and situational stress. *J Chron Dis* 1986;39:619–630.
62. Liu BA, Topper AK, Reeves RA, et al. Falls among older people: Relationship to medication use and orthostatic hypotension. *J Am Geriatr Soc* 1995;43:1141–1145.
63. Lipsitz LA, Storch HA, Minaker KL, et al. Intraindividual variability in postural blood pressure in the elderly. *Clin Sci* 1985;69:337–341.
64. Lipsitz LA, Fullerton KJ. Postprandial blood pressure reduction in healthy elderly. *J Am Geriatr Soc* 1986;34:267–270.
65. Vaitkevicius PV, Esserwein DM, Maynard AK, et al. Frequency and importance of postprandial blood pressure reduction in elderly nursing-home patients. *Ann Intern Med* 1991;115:865–870.
66. Robertson D, Wade D, Robertson RM. Postprandial alterations in cardiovascular hemodynamics in autonomic dysfunctional states. *Am J Cardiol* 1981; 48:1048–1052.
67. Micieli G, Martignoni E, Cavallini A, et al. Postprandial and orthostatic hypotension in Parkinson's disease. *Neurology* 1987;37:386–393.
68. Jansen RWMM, Kelley-Gagnon MM, Lipsitz LA. Intraindividual reproducibility of postprandial and orthostatic blood pressure changes in elderly nursing home patients: Relationship with chronic use of cardiovascular medications. *J Am Geriatr Soc* 1996 (in press).
69. Aronow WS, Ahn C. Postprandial hypotension in 499 elderly persons in a long-term health care facility. *Am J Geriatr Soc* 1994;42:930–932.
70. Jansen RWMM, Connelly CM, Kelley-Gagnon MM, et al. Postprandial hypotension in elderly patients with unexplained syncope. *Arch Intern Med* 1995; 155:945–952.
71. Jansen RWMM, Peeters TL, Lenders JWM, et al. Somatostatin analog octreotide (SMS 201–995) prevents the decrease in blood pressure after oral glucose loading in the elderly. *J Clin Endocrinol Metab* 1989;68:752-756.
72. Jansen RWMM, de Meijer PHEM, van Lier HJJ, et al. Influence of octreotide (SMS 201–995) and insulin administration on the course of blood pressure

after an oral glucose load in hypertensive elderly subjects. *J Am Geriatr Soc* 1989;37:1135–1139.

73. Hoeldtke RD. Postprandial hypotension. In: Low PA (ed): *Clinical Autonomic Disorders. Evaluation and Management.* Boston: Little, Brown and Co; 1993;701–711.

74. Kapoor W, Snustad D, Peterson J, et al. Syncope in the elderly. *Am J Med* 1986;80:419–428.

75. Lindroos K, Kupari M, Heikkila J, et al. Prevalence of aortic valve abnormalities in the elderly: An echocardiographic study of a random population. *J Am Coll Cardiol* 1993;21:1220–1225.

76. Schwartz LS, Goldfisher J, Sprague GJ, et al. Syncope and sudden death in aortic stenosis. *Am J Cardiol* 1969;23:647–658.

77. Selzer A. Changing aspects of the natural history of aortic valvular stenosis. *N Engl J Med* 1987;317:91–98.

78. Banning AP, Hall RJC. In: Kenny RA (ed): *Syncope in the Older Patient. Causes, Investigation and Consequences of Syncope and Falls.* Chapman & Hall Medical; 1996;201–218.

79. Petrin TJ, Tavel ME. Idiopathic hypertrophic subaortic stenosis as observed in a large community hospital: Relation to age and history of hypertension. *J Am Geriatr Soc* 1979;27:43–46.

80. Impallomemi MG, Arnot RN, Alexander MS. Incidence of pulmonary embolism in elderly patients newly admitted to an acute geriatric unit: A prospective study. *Clin Nucl Med* 1990;15:84–87.

81. Bass EB, Curtiss EI, Arena VC, et al. The duration of Holter monitoring in patients with syncope. Is 24 hours enough? *Arch Intern Med* 1990;150:1073–1078.

82. McIntosh S, de Costa D, Kenney RA. Benefits of an integrated approach to the investigation of dizziness, falls and syncope in elderly patients referred to a syncope clinic. *Age Ageing* 1993;22:53–58.

83. Mahony DO. Pathophysiology of carotid sinus hypersensitivity in elderly patients. *Lancet* 1995;346:950–952.

84. Morely CA, Sutton R. Carotid sinus syncope. *Int J Cardiol* 1984;6:287–293.

85. McIntosh SJ, Lawson J, Kenny RA, et al. Heart rate and blood pressure responses to carotid sinus massage in healthy elderly subjects. *Age Ageing* 1994; 23:57-61.

86. Wenthick JRM, Jansen RWMM, Hoefnagels WHL. The influence of age on the response of blood pressure and heart rate to carotid sinus massage in healthy volunteers. *Cardiology Elderly* 1993;1:453–459.

87. Brown KA, Maloney JA, Smith HC, et al. Carotid sinus reilex in patients undergoing coronary angiography: Relationship of degree and location of coronary artery disease to response to carotid sinus massage. *Circulation* 1980; 62:697–703.

88. Quest JA, Gillis RA. Effect of digitalis on carotid sinus baroreceptor activity. *Circ Res* 1974;35:247–255.

89. Reyes AJ. Propanolol and the hyperactive carotid sinus reflex syndrome. *Br Med J* 1973;2:662.

90. Bauerfiend X, Hall D, Denes P, et al. Carotid sinus hypersensitivity with alpha methyldopa. *Ann Intern Med* 1978;88:214–215.

91. Sra J, Jazayeri M, Avitall B, et al. Sequential catecholamine changes during upright tilt: Possible hormonal mechanisms responsible for pathogenesis of neurocardiogenic syncope. *J Am Coll Cardiol* 1991;17:216A.

92. Shalev Y, Gal R, Tchou P, et al. Echocardiographic demonstration of decreased left ventricular dimensions and vigorous myocardial contraction during syncope induced by head upright tilt. *J Am Coll Cardiol* 1991;18:746–751.

93. Grubb BP, Wolfe D, Samoil D, et al. Usefulness of floxetine hydrochloride for prevention of resistant upright tilt induced syncope. *Pacing Clin Electrophysiol* 1993;16:458–464.
94. Abboud FM, Aylward PE, Floras JS, et al. Sensitization of aortic and cardiac baroreceptors by arginine vasopressin in mammals. *J Physiol (Lond)* 1986; 377:251–265.
95. Fitzpatrick A, Banner N, Cheng A, et al. Vasovagal reactions may occur after orthotopic heart transplantation. *J Am Coll Cardiol* 1993;21:1132–1137.
96. Abi-Samra F, Malony JD, Fouad-Tarazi FM, et al. The usefulness of head-up tilt testing and hemodynamic investigations in the work up of syncope of unknown origin. *Pacing Clin Electrophysiol* 1988;11:1202–1212.
97. Grubb BP, Kosinski D, Samoil D, et al. Recurrent unexplained syncope: The role of head upright tilt table testing. *Heart Lung* 1993;22(6):502–508.
98. Hargreaves AD, Hag EO, Boon AN. Head-up tilt testing: The balance of evidence. *Br Heart J* 1994;72:216–217.
99. Grubb BP, Wolfe D, Samoil D, et al. Recurrent unexplained syncope in the elderly: The use of head-upright tilt table testing in evaluation and management. *J Am Geriatr Soc* 1992;40:1123–1128.
100. Wagshal AB, Scchuger CD, Habbal B, et al. Invasive electrophysiologic evaluation in octogenarians: Is age a limiting factor? *Am Heart J* 1993;126:1142–1146.
101. Krol RB, Morady F, Flacker GC, et al. Electrophysiologic testing in patients with unexplained syncope: Clinical and noninvasive predictors of outcome. *J Am Coll Cardiol* 1987;10:358–363.
102. Elayada MA, Hall RJ, Reul RM, et al. Aortic valve replacement in patients 80 years and older: Operative risks and long term results. *Circulation* 1993; 88(2):11–16.
103. Bernard Y, Etievent J, Mourand JL, et al. Long term results of percutaneous aortic valvuloplasty compared with aortic valve replacement in patients more than 75 years old. *J Am Coll Cardiol* 1992;20:796–801.

Recurrent Unexplained Syncope:

When All Else Fails

Andrew D. Krahn, MD, George J. Klein, MD,
and Raymond Yee, MD

Introduction

The etiology of recurrent syncope is often difficult to determine if the diagnosis is not evident from initial clinical and laboratory investigations.[1–4] The major obstacles to diagnosis are the periodic and unpredictable frequency of events and the high spontaneous remission rate.[5,6] Blood pressure and heart rate monitoring during spontaneous syncope constitute the "gold standard" for diagnosis of cardiovascular causes of syncope. This is usually an unattainable standard, although recent advances in long-term monitoring techniques have added a powerful tool to the diagnostic armamentarium. Despite these advances, clinicians must often rely on abnormal laboratory results to make inferential decisions regarding the etiology and treatment of this disorder.

Electrophysiological Testing

It is generally accepted that electrophysiological testing is the final arbitrator when noninvasive testing is negative or inconclusive.[1-2,7-9] This arises from the assumption that electrophysiological testing has a high sensitivity and specificity for determination of the cause of syncope. In the

From Grubb BP, Olshansky B (eds.). *Syncope: Mechanisms and Management.* Armonk, NY: Futura Publishing Co., Inc.; © 1998.

absence of a gold standard, this argument may be difficult to refute. However, it is clear that electrophysiological testing has a low sensitivity in patients with documented bradyarrhythmias associated with syncope.[10,11] Of eight patients with documented symptomatic sinus node dysfunction, electrophysiological testing of sinus node function was abnormal in only three.[10] In the same series, electrophysiological testing showed that only 2 of 13 patients with symptomatic atrioventricular block had abnormalities that suggested the correct diagnosis.

Electrophysiological testing is of low yield in patients without significant structural heart disease. This yield ranges from 16% to 64%,[9,12] although only 30% of patients in the latter sample had definite abnormalities. Doherty et al[13] identified absence of structural heart disease as an independent predictor of a negative electrophysiological test in recurrent syncope. Many of the abnormalities detected in these series do not reproduce the patient's spontaneous symptoms, and the relationship between the abnormality and the true cause of syncope remains unclear. This is born out by the 5% to 32% risk of recurrent syncope after a positive electrophysiological test, where therapy is directed at the abnormality that was detected at electrophysiological testing.[9,12-20]

Finally, electrophysiological testing is negative in 14% to 70% of the patients in major studies.[9,12-20] The wide variation in frequency of negative testing is largely explained by the differing prevalence of structural heart disease in each series. Table 1 summarizes the outcome of patients with negative electrophysiological testing. The overall recurrence risk for syncope is 11% per year after a negative study. In one series, 26% of patients

_____ **Table 1** _____

Recurrence Risk For Syncope After Negative Electrophysiological Testing

Author	N	% Negative EP	Recurrence (%)	Follow-up (months)	Incidence (% recurrence/ year)
Denniss[9]	111	67	24	20	14
Teichman[12]	137	25	47	31	18
Doherty[13]	85	34	24	27	11
Olshansky[14]	97	61	20	26	9
Click[15]	110	14	18	30	7
Twidale[16]	90	52	21	39	7
Denes[17]	82	29	7	47	2
Muller[18]	134	70	19	22	10
Lacroix[19]	98	52	27	23	14
Bachinsky[20]	140	69	18	24*	9
Total	**1084**	**47**	**22**	**29**	**11**

* Median.

referred to an electrophysiology group for syncope had a negative tilt table test and a negative electrophysiological test.[2] These patients had a 26% syncope recurrence rate over 18 months of follow-up. Despite this significant ongoing morbidity, mortality in these patients has been low. Cardiovascular mortality has a mean incidence of 2.4% per year, with a median of 1.4% per year, based on the literature.[9,12-20] The population of patients with recurrent syncope despite negative noninvasive and electrophysiological testing are said to have syncope of unknown etiology. Many of these patients are unable to drive, and they may suffer serious injuries associated with recurrent syncope.

Loop Recorders

Several recent advances in long-term cardiac arrhythmia monitoring have shown great promise for the difficult population of patients with syncope of unknown origin. The cardiac loop recorder continuously records and stores an external single modified limb-lead electrogram with a 1- to 4-minute memory buffer. After spontaneous symptoms occur, the patient activates an event button that stores the previous 1 to 4 minutes of recorded information, which can then be downloaded and analyzed. The leads and recording device can be worn for weeks or even months at a time, although long-term compliance is a problem. Compliance can be improved by patient education and careful routine follow-up, and is enhanced when patients are required to have a definitive diagnosis and treatment before being permitted to drive or return to work. Two reports from Duke University that detail use of the cardiac loop recorder have been published.[21,22] Linzer et al[22] report the use of a patient-activated loop recorder in 57 patients with syncope and nondiagnostic findings on history, physical, and 24-hour ambulatory monitoring. Despite recurrence of symptoms in 32 of 57 patients, a diagnosis was obtained in only 14. Device malfunction, patient noncompliance, and inability to activate the recorder were the three factors responsible for the lack of diagnosis in the remaining 18. Similar results are reported by Brown et al.[23] This device appears to have its greatest role in highly motivated patients with frequent syncope where spontaneous symptoms are likely to recur within 2 to 4 weeks. Further development of data acquisition and storage capabilities are likely to reduce patient-related difficulties in appropriate activation of the device after spontaneous symptoms.

Implantable Syncope Monitor

We recently reported on the use of an implantable loop recorder in patients with syncope of unknown etiology.[11] This is a pacemaker-sized device with two sensing electrodes 32 mm (1.25 in) apart within its shell (Figure 1). It continuously records a single-lead electrocardiogram (Medtronic USA, Inc.). The electrocardiographic signal is stored in a circular buffer that is capable of retaining either one 15-minute or two 7.5-minute segments of recorded rhythm. With use of a magnet, the patient, family member, or friend "freezes" the device during or after a spontaneous syncopal episode, storing the preceding 7.5- or 15-minute segment, which is retrievable at a later date. The syncope monitor has a battery life of approximately 2 years. While the patient is under local anesthesia, the device is implanted in the left pectoral region in the subcutaneous fat. It is placed within the pocket and rotated through 360° to optimize the magnitude of the recorded R-wave electrogram, and fastened to the underlying tissue.

Figure 2 summarizes the results of use of the syncope monitor during 2 years of recruitment and subsequent follow-up. Twenty-four patients with a mean age of 58.8±17.1 years had the device implanted. There were 17 males (71%). All but one patient had recurrent unexplained syncope; 1 patient had syncope that resulted in a motor vehicle accident. The mean number of preceding syncopal episodes was 7.6±5.9 during the preceding

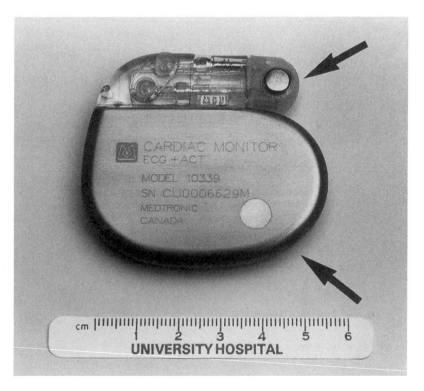

Figure 1. Photograph of an implantable syncope monitor. Arrows point to sensing electrodes.

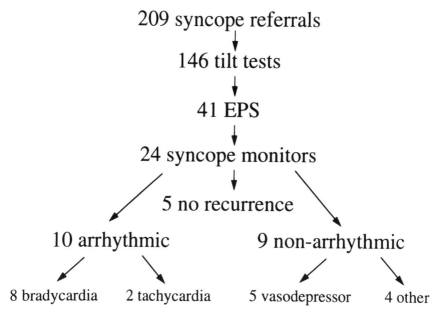

209 syncope referrals

146 tilt tests

41 EPS

24 syncope monitors

5 no recurrence

10 arrhythmic   **9 non-arrhythmic**

8 bradycardia   2 tachycardia   5 vasodepressor   4 other

Figure 2. Flow chart of patients referred to University Hospital for evaluation of recurrent syncope over a 2-year period. Twenty-four patients underwent syncope moniter implantation; 19 experienced recurrent syncope. EPS = electrophysiological studies. See text for details.

2 years. All patients underwent a clinical evaluation including ambulatory or in-hospital monitoring, and subsequently all had negative tilt and electrophysiological testing. Syncope recurred in 19 patients 4.6±3.8 months after device implantation. Syncope was arrhythmic in 10 patients (53%), with 8 of the 10 representing bradyarrhythmias. A representative rhythm strip frozen by a patient's spouse after an episode of syncope is shown in Figure 3. Syncope was nonarrhythmic in nine patients (47%). These patients underwent additional investigations tailored by clinical suspicion. Repeat tilt testing was performed in those patients whose history was compatible with vasodepressor syncope and whose rhythm strip showed mild slowing (rates 40 to 60 bpm) during spontaneous symptoms. Five of the nine patients had a final diagnosis of vasodepressor syncope with a positive repeat tilt test. It is possible that some of the bradycardic patients also had a cardioinhibitory form of neurally mediated syncope that was amenable to pacing. Of the remaining 4 patients, 1 had hypertrophic cardiomyopathy with sinus tachycardia during syncope with presumed obstructive symptoms that have resolved with β-blockade, 1 had psychogenic syncope that has resolved with counseling, and 2 are being investigated and followed by neurologists for possible atypical seizure disorder. The latter two patients

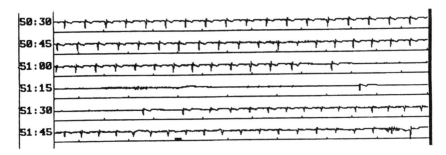

Figure 3. Syncope monitor rhythm strip in a patient during an episode of syncope. Note the 23-second period of asystole with a single junctional escape beat.

had sinus rhythm or sinus tachycardia during spontaneous syncope. Therapy specific to the underlying etiology has been implemented in all but the last two patients, with resolution of syncope during approximately 19.1 months of follow-up. The remaining five patients have not had a recurrence during 9.5±3.3 months of follow-up.

These data highlight the diverse etiology of syncope in this population. They also illustrate the limitations of conventional monitoring techniques. Only 3 of the 19 patients in this series had syncope within the first month after device implantation, a time window during which a conventional external loop recorder may have proven useful had it been complied with. The mean time for documentation of an arrhythmic etiology of syncope was 4.6 months. It is not surprising that the yield of symptom-rhythm correlation on routine ambulatory monitoring is very low. No patient in our series suffered significant morbidity or mortality as a result of recurrence of his or her syncope, consistent with the good prognosis seen in this population.

Cost Consideration

We analyzed the cost of investigations and treatment in the 24 patients receiving the syncope monitor in the 2 years prior to and after implantation of the device.[24] The cost of the device was arbitrarily set at $2000 (US dollars) for purpose of analysis, because due to their investigational nature, the devices were provided by the manufacturer at no cost. The cost of the investigations prior to implant was $12,175 per patient. Device implantation, follow-up, and explanation cost $7660 per patient. Since a diagnosis was obtained in most patients, we were able to calculate a mean cost of therapy of $4435 per patient (including pacing in eight patients). The subsequent cost of care fell dramatically to $605 per patient over the 2 years after therapy was initiated. The high cost of investigation of syncope and the apparent significant reduction in cost after a diagnosis was obtained with the syncope monitor led us to analyze the potential cost impact of the syncope monitor in patients with recurrent syncope.

A theoretical cohort of 100 patients with recurrent syncope undergoing a series of investigations was analyzed.[25] We created a typical diagnostic cascade in which patients were subjects to a series of investigations including Holter monitoring, echocardiography, head-up tilt testing, an external loop recorder, and electrophysiological testing. The diagnostic yield of each test was estimated from the published literature, and the test cost was based on median hospital and physician charges. The cost per diagnosis obtained ranged from $804 for the external loop recorder to $109,920 for electrophysiological testing in patients without structural heart disease. The syncope monitor had a cost per diagnosis of $7501.

Similar to the above-mentioned pilot study, use of the syncope monitor as a device of last resort after all previous investigations were negative resulted in an average cost per diagnosis of $4860, with a 96% yield. At the opposite extreme, use of the syncope monitor prior to all other investigations yielded a cost per diagnosis of $5926, with an 80% yield. Omission of echocardiography and electrophysiological testing in patients without structural heart disease further reduced the cost to $2851 per diagnosis without a significant fall in diagnostic yield (95%). These data are limited by their theoretical nature, but they highlight the potential for investigational tools such as the syncope monitor to be applied to this population in a cost-conscious manner.

Unfortunately, there were no clear baseline characteristics that would have predicted the etiology of syncope. For example, empirical pacing in those over age 60 would have resulted in inappropriate pacemaker implantation in 4 of the 10 patients who had recurrent syncope who were over 60, and it would have missed the 2 patients (out of 9) under age 60 who had a bradycardic etiology. Further development of implantable monitoring technology promises to involve much smaller devices, automatic rate detection parameters, and user-friendly data storage and retrieval systems, and perhaps it will eventually include monitoring of other physiological parameters such as blood pressure. As the device becomes smaller and requires a less invasive implantation procedure, it will likely prove useful at an earlier stage in the diagnostic work-up of patients with recurrent syncope. Use in larger patient populations is also likely to clarify clinical predictors of syncopal etiology in this difficult population.

When All Else Fails

Despite intensive investigations, some patients will continue to have recurrent syncope with associated morbidity. In order to lessen the severity of or even prevent attacks, patients should learn to recognize their prodrome and sit or lie down as quickly as possible to minimize injury during recurrences. Although patients may be hesitant to comply with this in public, recurrence of syncope will often draw more unwanted attention to the individual than will lying or sitting down to prevent injury. In patients who have a suspected vasomotor component to their syncope, adequate hydration (2 L/day) and regular meals with sufficient salt intake will minimize intravascular volume depletion. The patient's spouse or family member can be taught to monitor the radial or carotid pulse or to apply a rhythm transmission device to the patient's chest during symptoms. Patients without structural heart disease and their families should be assured that although a specific diagnosis has not been obtained, the prognosis is excellent. Finally, repeat tilt testing in those patients who are suspected to have neurally mediated syncope may be useful. In our own series, 5 of the 19 patients with recurrent syncope had a positive repeat tilt after being initially negative when this etiology was suspected from the history and nonspecific slowing on the rhythm strip. We used a 60° tilt for 30 minutes with isoproterenol during the last 15 minutes.[26] More aggressive tilt protocols may improve sensitivity while reducing the specificity. This may be an acceptable trade-off if the test is positive and if it reproduces the patient's symptom prodrome.

In the absence of a released long-term monitoring device such as the syncope monitor, empirical decisions based on a presumed etiology for syncope (a "therapeutic trial") may be considered. There is often significant pressure from the patient and family to arrive at a diagnosis, especially when recurrent physical injury or loss of occupation has occurred. In patients with "typical" Stokes-Adams attacks and failed attempts to document the presumed bradyarrhythmia, one may consider implantation of a permanent pacemaker. In a study of 104 patients with pacemaker implantation for syncope, Rattes et al[27] divided patients into those with syncope associated with documented bradycardia (Group 1), those with syncope and evidence to support a bradycardic etiology such as bradycardia without syncope during monitoring, bundle branch block, or first- or second-degree atrioventricular AV block (Group 2), and those with syncope and a clinical diagnosis of probable bradycardia without supportive evidence (Group 3). The 3-year recurrence of syncope was 6.3% and 7.3% in Groups 1 and 2 respectively, and 32% in Group 3 ($P<0.01$) (Figure 4). These data support the role of empirical pacing in patients with evidence to support a bradycardic etiology. Group 3 patients had experienced a mean of 4.6 syncopal episodes in the previous year before pacemaker implantation. Despite the absence of a control group, this provides the grounds for empirical pacing in selected patients with a typical history, but with no objective evidence to support bradycardia.

In patients with recurrent unexplained syncope and underlying structural heart disease, it is reasonable to be cautious and to consider that the underlying cause is a self-terminating ventricular arrhythmia. Electrophys-

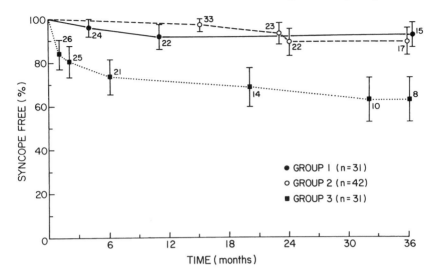

Figure 4. Cumulative proportion of patients free of syncope over time after pacemaker implantation. Group 1: syncope suspected to be bradycardic without supportive evidence. See text for discussion. Adapted from Reference 25.

iological testing is less likely to be positive in patients with dilated versus ischemic cardiomyopathy. There is concern that these patients in particular remain at high risk for lethal ventricular arrhythmias after a negative electrophysiological study, and that further delay in obtaining a diagnosis risks the chance of a fatal recurrence. Empirical therapy with antiarrhythmic drugs is a consideration, but it may provide less of a "safety net" in the event of ineffective therapy. It also does not address the possibility of a bradycardia etiology, and it may paradoxically aggravate it. Implantation of a cardioverter-defibrillator in this uncommon situation is appealing because it will effectively treat ventricular arrhythmias, pace bradyarrhythmias, and provide diagnostic information after a recurrent event. It is appreciated that "empirical" trials with pacemakers and implantable defibrillators are less than ideal as a strategy and that they represent a tactic of last resort.

Conclusions

Syncope of unknown etiology remains a challenging problem despite a large armamentarium of investigations available to the practicing cardiologist. Recent advances in external and implantable loop recorders demonstrate a diverse etiology for syncope once a diagnosis is established. These devices are powerful new tools that are useful for establishing or excluding a specific arrhythmic etiology in this patient population.

References

1. Kapoor WN, Hammill SC, Gersh BJ. Diagnosis and natural history of syncope and the role of electrophysiologic testing. *Am J Cardiol* 1989;63:730–734.
2. Sra JS, Anderson AJ, Sheikh SH, et al. Unexplained syncope evaluated by electrophysiologic studies and head-up tilt testing. *Ann Intern Med* 1991;114:1013–1019.
3. Morady F, Shen E, Schwartz A, et al. Long-term followup of patients with recurrent unexplained syncope evaluated by electrophysiologic testing. *J Am Coll Cardiol* 1983;2:1053–1059.
4. Kapoor WN, Karpf M, Weiand S, et al. A prospective evaluation and followup of patients with syncope. *N Engl J Med* 1983;309:197–204.
5. Manolis AS, Linzer M, Salem D, Estes NAM. Syncope: Current diagnostic evaluation and management. *Ann Int Med* 1990;112:850–863.
6. Kapoor WN. Evaluation and management of the patient with syncope. *JAMA* 1992;268:2553–2560.
7. Akhtar M, Shenasa M, Denker S, et al. Role of cardiac electrophysiologic studies in patients with unexplained syncope. *Pacing Clin Electrophysiol* 1983;6:192–201.
8. Sharma AD, Klein GJ, Milstein S. Diagnostic assessment of recurrent syncope. *Pacing Clin Electrophysiol* 1984;7:749–759.
9. Denniss AR, Ross DL, Richards DA, Uther JB. Electrophysiologic studies in patients with unexplained syncope. *Int J Cardiol* 1992;35:211–217.
10. Fjuimara O, Yee R, Klein GJ, et al. The diagnostic sensitivity of electrophysiologic testing in patients with syncope caused by transient bradycardia. *N Engl J Med* 1989;321:1703–1707.
11. Krahn AD, Klein GJ, Norris C, Yee R. The etiology of syncope in patients with negative tilt table and electrophysiologic testing. *Circulation* 1995;92(7):1819–1824.
12. Teichman SL, Felder SD, Matos JA, et al. The value of electrophysiologic studies in syncope of undetermined origin: Report of 150 cases. *Am Heart J* 1985;110:469–479.
13. Doherty JU, Pembrook-Rogers D, Grogan EW, et al. Electrophysiologic evaluation and followup characteristics of patients with recurrent unexplained syncope and presyncope. *Am J Cardiol* 1985;55:703–708.
14. Olshansky B, Mazuz M, Martins JB. Significance of inducible tachycardia in patients with syncope of unknown origin: A long-term followup. *J Am Coll Cardiol* 1985;5:216–223.
15. Click RL, Gersh BJ, Sugrue DD, et al. Role of invasive electrophysiologic testing in patients with symptomatic bundle branch block. *Am J Cardiol* 1987;59:817–823.
16. Twidale N, Heddle WF, Ayres BF, Tonkin AM. Clinical implications of electrophysiologic study findings in patients with bifascicular block and syncope. *Aust N Z J Med* 1988;18:841–847.
17. Denes P, Uretz E, Ezri MD, Borbola J. Clinical predictors of electrophysiologic findings in patients with syncope of unknown origin. *Arch Intern Med* 1988;148:1922–1928.
18. Muller T, Roy D, Talajic M, et al. Electrophysiologic evaluation and outcome of patients with syncope of unknown origin. *Eur Heart J* 1991;12:139–143.
19. Lacroix D, Dubuc M, Kus T, et al. Evaluation of arrhythmic causes of syncope: Correlation between Holter monitoring, electrophysiologic testing, and body surface potential mapping. *Am Heart J* 1991;122:1346–1354.

20. Bachinsky WB, Linzer M, Weld L, Estes NAM. Usefulness of clinical characteristics in predicting the outcome of electrophysiologic studies unexplained syncope. *Am J Cardiol* 1992;69:1044–1049.
21. Cumbee SR, Pyor RE, Linzer M. Cardiac loop recording: A new noninvasive diagnostic test in recurrent syncope. *South Med J* 1990;83(1):39–43.
22. Linzer M, Pritchell ELC, Pontinen M, et al. Incremental diagnostic yield of loop electrocardiographic recorders in unexplained syncope. *Am J Cardiol* 1990;66:214–219.
23. Brown AP, Dawkins KD, Davies JG. Detection of arrhythmias: Use of a patient-activated ambulatory electrocardiogram device with a solid state memory loop. *Br Heart J* 1987;58:251–253.
24. Krahn AD, Klein GJ, Norris C, Yee R. The high cost of syncope: Use of a new insertable loop recorder in recurrent syncope of unknown etiology. *Eur Heart J* 1996;17,P3140.
25. Krahn AD, Klein GJ, Yee R, et al. Cost effective analysis of diagnostic strategies in syncope of unknown etiology. *Circulation* 1996;94(8):I–624.
26. Morillo CA, Klein GJ, Zandri S, Yee R. Diagnostic accuracy of a low-dose isoproterenol head-up tilt protocol. *Am Heart J* 1995;129(5):901–906.
27. Rattes MF, Klein GJ, Sharma AD, et al. Efficacy of empirical cardiac pacing in syncope of unknown cause. *Can Med Assoc J* 1989;140:381–385.

Driving and Syncope

Brian Olshansky, MD and Blair P. Grubb, MD

I want to die peacefully in my sleep like my grandfather did, not screaming like the passengers who were in his car.

-George Burns

Motor vehicle accidents are one of the leading causes of death and disability in the western world. While it would seem self evident that syncope and driving do not mix, this can be a source of conflict between the physician and the patient. The ability to drive is enjoyed by adults worldwide, and while perceived as a luxury by some, it is felt to be a necessity by others. For patients who reside in North America in particular, the inability to drive may be so confining that it can be considered a form of complete disability. Thus, for many people, any restrictions on their ability to drive are viewed as barbaric in nature. Amputation may be more acceptable to a patient, because after amputation, driving may not always be restricted.

As mentioned in previous chapters, recurrent episodes of syncope can be quite disabling and may produce a level of functional impairment similar to that caused by chronic debilitating diseases, such as rheumatoid arthritis, that can severely restrict social, educational, and occupational activities. Frequently, even if a physician attempts to restrict a patient's driving, the patient will continue to drive or may seek another physician. Indeed, the conflict over driving may severely compromise the patient-doctor relationship and may cause the patient to go "doctor hopping" until he or she finds one who is willing to place less restrictions on his or her activities. Frequently, the patient will simply ignore the physician's advice and continue to drive [for example, our first Loyola implantable defibrillator patient with malignant ventricular arrhythmias and syncope had a custom-

From Grubb BP, Olshansky B (eds.). *Syncope: Mechanisms and Management.* Armonk, NY: Futura Publishing Co., Inc.; © 1998.

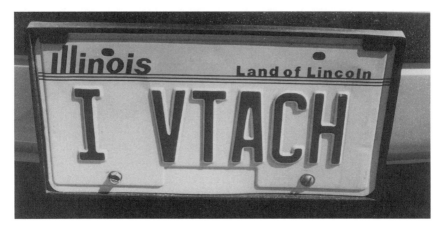

Figure 1. A customized license plate on the car of a cardiac patient at Loyola University Medical Center.

ized license plate that read: "AICD-1," while another had a plate made that stated: "I VTACH" (Figure 1)].

Individuals who experience recurrent unpredictable periods of loss of consciousness, but who continue to drive, risk not only their own lives but the lives of others as well. Even a momentary lapse in orientation while driving under slow and relatively safe conditions may lead to a disaster, resulting in injury and death. This unique situation places a considerable burden on the physician, who must balance the needs of the patient against those of society, and somehow come up with recommendations that are appropriate to the patient with syncope. Although there is no uniform consensus about syncope, similar conditions that may impair driving, such as epilepsy, have been addressed by the creation of legal statutes (see Chapter 18). Conditions such as the presence of arrhythmias in relation to alteration in levels of consciousness were the subject of an organized policy conference. The report was published as "official" recommendations.[1] It is important to remember, however, that these recommendations are not legally binding, and they potentially reflect views of a small, but vocal, minority with strong opinions on the subject. There is often an issue of fairness to consider as well. Individuals who suffer from advanced congestive heart failure or cardiomyopathy (even if they have not passed out) may be considered to be at a similar risk for cardiac arrest or syncope while driving; this issue, however, has never been considered in a formal way.

Regarding the patient with recurrent syncope who wishes to drive, there are several key issues that must be addressed: 1) What is the likelihood of syncope while driving? 2) What is the potential recurrence rate of the syncope? 3) What are the circumstances under which syncope is most likely to occur? 4) How much, if any, warning does the patient have prior to syncope? 5) How long does a typical episode last? 6) How often, and under what circumstances, does the patient drive? 7) How frequent are the episodes? 8) What are the legal implications of the physician's recommendations? 9) How likely is the patient to follow the physician's recommendations?

At his point, it is important to stress that the physician must become aware of the local legal requirements. The local statutes are highly varied and are subject to continuous change (Table 1). The medical-legal aspects of syncope are addressed in greater detail in Chapter 18. This chapter, while not a legal treatise, attempts to provide some insight and perspective into the problem of patients with syncope who wish to drive. In addition, some prudent recommendations for patients who have experienced syncope, with respect to their return to driving, are provided.

The Epidemiology of Driving

It goes without saying that the act of driving is never completely safe. In the United States alone, nearly 40,000 people die each year from traffic accidents, and an even greater number are injured. Although deaths due to firearms have recently exceeded those due to traffic accidents, this has not been due to a dramatic increase in road safety or innovations in automobile technology. Indeed, nearly all traffic accidents are not due to any specific medical condition, and even fewer are attributed to syncope. It is presently estimated that <0.1% of reported auto accidents are due to a preexisting medical condition; the majority of these are related to cardiac conditions.[2–27] There would be much greater impact if people wore seatbelts or if alcoholics were prevented from driving, than if all patients with syncope were restricted from driving. A large number of serious accidents would also be prevented if adolescent drivers were prohibited to drive, but such restriction is considered unfeasible (Figure 2). It is likely, however, that younger-aged drivers are at an even higher risk of causing a serious accident than are drivers who have experienced syncope. There are many other factors that may be involved.[28–46]

Data on the relationship between syncope and driving are difficult to obtain. In the confusion that surrounds an accident, stories are often altered. For example, a patient who suffered a syncopal event may report that they "fell asleep at the wheel," or vice versa. As discussed in other chapters, there is often an amnesia that surrounds the event, especially if the episode is compounded by trauma associated with the accident. Some, fearful that their license may be revoked, may lie, saying "I lost control of the car," or "I was trying to beat the red light," in order to hide syncope as a cause.

_____ Table 1 _____

Driving Recommendations by State

State	Seizure	Syncope	Arrhythmia	Mandatory Physician Reporting
		Months' restriction		
Alabama	6	6	0	No
Alaska	6	6	0	No
Arizona	3	3	0	No
Arkansas	12	0	0	No
California	Review	Review	Review	Yes
Colorado	Review	Review	Review	Yes
Connecticut	3	3	0	No
Delaware	Review	0	0	Yes
Florida	6	Review	Review	Unknown
Georgia*	12	12	0	Unknown
Hawaii	Review	Review	Review	No
Idaho	6	0	0	No
Illinois	Review	Review	Review	No
Indiana	Review	Review	Review	No
Iowa[LC]	6	6	6	No
Kansas	6	6	Review	No
Kentucky	3	3	0	No
Louisiana	6	Review	Review	No
Maine	3	6	6 (with ICD)	No
Maryland	3	3	3	No
Massachusetts	6	Review	Review	No
Michigan[LC]	6	6	0	No
Minnesota	6	6	0	No
Mississippi	12	0	0	No
Missouri	6	6	0	No
Montana[LC]	6	6	0	No
Nebraska	3	3	0	No
Nevada	3	3	3	Yes
New Jersey	12	12	Review	Yes
New Mexico	12	12	0	No
New York	6	LC	Review	No
North Carolina	12	Review	Review	No
North Dakota	3	Review	Review	No
Ohio	Review	Review	Review	No
Oklahoma	12	12	Review	No
Oregon	6	6	6–12	Yes
Pennsylvania	6	Review	Review	Yes
Rhode Island	Review	Review	Review	No
South Carolina	6	0	0	No
South Dakota	12	12	0	No

continues

_____ Table 1 Continued _____

Driving Recommendations by State

State	Seizure	Syncope	Arrhythmia	Mandatory Physician Reporting
		Months' restriction		
Tennessee[LC]	0	0	0	No
Texas	6	12	6	No
Utah	3	3	3	No
Vermont	6	6	Review	No
Virginia	6	Review	Review	No
Washington	6	6	0	Unknown
Washington D.C.	12	Review	Review	No
West Virginia	12	12	Review	No
Wisconsin	3	Review	Review	No
Wyoming	3	3	0	No

1995 data. Review = Each person is evaluated based on the recommendation of a state medical review board, a nonmedical review unit, or the patient's physician; LC = loss of consciousness, which enacts a specified driving restriction; *1991 data. Data reprinted by permission, Medtronic, Inc.[90]

CASE: A 67-year-old man is driving down the road and finds himself and his car in a stream alongside the road. The patient has a history of an ischemic cardiomyopathy and a left bundle branch block. At electrophysiological testing, he has inducible ventricular tachycardia as well as evidence for infra-Hisian block. An implantable cardioverter defibrillator (ICD) is placed with back-up ventricular pacing. Several months later he returns, complaining of fatigue, VVI pacemaker dependent (his ICD had not fired). He later receives a DDD pacemaker, has remained asymptomatic, and is allowed to return to driving in 6 months.

Rehm et al[47,48] prospectively studied drivers involved in road crashes over a 1-year period. Of 84 elderly individuals involved in accidents at a level I trauma center, 67 of the elderly were deemed at fault. Twelve accidents of the 67 were thought to be due to syncope, 53 patients had significant underlying medical problems, and 4 were intoxicated. Syncope appears to be a significant cause of serious driving accidents in the elderly. Linzer, et al[49] showed that the presence of syncope often leads to restriction in daily activities in up to 76% of individuals. Sixty-four percent will have some restriction in driving.[49] In 1958, Norman[50] began collecting information from London Transport bus drivers to determine which medical conditions lead to accidents.[4,51] Data were subsequently collected until 1972.[51] In that period, there were 108 incidents of acute illness, causing 54 accidents. This calculates to one accident every 115,000,000 miles. This small population is highly select and the accu-

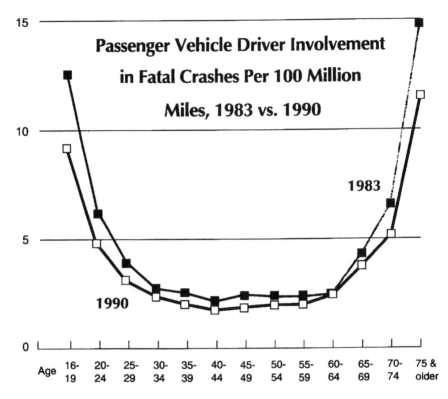

Figure 2. Risks of driving have been positively correlated with the age of the driver, previous driving record, time of driving, and conditions of driving. These risks have remained similar over the past few years. Fatal crashes are related more to these risks than to medical conditions, particularly syncope. From The Insurance Institute for Highway Safety.

racy of the data cannot be guaranteed. During that time, syncope of undetermined etiology contributed to 14 of these accidents, of which 10 resulted in a collision. Other conditions diagnosed included: vasovagal attacks in 20, causing 12 collisions, transient ischemic attacks in 3, with one collision, and epilepsy in 18, causing 14 collisions. Acute ischemic heart disease was responsible for 32 accidents, but only 8 resulted in a collision. The bulk of the episodes occurred in males over the age 50 years. Regarding drivers of cars, the casualty rates in the 20- to 29-year-old age group is 2.5 times that of the 50- to 59-year-old age group. This suggests that acute illness, including syncope, is unlikely to be a major cause of serious accidents. Raffle, in his 1974 paper, *Fitness to Drive*[51] considered the following equation:

$$Risk = hours + route\text{-}weight\ (of\ the\ bus) + experience + \text{``unfitness''}$$

While fitness is an important consideration, it appears that unfitness, representing many types of medical conditions, is only a minor aspect. Grattan[52] reviewed 9390 accidents and found that 15 were caused by an acute illness, 6 of which were due to transient loss of consciousness. Herner and Ysander[5] studied 612 drivers with diabetes, cardiovascular disease, and other problems. Drivers in the medically ill group had a 4.1% incidence of accidents compared to 7.7% in a control group. Forty one of 44,255 road accidents in Sweden were probably caused by illness over a 4-year period, but syncope was not a major cause of accidents in these individuals.[5]

There is a widely held view in the community that elderly and medically unfit drivers are a hazard in the road system. It is important, therefore, that the true position regarding these drivers should be put before the public, because it appears from available evidence that this group does not provide a greater risk on the road than do the general cross section of drivers.[13] Voigt[53] reported 47 cases of death behind the wheel. In 36 cases, the driver stopped the car before dying. Thirty-five deaths resulted in a collision, but injuries were present in only two, and they were minor injuries. Similarly, Peterson and Petty[2] reported that of 871 individuals who died suddenly in Baltimore over a 4-year period, more than half of the drivers were able to stop their cars before dying. Based on this information, it appears unlikely that patients with serious medical disorders are the cause of a significant number of traffic accidents. In a study by Hossack,[13] of 54 individual drivers who died while driving, 53 died suddenly. This represents a population of 600 consecutive drivers who died in accidents, but not before the accidents. These data, alternatively, suggest that there may be some concern that medical illness could be the cause of a significant number of car accidents, but it would be difficult to identify the individuals at highest risk. It still appears that intoxicated males between 20 and 30 years of age are responsible for the great majority of car accidents, especially those that cause significant injury.

Sheldon[54] evaluated patients with neurocardiogenic mechanisms as the suspected cause of syncope. In this report, a total of 217 adults with at least one syncopal spell thought to be due to neurocardiogenic causes were evaluated. Seven patients had stopped driving after their first syncopal spell. One individual had an estimated 6000 spells, but never had a motor vehicle accident! The remaining 209 patients had a mean age of 42 with a median of 4 syncopal spells before further evaluation with tilt table testing. Five patients lost consciousness while driving, 4 of which had motor vehicle accidents, and 2 caused driver injury. No one was killed and no bystanders were injured. Sheldon[54] estimates the risk of syncope of this population to be 0.33%/driver/year. The risk of harm from syncope due to neurocardiogenic causes in this population was even less—it was 2 /1534/year, or 0.13% per year. In contrast, other data[4] suggest that the risk of syncope is 0.02%. The Canadian Cardiovascular Society estimates an that acceptable risk of death and injury to others while driving due to syncope is 0.005%.[55]

Sheldon suspects that counseling and proper treatment may reduce the risk of syncope while driving by 90%, and that the risk may become as low as 0.026%. This may be an acceptable risk.[54] While the risk may be low, Sheldon[54] advises that if there are recurrent symptoms, and especially if there is no prodrome for syncope, driving should be restricted for at least 3 months. This number is similar to restrictions placed on driving, lasting a mean of 4.3±4.9 months, in several states. Only eight states have regulations regarding syncope due to ventricular arrhythmias (see Table 1). It is of note that any cause of alteration in consciousness, including supraventricular tachycardia, cough syncope, or vasovagal syncope, may increase the risk of motor vehicle accidents.[56-58]

An editorial by Sowton[59] reviews several reports and personal communications concerning patients with permanent pacemakers and driving. This report is over 25 years old. Even based on the data of the times, and not considering the major advances in pacemakers (and refinements of indications to implant pacemakers) made over the years, it appears that patients with pacemakers are not at substantially increased risk of motor vehicle accidents. Based on the data at that time, it did not appear that pacemakers were responsible for motor vehicle accidents.[59,60]

In another report, 71 of 1348 (5%) coronary deaths occurred while driving.[60a] Accidents were subsequently caused in 24. In an even larger study,[60b] 98 of 9330 (1%) sudden deaths occurred while driving. Based on these and similar data, the actuarial risk of sudden death in the United States has been estimated at 4.5 x 10^6 hours.[60c] The projected net rise in fatal accidents, if all individuals were allowed to drive freely, has been estimated to be 0.001%.[71]

The risk of driving is clearly dependent on the frequency and the length of the driving. Highway driving and city driving have different risks.[61] The expertise, the mood of the individuals, and other noncardiac medical conditions all play a role in the outcome of driving.[61,62] The cause of loss of consciousness is also important. This issue has been most notably addressed regarding epilepsy.[3,63-68] For a patient who has an implanted defibrillator for malignant ventricular arrhythmias, the risk varies tremendously based on the type of arrhythmias for which the ICD was implanted, the underlying cardiac condition, the hemodynamic response to the arrhythmia, and the patient's reaction to a shock.[69-74] The risk that an ICD patient will cause an accident while driving is probably similar to that posed by a teenage male driving. There are other disease conditions that can impact on driving.[75-81]

Restrictions to Driving: What Does the Law Say?

Restrictions to driving vary from state to state. It is important for physicians caring for patients to know what the local laws are and what their own responsibilities concerning individual patients are. These laws are continuously subject to change, and they do change. In some states, it is considered an imposition on the right to privacy to notify the Motor Vehicle Bureau about a patient who may pass out behind the wheel or one who is likely to sustain a motor vehicle accident due to an underlying heart condition or other medical condition. In other states, however, it is mandatory that the physician report the patient to the Department of Motor Vehicles. Alternatively, no physicians have been prosecuted due to negligence in reporting an individual who may pose a risk by driving a car. Furthermore, no specific guidelines exist regarding syncope or transient loss of consciousness, as they do for patients who have seizure disorders.

In Illinois, the law (Motor Vehicle Code) states that it is the duty of every driver who has a medical condition likely to cause loss of consciousness, or who has any loss of ability to safely operate a motor vehicle, to report this to the Illinois Department of Motor Vehicles within 10 days of becoming aware of such a condition. Then, a form is sent to the responsible physician who must fill it out. There is a review board that assesses the driver's ability to continue to drive. While under no obligation, and at no risk to him- or herself, a physician may report an individual patient in Illinois who may pose a risk by driving.

In any event, most physicians do not know their local state laws.

Pathophysiology of Driving

Even though driving is a relatively sedentary activity, operating a motor vehicle can have a major impact on physiology and may actually exacerbate some underlying medical conditions.[78–86] The mental stress caused by driving cannot be underestimated.[62,87-89] Similar to performing complex mathematics, driving can provoke ischemia and can alter autonomic tone. This is dependent on the driver, as well as the driving locale (rush hour traffic versus driving on an isolated interstate), the time of day, the abilities of the driver, the driver's mood, and the use of radar in the area, among other factors. Holter monitors have been applied to drivers to assess their heart rate response.[83,86-87] It appears that race car driving can increase the heart rate so that it exceeds 200 bpm. Even normal driving can lead to an increase in heart rate, exceeding 140 bpm. ST segment depression has been observed by continuous Holter recordings in 3 of 32 normal patients and 13 of 24 patients with known coronary artery disease.[83,86] Driving has been associated with the presence of extrasystoles, but it has not been clearly correlated with the presence of sustained tachyarrhythmias or bradyarrhythmias.

The actual pathophysiological risk regarding transient loss of consciousness behind the wheel is actually unknown. In fact, it can be hard to determine when an individual actually passes out, or when he or she simply goes to sleep behind the wheel. It is also likely that reports of transient loss of consciousness may be ready explanations for other potential etiologies for motor vehicle accidents. It appears, however, that even in a population of patients with syncope, the risk for driving is relatively small. The risk posed by drivers who experience syncope is also dependent on the frequency and the length of driving. For some individuals such as those patients who have potentially malignant ventricular tachyarrhythmias and who have an ICD, the risk of an accident due to transient loss of consciousness from a malignant ventricular arrhythmia that is corrected by an ICD shock is low, but it is higher than the risk of an accident in the general population. The chances of these patients having an accident are at a level similar to those of a teenage male, but teenage males are not generally restricted from driving (see Figure 2).

For many relatively sedentary individuals, driving may be one of the most stressful activities of the day. Therefore, in patients who have a potentially ischemically mediated tachyarrhythmia, or in those who have a catecholamine-sensitive ventricular tachycardia, driving may trigger an episode. Alternatively, driving does not appear to be a potent stimulus for vasodepressor episodes. Recommendations for driving for patients with syncope depend on the suspected cause of syncope. In patients with arrhythmic causes of syncope in whom the problem is completely treated, it may not be appropriate to restrict driving activities. For example, if a patient had lost consciousness due to asystole from complete heart block but had this problem effectively treated with a pacemaker, after proper recovery from the pacemaker implant, it is difficult to restrict driving further. On the other hand, most patients who pass out have, at best, a suspected cause of syncope or a cause that is multifactorial. In such cases, it is prudent to have the patient not drive for a period of time in order to assess the adequacy of treatment. Firm recommendations regarding this time limit are difficult to quantitate, and must be considered on a case by case basis.

In consideration of three broad categories of cause of syncope, several precedents have been set. Some of these are based on guidelines for patients with seizure disorders. Others are based on data from patients with malignant arrhythmias. In these patients, Larsen[73] has found that at 6 months, the incidence of recurrence of ICD shocks for patients who have an ICD for a malignant ventricular arrhythmia levels off. Some patients who have malignant arrhythmia declare that they are at high risk for an ICD shock early after device implantation. Others do not fit into this category. As there is always the possibility of loss of consciousness with the development, even transiently, of a ventricular arrhythmia, many physicians temporarily or even prematurely restrict patients with ICD. Restrictions vary substantially between Europe and the United States (see Table 1). It is uncertain whether similar guidelines can be applied to other patients with syncope, but they are probably inappropriate. Consider a young patient with vasodepressor syncope, the most common cause of syncope. For one episode of loss of consciousness, driving restriction may be harsh, but there is a spectrum to consider in this regard. For a patient with "malignant" neurocardiogenic syncope in whom a tilt table test is positive, and in whom the episodes occur without obvious cause, driving restriction, at least temporarily, may be appropriate. A 3-month period of driving restriction would seem to be appropriate, but this depends on the clinical situation, because even for this patient, the risk of recurrence of syncope is rare, and the risk posed by driving is even more rare considering the time spent behind the wheel. Patients with a single unexplained episode of syncope despite a complete and appropriate evaluation will have a low incidence of recurrence (perhaps <20%) in the next several years. Such patients cannot be restricted from driving unless episodes recur and are relatively frequent.

> CASE: An 82-year-old male has episodes of profound fatigue and near syncope. An ECG shows complete heart block with a response rate of 35 bpm. A permanent pacemaker is placed. He quickly becomes pacemaker dependent. Is it safe for him to drive?

> CASE: A 17-year-old female athlete just started college. She has recurrent syncope without an obvious prodrome. A tilt table test is positive at 10 minutes, reproducing her symptoms. She wants to drive like all her friends. What do you recommend?

> CASE: A 55-year-old truck driver, after a hard night of drinking, falls face first into his oatmeal. A tilt table test is markedly positive at 5 minutes. He undergoes therapy with a β-blocker. He drives toxic waste around the city in a truck as part of his job. Do you let him drive . . . ever? He has been taking disopyramide and a β-adrenergic blocker for 5 years, continues to drive as part of his job, and never passes out again.

> CASE: A 78-year-old male has syncope and a dilated cardiomyopathy and undergoes an electrophysiological test that shows inducible sustained ventricular tachycardia. An ICD is implanted, but a recommendation is made that he wait 6 months to drive. He does not drive for 6 months, but then he starts driving. He receives an occasional ICD shock without loss of consciousness. Then, 6 years later, he loses consciousness, followed by an ICD shock, while driving. He drives into a tree, narrowly missing children sledding down a nearby hill.

The recommendation for driving for syncope patients remains clouded. In part, this is related to the multitude of causes for syncope and the wide variation in presentations. Based on present data, it appears that physicians should be assuaged that the legal risks regarding driver recommendation for syncope are minimal as long as the issues are discussed (and documented) with the patient and if necessary, with the proper legal channels. It is best to concentrate efforts on proper treatment of the cause of syncope, and while prudent guidelines for driving can be established based on common sense, these guidelines must be individualized for each patient. It appears that this will not change in the near future.

References

1. Epstein AE, Miles WM, Benditt DG, et al. Personal and public safety issues related to arrhythmias that may affect consciousness: Implications for regulation and physician recommendations. An AHA/NASPE Medical Scientific Statement. *Circulation* 1996;94:1147–1166.
2. Peterson BJ, Petty CS. Sudden natural death among automobile drivers. *J Forensic Sci* 1962;7:274–284.
3. Parsons M. Fits and other causes of loss of consciousness while driving. *Q J Med* 1986;58:295–303.
4. Norman LG. Medical aspects of road safety. *Lancet* 1960;1:989–994, 1039–1045.
5. Herner B, Smedby B, Ysander L. Sudden illness as a cause of motor vehicle accidents. *Br J Indust Med* 1966;23:37–41.
6. West I, Nielsen GL, Gilmore AE, Ryan JR. Natural death at the wheel. *JAMA* 1968;205:266–271.
7. Kerwin AJ. Sudden death while driving. *Can Med Assoc J* 1984;131:312–314.
8. Hossack DS. Death at the wheel: A consideration of cardiovascular disease as a contributory factor to road accidents. *Med J Aust* 1974;1:164–166.
9. Ostrum M, Eriksson A. Natural death while driving. *J Forensic Sci* 1987;32:988–998.
10. Christian MS. Incidence and implications of natural deaths of road users. *Br Med J* 1988;297:1021–1024.
11. Waller JA. Cardiovascular disease, aging, and traffic accidents. *J Chronic Dis* 1967;20:615–620.
12. Anecol DH, Roberts WC. Sudden death behind the wheel from natural disease in drivers of four-wheeled motorized vehicles. *Am J Cardiol* 1990;66:1329–1335.
13. Hossack M. Medical catastrophe at the wheel. *Med J Aust* 1980;1:327–328.
14. Ryan GA. Casualty care in car crashes. *Int J Epidemiol* 1974;3:31–35.
15. Parsons M. Fits and other causes of loss of consciousness while driving. *Q J Med* 1986;58:295–303.
16. Anonymous. Natural death at the wheel. *Br Med J* 1969;1:332.
17. Baker SP, Spitz WU. An evaluation of the hazard created by natural death at the wheel. *N Engl Med* 1970;283:405–409.
18. Brandaleone H, Katz R, Tebrock HE, Wheatley GM. Study of the relationship of health impairments and motor vehicle accidents. *J Occup Med* 1972;14:854–859.
19. Brouwer WH, Ponds RW. Driving competence in older persons. *Disability & Rehabilitation* 1994;16:149–161.
20. Copeland AR. Sudden natural death 'at the wheel' revisited. *Med Sci Law* 1987;27:106–113.
21. Waller PF. The older driver. *Hum Factors* 1991;33:499–505.
22. Waller JA. Medical conditions: What role in crashes? *N Engl J Med* 1970;283:429–430.
23. Williams AF, Preusser DF, Ulmer RG, Weinstein HB. Characteristics of fatal crashes of 16-year-old drivers: Implications for licensure policies. *J Public Health Policy* 1995;16:347–360.
24. Schmidt P, Haarhoff K, Bonte W. Sudden natural death at the wheel: A particular problem of the elderly? *Forensic Sci Int* 1990;48:155–162.
25. Retchin SM, Anapolle J. An overview of the older driver. *Clin Geriatr Med* 1993;9:279–296.
26. McLean AJ. Death at the wheel. *N Engl J Med* 1970;283:1234.

27. Baldwin RW, Schoolman LR, Whittlesey P, et al. Medical conditions constituting a hazard in driving. *Md Med J* 1966;15:55–58.
28. Grimmond BB. Suicide at the wheel. *N Z Med J* 1974;80:90–94.
29. Simon F, Corbett C. Road traffic offending, stress, age, and accident history among male and female drivers. *Ergonomics* 1996;39:757–780.
30. Sorock GS, Ranney TA, Lehto MR. Motor vehicle crashes in roadway construction workzones: An analysis using narrative text from insurance claims. *Accid Anal Prev* 1996;28:131–138.
31. Mayou R, Simkin S, Threlfall J. The effects of road traffic accidents on driving behaviour. *Injury* 1991;22:365–368.
32. Pakola SJ, Dinges DF, Pack AI. Review of regulations and guidelines for commercial and noncommercial drivers with sleep apnea and narcolepsy. *Sleep* 1995;18:787–796.
33. Ray WA, Thapa PB, Shorr RI. Medications and the older driver. *Clin Geriatr Med* 1993;9:413–438.
34. Knight B. The drinking driver. *Practitioner* 1972;209:294–301.
35. Logan BK. Methamphetamine and driving impairment. *J Forensic Sci* 1996;41:457–464.
36. Marottoli RA, Drickamer MA. Psychomotor mobility and the elderly driver. *Clin Geriatr Med* 1993;9:403–411.
37. Marshall C, Boyd KT, Moran CG. Injuries related to car crime: The joy-riding epidemic. *Injury* 1996;27:79–80.
38. Hanning CD, Welsh M. Sleepiness, snoring and driving habits. *J Sleep Res* 1996;5:51–54.
39. Hemenway D, Solnick SJ. Fuzzy dice, dream cars, and indecent gestures: Correlates of driver behavior? *Accid Anal Prev* 1993;25:161–170.
40. Corfitsen MT. Enhanced tiredness among young impaired male nighttime drivers. *Accid Anal Prev* 1996;28:155–162.
41. Deichmann WB. Backward driving. *JAMA* 1972;221:1517.
42. Gillberg M, Kecklund G, Akerstedt T. Sleepiness and performance of professional drivers in a truck simulator: Comparisons between day and night driving. *J Sleep Res* 1996;5:12–15.
43. Gregersen NP. Young drivers' overestimation of their own skill: An experiment on the relation between training strategy and skill. *Accid Anal Prev* 1996;28:243–250.
44. Brown ID. Driver fatigue. *Hum Factors* 1994;36:298–314.
45. Brown ID. Effect of a car radio on driving in traffic. *Ergonomics* 1965;8:475–479.
46. Schenck CH, Mahowald MW. A polysomnographically documented case of adult somnambulism with long-distance automobile driving and frequent nocturnal violence: Parasomnia with continuing danger as a noninsane automatism? *Sleep* 1995;18:765–772.
47. Rehm CG, Ross SE. Elderly drivers involved in road crashes: A profile. *Am Surg* 1995;61:435–437.
48. Rehm CG, Ross SE. Syncope as etiology of road crashes involving elderly drivers. *Am Surg* 1995;61;1006–1008.
49. Linzer M, Varia I, Pontinen M, et al. Medically unexplained syncope: Relationship to psychiatric illness. *Am J Med* 1992;92:1A–18S1A–25S.
50. Norman LG. The Health of bus drivers: A study in London transport. *Lancet* 1958;805–812.
51. Raffle PA. Fitness to drive. *Trans Med Soc Lond* 1974;90:197–205.
52. Grattan E, Jeffcoate GO. Medical factors and road accidents. *Br Med J* 1968;1:75–79.

53. Voigt J. Road traffic deaths from natural causes. International Association for Accident and Traffic Medicine. *Proceedings of the Third Triennial Congress on Medical and Related Aspects of Motor Vehicle Accidents. 5/29–6/4, 1969.* Ann Arbor: University of Michigan Highway Safety Research Institute; 1969:71.

54. Sheldon R, Koshman ML. Can patients with neuromediated syncope safely drive motor vehicles? *Am Heart J* 1995;75:955–956.

55. Consensus Conference, Canadian Cardiovascular Society. Assessment of the cardiac patient for fitness to drive. *Can J Cardiol* 1992;8:406–412.

56. Decter BM, Goldner B, Cohen, TJ. Vasovagal syncope as a cause of motor vehicle accidents. *Am Heart J* 1994;127:1619–1621.

57. Haffner HT, Graw M. Cough syncope as a cause of traffic accident. [German: Hustensynkope als Unfallursache]. *Blutalkohol.* 1990;27:110–115.

58. Dhala A, Bremner S, Blanck Z, et al. Impairment of driving abilities in patients with supraventricular tachycardias. *Am J Cardiol* 1995;75:516–518.

59. Sowton E. Driving licences for patients with cardiac pacemakers. *Br Heart J* 1972;34:977–980.

60. Brandaleone H. Motor vehicle driving and cardiac pacemakers. *Ann Intern Med* 1974;81:548–550.

60a. Myerburg RJ, Davis JH. The medical ecology of public safety I: Sudden death due to coronary heart disease. *Am Heart J* 1964;68:586–595.

60b. Bowen DA. Deaths of drivers of automobiles due to trauma and ischemic heart disease: A survey and assessment. *Forensic Sci* 1973;2:285–290.

60c. Gillum RF. Sudden coronary death in the United States 1980–1985. *Circulation* 1989;79:756–765.

61. Rutley KS, Mace DG. Heart rate as a measure in road layout design. *Ergonomics* 1972;15:165–173.

62. Somerville W. Emotions, catecholamines and coronary heart disease. *Adv Cardiol* 1973;8:162–173.

63. Taylor J, Chadwick D, Johnson T. Risk of accidents in drivers with epilepsy. *J Neurol Neurosurg Psychiatry* 1996;60:621–627.

64. Gustaysson P, Alfredsson L, Brunnberg H, et al. Myocardial infarction among male bus, taxi, and lorry drivers in middle Sweden. *Occup Environ Med* 1996;53:235–240.

65. Spudis EV, Penry JK, Gibson P. Driving impairment caused by episodic brain dysfunction. Restrictions for epilepsy and syncope. *Arch Neurol* 1986;43:558–564.

66. Anonymous. Consensus conference on driver licensing and epilepsy: American Academy of Neurology, American Epilepsy Society, and Epilepsy Foundation of America. Washington, D.C., May 31–June 2, 1991. Proceedings. [Review] *Epilepsia* 1994;35:662–705.

67. Stock MS, Burg FD, Light WO, Douglass JM. Licensing the driver with alterations of consciousness. *Arch Neurol* 1970;23:210–211.

68. Krumholz A, Fisher RS, Lesser RP, et al. Driving and epilepsy: A review and reappraisal. *JAMA* 1991;265:622–626.

69. Cambre S, Silverman ME. It is safe to drive with an automatic implantable cardioverter defibrillator or a history of recurrent symptomatic ventricular arrhythmias? *Heart Dis Stroke* 1993;2:179–181.

70. Beauregard LM, Barnard PW, Russo AM. Perceived and actual risks of driving in patients with arrhythmia control devices. *Arch Intern Med* 1995;155:609–613.

71. Anderson MH, Camm AJ. Legal and ethical aspects of driving and working in patients with an implantable cardioverter defibrillator. *Am Heart J* 1994;127:1185–1193.

72. Strickberger SA, Cantillon CO, Friedman PL. When should patients with lethal ventricular arrhythmia resume driving? *Ann Intern Med* 1991;15;560–562.

73. Larsen GC, Stupey MR, Walance CG, et al. Recurrent cardiac events in survivors of ventricular fibrillation or tachycardia: Implications for driving restrictions. *JAMA* 1994;17:1335–1339.
74. Curtis AB, Conti JB, Tucker KJ, et al. Motor vehicle accidents in patients with an implantable cardioverter-defibrillator. *J Am Coll Cardiol* 1995;26:180–184.
75. Brandaleone H. Driving and the coronary patient. *J Rehabil* 1966;32:97.
76. Anonymous. Highway travel and angina pectoris. *Can Med Assoc J* 1973;108:1095.
77. Douglass JM, Stock MS, Light WO, Burg FD. Licensing the driver with cardiovascular dysfunction. *Am Heart J* 1970;80:197–201.
78. Kushnir B, Fox KM, Tomlinson IW, et al. Primary ventricular fibrillation and resumption of work, sexual activity, and driving after first acute myocardial infarction. *Br Med J* 1975;4:609–611.
79. Wielgosz AT, Azad N. Effects of cardiovascular disease on driving tasks. *Clin Geriatr Med* 1993;9:341–348.
80. Somerville W. Heart disease and fitness to drive motor vehicles. *Med Leg J* 1970;38:42–50.
81. McCue H. Cardiac arrhythmias in relation to automobile driving. Presented at the Scientific Conference on Personal and Public Safety Issues Related to Arrhythmias. Washington DC: January 12–13, 1995.
82. Littler WA, Honour AJ, Sleight P. Direct arterial pressure and electrocardiogram during motor car driving. *Br Med J* 1973;2:273–277.
83. Lauwers P, Aelvoet W, Sneppe R, Remion M. Effect of car driving on the electrocardiogram of patients with myocardial infarction and an E.C.G. at rest devoid of dysrhythmia and repolarisation abnormalities: Comparison with the E.C.G. changes obtained during exercise. *Acta Cardiol* 1973;28:27–43.
84. Taggart P, Carruthers M. Hyperlipidaemia induced by the stress of racing driving. *Lancet* 1971;1:854.
85. Falkner F. The stress of racing driving. *Lancet* 1971;1:650.
86. Taggart P, Gibbons D, Sommerville W. Some effects of motor car driving on the normal and abnormal heart. *Br Med J* 1969;4:130–134.
87. Bellett S, Roman L, Kostis J, Slater A. Continuous electrocardiographic monitoring during automobile driving: Studies in normal subjects and patients with coronary disease. *Am J Cardiol* 1968;22:856.
88. Sartory G, Roth WT, Kopell ML. Psychophysiological assessment of driving phobia. *J Psychophysiol* 1992;6/4:311–320.
89. Cocco G, Iselin HU. Cardiac risk of speed traps. *Clin Cardiol* 1992;15:441–444.
90. Medtronic, Inc. When may patients with implanted defibrillators drive? *Follow-Up Forum* Winter 1995/1996;1(3):8–10.

Syncope and the Law

Mark Jay Zucker, MD, JD, FACC
and Gerald J. Bloch, LLB

Introduction

It is well recognized that syncope, regardless of the etiology, can affect not only the patient, but third parties as well. For this reason, physicians should naturally be concerned with the accuracy and implications of their diagnoses and treatment plans, including the consequences of either permitting or restricting the patient from participating in certain activities. In general, however, medical professionals can derive some comfort from the knowledge that as long as a decision made by the practitioner is based upon solid medical reasoning and made in good faith, medical-legal implications should be minimal.

The most significant medical-legal concern in the management of the patient presenting with syncope is the possibility that the failure to restrict activity may jeopardize the patient's life or the life of an innocent third party. Although this is of particular concern for physicians treating competitive athletes, drivers of motor vehicles, pilots of aircraft, operators of heavy equipment, handlers of hazardous materials, and the elderly, there are a myriad of circumstances in which the failure to prevent or warn about potential recurrence can prove disastrous.

While the medical evaluation and treatment of syncope can be tedious and occasionally unrewarding, the medical-legal principles addressing the issues surrounding loss of consciousness are fairly straightforward. In the absence of specific statutes or regulations governing the reporting of these conditions, the liability of a physician is based solely upon common law rules of negligence.

From Grubb BP, Olshansky B (eds.). *Syncope: Mechanisms and Management.* Armonk, NY: Futura Publishing Co., Inc.; © 1998.

Negligence law addresses "conduct," and embraces acts of commission as well as acts of omission; ie, what an individual did or failed to do. In general, the law imposes on an individual a duty to conduct oneself in a manner that does not expose others to an unreasonable risk of harm. A breach of that duty that proves to be the proximate cause of a subsequent harm constitutes negligence. Basic to any consideration of negligence is the idea or concept that the harm was "foreseeable."[1] Foreseeability, although a key factor in determining whether a duty exists, is not the only factor. The question of duty in a negligence action should also take into account the likelihood of injury, the magnitude of the burden of guarding against it, and the consequences of placing that burden on the defendant.[2,3]

A physician is thus charged with the duty of providing care and treatment in a manner that does not "unreasonably" threaten the safety of the patient or others. Unreasonably may be defined as conduct that falls below the standard established by law for the protection of others against unreasonable risk of harm.[4] What is reasonable depends on the state of medical knowledge and the unique characteristics and factors associated with that particular individual.

Medical Considerations: Standard of Care

The differential diagnosis of syncope includes both cardiovascular and noncardiovascular etiologies. History and physical examination alone, however, can provide a diagnosis in only about half of the cases.[5] Unfortunately, establishing a definitive diagnosis is critical to the prediction of recurrence. Liability exists only when the physician, presented with a patient with loss of consciousness, fails to meet the reasonable standard of care, described in detail elsewhere in this chapter. A brief restatement of the work-up focusing on documentation, however, is in order.

Particular attention should be paid to the patient's history, physical examination, and observations made by individuals who may have witnessed the event. At a minimum, the history must include a chronological record from the initial onset of symptoms until presentation for medical evaluation. Documentation of premonitory symptoms (such as palpitations), association with activity or positional changes, existence of triggers, changes in dietary habits and/or medications, and the presence or absence of emotional stress should be included. Further, a thorough inquiry into any past medical illnesses that might be of significance to the present loss of consciousness (such as chest pain, palpitations, lightheadedness, etc.) should be conducted. In many cases, obtaining an adequate history for a patient with syncope may require going beyond interviewing the patient; information available from family and friends is sometimes crucial.[6]

When a careful history and physical examination do not establish the etiology of the syncopal episode, further diagnostic testing is indicated.

Ambulatory electrocardiographic recording is frequently unrevealing. Event recorders, by increasing the electrocardiographic sampling time, are somewhat more useful. Tilt table testing has been used to assess patients at risk for vasovagal syncope, but it is highly nonspecific. Treadmill testing to rule out exercise-induced arrhythmias should be considered for an individual with exercise-induced syncope. Ultimately, if the etiology remains elusive, formal electrophysiological testing may be indicated.[7]

Obtaining a detailed and accurate medical history can be a time-consuming and admittedly frustrating process. The use of a checklist or outline may facilitate the process. The history and physical examination are essential to ensuring that a proper diagnosis is made, appropriate laboratory evaluations are ordered, and correct therapy is instituted. The failure to order a test generally considered critical to the work-up may represent a breach of the standard of care and may constitute negligence, unless the physician has determined that either the yield is unacceptably low, the test will not provide the needed information, or the test is not safe for the particular patient.[8]

The importance of adequate documentation in the medical record cannot be overemphasized, as documentation represents the only credible evidence that logical appropriate questions were asked in order to differentiate between those in need of an extensive work-up and those in whom the syncope was of a benign origin.

Statutory and Administrative Considerations

Typically, patients seek initial guidance from their physician with respect to activity restrictions. For this reason, a physician should be familiar with the applicable statutory or administrative requirements of his or her own jurisdiction that may apply to the operation of motor vehicles, aircraft, or any other activity that requires state licensing. Familiarizing oneself with applicable state regulations takes nothing more than a telephone call to the appropriate licensing agency. Nevertheless, a recent survey of randomly sampled cardiologists[9] revealed that only 26% correctly understood their state's restrictions on driving. Moreover, although 44% of arrhythmia specialists were familiar with their state's regulations, the same could be said of only 8% of the general cardiologists. Most physicians rely instead upon their own observations and the prevailing standard of care in the community.[9]

Although driving restrictions are highly variable, virtually all states either review on a case-by-case basis or restrict privileges when an individual experiences a syncopal episode secondary to a seizure disorder. Many states also restrict driving by patients who have lost consciousness for reasons other than a seizure. Probably to the surprise of most physicians, more than half of the states will also review on a case-by-case basis or restrict driving privileges of individuals with "arrhythmias" [10] (see Table 1). As of 1992, eight states (California, Colorado, Delaware, Nevada, New Hampshire, New Jersey, Oregon, and Pennsylvania) required physicians to report, in good faith, patients who have a physical or mental condition which, in the physician's judgment, impairs the patient's ability to exercise reasonable and ordinary control over a motor vehicle. The report may be made without the patient's informed consent. By way of example, see Wisconsin Statute § 146.82(3), which provides in pertinent part:

> REPORTS MADE WITHOUT INFORMED CONSENT. (a) Notwithstanding sub.(1), a physician who treats a patient whose physical or mental condition in the physician's judgment affects the patient's ability to exercise reasonable and ordinary control over a motor vehicle may report the patient's name and other information relevant to the condition to the Department of Transportation without the informed consent of the patient.

Many states will grant a physician immunity from liability for either reporting or failing to report, in good faith, a physical and/or mental condition that did or did not, in the physician's judgment, impair the patient's ability to operate the motor vehicle.[11] For example, see Wisconsin Statute 448.03(5)(b), which states:

> (b) No physician shall be liable for any civil damages for either of the following:
>   2) Reporting in good faith to the Department of Transportation under § 146.82(3) a patient's name and other information relevant to a physical or mental condition of the patient which

_____ Table 1 _____

States' Driving Regulations Regarding Patients with Arrhythmias

Restrict Driving Privileges (Months)		Review on a Case-by-Case Basis	
Iowa	6	California	North Carolina
Maine	6 (with ICD)	Colorado	North Dakota
Maryland	3	Florida	Ohio
Nevada	3	Hawaii	Oklahoma
Oregon	6–12	Illinois	Pennsylvania
Texas	6	Indiana	Rhode Island
Utah	3	Kansas	Vermont
		Louisiana	Virginia
		Massachusetts	Washington D.C.
		New Jersey	West Virginia
		New York	Wisconsin

in the physician's judgment impairs the patient's ability to exercise reasonable and ordinary control over a motor vehicle.

3) In good faith, not reporting to the Department of Transportation under § 146.82(3) a patient's name and other information relevant to a physical or mental condition of the patient which in the physician's judgment does not impair the patient's ability to exercise reasonable and ordinary control over a motor vehicle.

Note that the Wisconsin statute would not provide immunity to a physician for failing to report an individual whose ability to exercise reasonable care and ordinary control is, in the physician's judgment, impaired. Liability under these circumstances would be subject to the defense of "good faith."

In summary, physicians should recognize that statutory requirements may place the burden of reporting primarily on the physician. Moreover, the physician-patient privilege, although professionally and statutorily based, is not absolute. In those circumstances, where the "public interest" so demands, exceptions to the privilege are permitted, if not outright required.

Syncope and the Athlete

Syncope in the competitive athlete represents a unique and difficult problem.[7,12] The physician caring for such an athlete with a history of syncope, or for that matter, any significant cardiovascular disorder, may be subjected to enormous pressure from the individual, institution, family, and friends to provide a "clean" bill of health, thereby permitting a return to the prior activity. No cases highlight the problem better than those of basketball players Hank Gathers and Reggie Lewis. In each instance, the athlete obtained medical clearance despite an initial diagnosis of a cardiac condition.

Gathers, playing for Loyola Marymount, first collapsed on December 9, 1989. Seventeen days later, physicians had him play one-on-one basketball with a Holter monitor attached to his heart. 188 episodes of ventricular tachycardia with rates of almost 200 bpm were recorded. Gathers was started on a β-blocker (propanolol), and the Holter monitor was repeated. The frequency and complexity of the ventricular ectopic activity was greatly reduced. Unfortunately, due to side effects, and reportedly upon Gathers request, the dosage of propanolol was decreased gradually from 240 mg/day to 40 mg/day. The last dosage change occurred 6 days before his death, and was made with the understanding that he would return 2 days later to see if the lower dosage was safe and effective prior to playing in an upcoming postseason game. Gathers did not appear for the appointment, dodged calls from the physician, and ultimately convinced the physician to delay the test until after the game. Gathers died during that postseason game.

An autopsy listed the cause of Gathers's death as cardiomyopathy of unknown etiology. His death, at age 23, reverberated among team physicians and athletic directors who imagined themselves on the damage end of a lawsuit where the claim involved the loss of earnings of someone who was likely to be a professional athlete capable of commanding astronomically high salaries.

Indeed, Gathers's mother, minor son, and other heirs subsequently filed a multimillion dollar suit against Loyola Marymount, the coach, the trainers, and seven physicians involved with the case.[13] Not only did the plaintiffs contend that the physicians' treatment was negligent, but claimed further that the defendants had conspired and fraudulently failed to inform Gathers of the seriousness of his heart condition and the dangers associated with continuing to play competitive basketball. Finally, the plaintiffs alleged that the dosage reduction was made to ensure that Gathers playing ability and stamina were not compromised.[14,15,16]

The Gathers suit was eventually settled out of court for nearly $2.4 million. Lawsuits along these lines, however, are frequently filed. In 1986, Anthony Penny, a Central Connecticut State University basketball player, was diagnosed with hypertrophic cardiomyopathy. His physician recommended that he discontinue playing competitive basketball and imposed a restriction of 2 years. Not satisfied with that recommendation, he sought additional opinions, and was ultimately permitted to remain on the University's team. After completing his college basketball career, he filed a malpractice suit questioning the competence of the cardiologist who first made the diagnosis.[17] Penny claimed damages of $1,000,000, based in part on the lost future income from professional basketball and the lost enjoyment of life resulting from the 2-year restriction imposed upon him by the physician. Penny subsequently died during a competitive basketball game in England. The lawsuit was voluntarily dismissed.

Perhaps no case has created as much publicity as that of Reggie Lewis, captain of the Boston Celtics basketball team, who died in May 1993 while shooting baskets at a gymnasium. Two months earlier, Lewis had fainted during a Celtics game. A "team" of 12 cardiologists assembled by the Celtics' physician diagnosed his condition as "cardiomyopathy" and recommended that he not play competitive basketball again. A second medical opinion, requested by Lewis, concluded that he had the heart of a normal athlete and that the syncopal episode was due to a benign neurological condition. A third consultant found evidence to support each of the former consultant's opinions. Regardless, the autopsy confirmed the diagnosis of cardiomyopathy.[18,19]

Physicians should recognize that statutes designed to prevent discrimination against handicapped individuals may provide legal redress for athletes precluded from participation in competitive sports. Section 504(a) of the Rehabilitation Act (29 USCA 794 (West Supp. 1992)) states in pertinent part that:

> "no otherwise qualified individual with handicaps in the United States, as defined in 706(8) of this title, shall, solely by reason of her or his handicap, be excluded from the participation in, be denied the benefits of, or be subjected to discrimination under any program or activity receiving Federal financial assistance."

Most high schools and colleges receive some federal funding that makes these institutions subject to the rules and regulations of the Act. As well, the Amateur Sports Act of 1978 (36 USC §371 et seq. (1988)) also ensures equal opportunities in athletics programs for handicapped individuals.

It is at least arguable that ventricular arrhythmias and/or syncope constitute a "handicap," which under specific circumstances, may invoke the protection of these statutes. In such cases, the court will be charged with striking a balance between the statutory rights of the athlete and the desire of the school or team to not permit the "handicapped" athlete to play. How a court will rule is fact-sensitive and will depend upon whether the plaintiff can establish that his or her handicap constitutes the type of physical "impairment" contemplated by the Act. In *Larkin v Archdiocese of Cincinnati*, for example, the federal district court upheld a private high school's refusal to permit an athlete with hypertrophic cardiomyopathy to play football.[20,21]

The cases of Gathers, Lewis, Penny, and Larkin demonstrate that providing medical clearance for sports participation and treating athletic injuries may involve not only complex medical issues, but complex legal issues as well. Surprisingly, the number of reported judicial opinions involving litigation between team physicians, the specialists to whom the athletes are referred, and the competitive athlete is small.[21,22,23]

Standards for Athletic Participation

Physicians involved in the treatment of athletes, whether primary care providers, team or sports medicine physicians, or specialists, often have the responsibility for medically clearing athletes prior to their returning to play. Coincident with the responsibility for the medical decisions is the legal responsibility for harm to an athlete resulting from the failure to conform to accepted medical practices.

In contrast to the "normal" patient, the competitive athlete is psychologically and economically intent upon returning to the game. The team, the treating physician, or the consulting physician may find him- or herself under extreme pressure from the coach, management, friends, or the athlete to "clear" the athlete.[24] Nowhere is the documentation of advice and the reasons behind the advice more important. If the athlete is properly advised such that he or she understands the risks and benefits, and he or she chooses to disregard the physician's recommendation, legal liability will probably be avoided. At the least, the defense of contributory negligence and assumption of risk can be raised.

It must be recognized that competitive athletes are often young, and are occasionally lacking in understanding. The conveyance of information must be made in a form capable of being understood and acknowledged. Options should be provided and opportunities to minimize risk should be discussed.

In 1985, The American College of Cardiology convened the 16th Bethesda Conference, which formulated recommendations for sports participation by athletes with cardiovascular abnormalities. The participants at that conference appreciated that "*many decisions regarding disqualification from sports involve circumstances in which definitive scientific answers are conspicuously lacking.*" Nevertheless, the Bethesda conference's nationally accepted recommendations provided, for the first time, guidance to physicians who are charged with the responsibility for making eligibility decisions.[25]

Nine years later, at the 26th Bethesda Conference, the ethical, legal, and practical considerations affecting medical decision making in competitive athletes were readdressed. Updated, objective, scientifically based consensus guidelines were published in October of 1994, and are now accepted as the medical, and "legal" standard of care.[26] It is likely that these guidelines would be used by a court in resolving a malpractice claim or athletic participation dispute.

In the final analysis, however, the physician should provide a participation recommendation consistent with his or her best medical judgment. Nonmedical factors should not influence that decision. The physician must act reasonably, in good faith, and in such a manner as to not create an unreasonable risk of harm to the patient. If reasonable care dictates that an athlete with a potentially lethal condition not be allowed to play, then it is the physician's obligation to so inform the patient.[27]

Whether the physician must inform others is situation-specific, and probably depends upon whether the physician is the athlete's physician or the team physician. Certainly, in the former case, the law would be quite protective of the patient-physician relationship. Whether a team physician may assert the physician-patient privilege, however, is less clear-cut. Hence, a prudent team physician should disclose prior to starting an examination that the he or she is also acting on behalf of the team, and obtain permission to release pertinent medical information to team officials.[27]

While it may be true that competitive athletes are motivated, stoic, and driven to succeed, most athletes will act reasonably in response to a trusted physician's recommendation regarding athletic participation. Winning that trust is as much a function of "bedside manner" as is imparting the scientific and medical information.

Fortunately or unfortunately, there have been no cases of cardiac death involving a high-profile athlete that have ever created judicial precedent. Where such cases have been brought, they have been settled, dismissed, or not gone to trial. Thus, in the absence of "on-point" case law, physician liability remains based on the traditional rules of law, that is, did the physician exercise reasonable care under the circumstances? Physicians are held to a standard no greater than this.

Syncope and Driving

Probably coincident with the introduction of the motor car in the late 1800s was the recognition that certain medical conditions were not compatible with driving. The first traffic accidents attributable to epilepsy, for example, were reported in 1906. Individuals with seizure disorders were subsequently not granted driving privileges in the United States until 1949. Today, all states permit people with controlled seizure disorders to drive. Control is generally determined by a legally prescribed seizure-free interval.[28]

Syncope, whether neurally mediated or cardiovascular, also compromises the safety of activities such as flying and driving. In recognition of this, the United States Federal Aviation Administration (FAA) has promulgated guidelines that are used by the FAA Aeromedical Certification Division when evaluating an applicant with known supraventricular or ventricular arrhythmias. Similar comprehensive medical standards addressing eligibility for flying were also adopted by the Joint Aviation Authorities, an international agency encompassing 26 European nations, in 1996.

In contrast to flying, medical criteria for driving fitness are less formal, probably less strict, and generally determined by the individual states. Indeed, a distinction should be made between personal drivers and commercial operators such as bus drivers and truckers. Whereas the former are licensed solely by the state, the latter are regulated in part by United States Department of Transportation through the Federal Motor Carrier Safety Regulation. *"It is the intent of the Federal Motor Carrier Safety Regulation to disqualify a driver who has a current cardiovascular disease which is accompanied by and/or likely to cause symptoms of syncope, dyspnea, collapse, or congestive heart failure . . ."*[29]

Although the actual incidence of medically related automobile accidents is not known, at least two facts, are well accepted. First, sudden death while driving is rare.[30,31] Second, the impairment of driving ability appears to increase with age and the concomitant increased prevalence of underlying medical disorders. By way of example, an analysis of 67 motor vehicle accidents in New Jersey occurring in patients age 60 years and over, revealed 12 instances attributable to syncope.[32] A follow-up study by the same investigators demonstrated a positive work-up for syncope in 25 of 33 elderly drivers, where no external cause for the road crash could be found. Thirteen drivers had history of syncope.[33]

Loss of consciousness during driving has been reported not only in patients with malignant ventricular arrhythmias, bradyarrhythmias, and heart block, but in 19% to 36% of patients with supraventricular tachyarrhythmias as well.[34] Moreover, so called "benign" events such as vasovagal syncope have also resulted in motor vehicle accidents, prompting some physicians to advise their patients with this diagnosis not to drive because of the possibility of a recurrence despite treatment.[35]

Of course, the rhythm disturbances of greatest concern are ventricular tachycardia and ventricular fibrillation. Treatment of these rhythm abnormalities increasingly includes implantation of a cardioverter defibrillator. The degree of risk posed by allowing individuals with implantable cardioverter defibrillators (ICDs) to drive must be addressed. Certainly, across-the-board driving restrictions, as prescribed by many electrophysiologists,[30] may be inappropriate. Instead, each patient should be evaluated individually with respect to risk of arrhythmia recurrence and risk of postshock syncope. Unfortunately, although most patients do not experience syncope after implantation of an ICD, there are probably no historical or clinical variables that can be used to predict loss of consciousness. In fact, nearly two thirds of those who lost consciousness during or after an ICD shock had never experienced a syncopal episode with previous shocks.[36]

In general, most hemodynamically significant rhythm disturbances occur in the first month after ICD implantation.[37] The hazard rate then remains moderate until 7 months, after which it decreases substantially.[38] Even at that, spontaneous shocks have been reported to occur during driving in up to 18% of patients with ICDs in place.[39]

Regardless of physician driving recommendations, the majority of patients who receive ICDs do not modify their driving habits.[40] Thankfully, the actual frequency of motor vehicle accidents in this patient population is low, with an injury and fatality rate per 100,000 comparable to that seen in the general US population.[34]

In 1996, the American Heart Association and The North American Society of Pacing and Electrophysiology published a medical/scientific statement on safety issues related to arrhythmias.[31] For the considerations outlined above, it was recommended that noncommercial drivers with ICDs in place refrain from driving for a minimum of 6 months after device implantation. Commercial driving should be prohibited permanently.

The above observations notwithstanding, a review of the reported case law as of January, 1997 revealed no cases involving a physician's failure to impose driving restrictions on a patient with a pacemaker or defibrillator. That such cases will occur is perhaps inevitable.

Liability of a Physician for Injury or Death of a Third Party: Case Law

Section 315 of the Restatement of Torts 2d[41] provides that there is no duty to control the conduct of a third person so as to prevent him from causing physical harm to another unless either a special relationship exists between the actor and the third person which imposes a duty on the actor to control a third person's conduct, or a special relationship exists between the actor and the other which gives the other a right to protection.

As to a physician, it was historically held at common law that no duty existed that would extend liability beyond that of the patient. During the past 20 years, however, this traditional analysis has been revisited, most notably in *Tarasoff v Regents of University of California*.[42] In this case, the court imposed a duty on psychotherapists to protect third parties from harm. The court's holding was grounded on Section 319 of the Restatement of Torts, which provides that one who "takes charge" of a third person, whom he knows or should know to be likely to cause bodily harm to others if not controlled, is under a duty to exercise reasonable care to control the third person to prevent him from doing such harm. The application of Section 319 to physicians is now generally accepted, and several jurisdictions have since allowed a cause of action by a third party against a physician for negligence in the treatment of a patient.[41,43]

The above comments notwithstanding, there are few reported cases involving injury or death to a third party caused by a patient, previously treated for syncope, who suffered a recurrent loss of consciousness resulting in a motor vehicle or industrial accident. Nevertheless, the extent of a physician's liability for injury to a third party can be inferred from existing case law.

In *Freese v Lemon*,[44] the Iowa Supreme Court, in a 5 to 4 decision, held that if a pedestrian could prove that a physician, who was treating a motorist who suffered a seizure while driving and lost control of his automobile, negligently failed to advise the motorist not to drive an automobile and failed to advise the motorist who had suffered an earlier seizure of the dangers involved in driving an automobile, the physician could be held liable for injuries sustained by the pedestrian, and that allegations to this effect sustained a cause of action against the physician. The case was subsequently tried, and resulted in a verdict for the physician. It must be noted, however, that the verdict, ultimately sustained by the Iowa Supreme Court, was based primarily on the grounds that the injured party failed to prove the applicable standard of care. One can surmise that had the plaintiff met the burden of proof, physician culpability could have been found.

By way of contrast, in *Kaiser v Suburban Transportation Systems*,[45] the plaintiff was successful. Mrs. Kaiser, a passenger on a Suburban Transportation System bus, was injured when the driver lost consciousness and the bus struck a telephone pole. The lapse of consciousness was attributed to the side effects of a drug (pyribenzamine), which had been prescribed by the driver's physician for treatment of a nasal condition. The driver testified that the doctor gave him no warning of the possible side effects of the drug and that he had taken the first pill on the morning of the accident. Four doctors, including the defendant, testified that, in view of the known side-effect, a warning should be given when the drug is prescribed.

A similar fact pattern was presented to the Texas courts in *Gooden v Tips*,[46] a claim by a third-party vehicular accident victim against a physician for failure to warn a patient about the risks of driving under the influence of a drug prescribed by the physician. The court upheld the victim's right to sue the physician, stating in pertinent part that the duty being imposed was not a duty to control the patient's actions, but rather a duty to warn the patient that his or her driving ability might be impaired, and in what manner. The court in *Gooden* went on to note that while the third party's suit could not be maintained as a malpractice action due to the absence of a patient-physician relationship, the suit could be maintained as an ordinary negligence action.

Physicians are frequently called on to conduct physical examinations of airline pilots, truck drivers, firefighters, police officers, etc, and to certify that these individuals are physically fit to perform the duties of their employment. In that regard, the Tennessee Supreme Court, in *Wharton Transport Corp. v Bridges*,[47] was asked to determine whether a third party could assert a claim against a physician for the failure to identify bilateral chorioretinitis, which severely impaired a commercial trucker's depth perception and resulted in injury to the plaintiffs. The court held that the injuries suffered, in the manner in which they occurred, were reasonably foreseeable to the physician who negligently performed the pre-employment examination, and the court reversed a directed verdict for the defense.

As noted, however, there are few cases that specifically address injury or death to a third party caused by the conduct of an individual with a history of syncope who suffers a recurrent loss of consciousness that results in a motor vehicle or industrial accident. In *Simmons v Aldi-Brenner Company*,[48] the court addressed the admissibility of "prior occurrences" to establish notice of a dangerous condition. Store customers and relatives of a deceased victim brought a negligence action against a motorist who lost consciousness and drove her car through a storefront. The etiology of the defendant's syncopal episode was atrioventricular block. Plaintiffs argued that the existence of vertigo in the past should have placed the defendant on notice that it was negligent for her to drive. The court, in relying on *Grant v Joseph J. Duffy Co.*,[49] observed that the crucial factor to determine admissibility of prior episodes is whether those episodes are "reasonably" similar. In the case at hand, the court noted that there was no suggestion from the plaintiff's counsel of a clear connection between an episode of syncope related to atrioventricular block and the previous episodes of vertigo.

Admittedly, there is a settled body of law creating a basis for imposing liability on a physician for foreseeable injuries to third parties. Thus, if there is negligence in the failure to properly diagnose, treat, or restrict the activities of patients with syncope, the potential liability of a physician may well extend to injuries or death caused by the patient. While such exposure properly should be of concern to a physician treating patients with syncope, the fact remains that historically, such cases appear to be few and far between.

Conclusions

Physicians involved in the treatment of patients with syncope or other similar disorders should always be cognizant of the activities in which the patient engages, and must carefully assess whether continuation of those activities will place the patient or others at an unreasonable risk of harm. Such assessment requires knowledge of applicable rules, regulations, and statutes, as well as maintaining familiarity with current practice modalities and guidelines. Reasoned and appropriate care will greatly minimize, and perhaps even eliminate, physician liability in these cases.

References

1. Prosser, Keeton. *Law of Torts, 5th Ed.* 1984.
2. *Lance v Senior,* 36 Ill2d 516, 224 NE2d 231 (1967).
3. *Kirk v Michael Reese Hospital and Medical Center,* 17 Ill2d 507, 111 Ill Dec 944, 513 NE2d 387, *cert denied,* (US) 99 LEd 2d 236 (1987).
4. Speiser, Krause, Gans. *American Law of Torts,* 1985.
5. Manolis AS, Linzer M, Salem D, Estes III M. Syncope: Current diagnostic evaluation and management. *Ann Int Med* 1990;112:850–863.
6. Benditt DG, Remole S, Milstein S, Bailin S. Syncope: Causes, clinical evaluation, and current therapy. *Ann Rev Med* 1992;43:283–300.
7. Zipes DP, Garson A Jr. 26th Bethesda Conference: Recommendations for determining eligibility for competition in athletes with cardiovascular abnormalities: Task force 6: Arrhythmias. *Med Sci Sport Exerc* 1994;26(10 suppl):S276–S283.
8. Pegalis, Wachsman. *American Law of Medical Malpractice, 2nd Ed.* 1992.
9. Strickberger SA, Cantillon CO, Friedman PL. When should patients with lethal ventricular arrhythmias resume driving? *Ann Int Med* 1991;115:560–563.
10. Medtronic, Inc. When may patients with implanted defibrillators drive? *Follow-Up Forum* Winter 1995/1996;1(3):8–10.
11. Wisconsin Statutes § 448.03(5)(b), 1995.
12. Williams CC, Bernhardt DT. Syncope in athletes. *Sports Med* 1995;19:223–234.

13. *Gathers v Loyola Marymount University,* No. C 759027 (CA Super Ct, filed Apr 20, 1990).
14. Hudson MA. Gathers collapse is issue. *The Los Angeles Times* August 16, 1992.
15. Hudson MA. A legacy on court, in court. *The Los Angeles Times* Oct 6, 1992.
16. Maron BJ. Sounding Board. Sudden death in young athletes: Lessons from the Hank Gathers Affair. *N Engl J Med* 1993;329:55–57.
17. *Penny v Sands,* No. H89–280 (D Conn, filed May 3, 1989).
18. Fainaru S. Legal advice given: Lewis side told suit not worth it. *The Boston Globe* August 10, 1993.
19. Johnson WO. Heart of the matter. *Sports Illustrated* May 24, 1993.
20. Partial Transcript of Proceedings at 25–26, *Larkin v Archdiocese of Cincinnati,* No. C-1-90-619 (SD Ohio, filed Aug 31, 1990).
21. Mitten MJ. Team physicians and competitive athletes: Allocating legal responsibility for athletic injury. *Univ Pitt L Rev* 1993;55:129–160.
22. Mitten MJ. Amateur athletes with handicaps or physical abnormalities: Who makes the participation decision? *Neb L Rev* 1992;71:987–1032.
23. Altman LK. The doctor's world: An Athlete's health and a doctor's warning. *The New York Times* March 13, 1990.
24. Manno A. A high price to compete: The feasibility and effect of waivers used to protect schools from liability for injuries to athletes with high medical risks. *Ky L J* 1991;79:867.
25. Mitchell JH, Maron BJ, Epstein SE. Sixteenth Bethesda conference: Cardiovascular abnormalities in the athlete: Recommendations regarding eligibility for competition. *J Am Coll Cardiol* 1985;6:1186–1232.
26. Maron BJ, Mitchell JH. Twenty-sixth Bethesda conference: Recommendations for determining eligibility for competition in athletes with cardiovascular abnormalities. *J Am Coll Cardiol* 1994;24:846-899.
27. Maron BJ, Brown RW, McGrew CA. Ethical, legal, and practical considerations affecting decision making in competitive athletes. *J Am Coll Cardiol* 1994;24:854–860.
28. Krumholz A, Fisher RS, Lesser RP, Hauser WA. Driving and epilepsy: A review and reappraisal. *JAMA* 1991;265:622–626.
29. Medical regulatory criteria for evaluation. § 391.41(b)(4). *Federal Register* November 23, 1977; amended October 1983.
30. Curtis AB, Conti JB, Reilly RE, Tucker KJ. Implantable cardioverter defibrillators: Should patients be allowed to drive? *J Am Coll Cardiol* 1994;23:206A.
31. Epstein AE, Miles WM. Personal and public safety issues related to arrhythmias that may affect consciousness: Implications for regulation and physician recommendations. *Circulation* 1996;94:1147–1166.
32. Rehm CG, Ross SE. Elderly drivers involved in road crashes: A profile. *Am Surg* 1995;61:435-437.
33. Rehm CG, Ross SE. Syncope as etiology of road crashes involving elderly drivers. *Am Surg* 1995;61:1006–1008.
34. Dhala A, Bremner S, Blanck Z, et al. Impairment of driving abilities in patients with supraventricular tachycardias. *Am J Cardiol* 1995;75:516–518.
35. Decter BM, Goldner B, Cohen TJ. Vasovagal syncope as a cause of motor vehicle accidents. *Am Heart J* 1994;127:1619–1621.
36. Kou WH, Calkins H, Lewis RR, et al. Incidence of loss of consciousness during automatic implantable cardioverter defibrillator shocks. *Ann Intern Med* 1991;115:942–945.
37. Larsen GC, Stupey MR, Walance CG, et al. When should survivors of ventricular tachycardia/fibrillation resume driving? *Circulation* 1990;82 (suppl III): III–83.

38. Larsen GC, Stupey MR, Walance CG, et al. Recurrent cardiac events in survivors of ventricular fibrillation or tachycardia: Implications for driving restrictions. *JAMA* 1994;271:1335–1339.

39. Zilo P, Luceri RM, Vardeman LL. Driving after implantation of a cardioverter defibrillator. *Pacing Clin Electrophysiol* 1994(part II);17:781.

40. Tucker KJ, Conti JB, King LC, et al. Driving behavior after implantation of cardioverter defibrillators. *Pacing Clin Electrophysiol* 1994(part II);17:781.

41. Restatement of Torts 2d, 1964.

42. *Tarasoff v Regents of University of California,* 17 Cal 3d 425, 131 Cal Rptr 14, 551 P2d 334 (Cal 1976).

43. Sarno GG. Liability of physician, for injury to or death of third party, due to failure to disclose driving related impairment. 43 ALR 4th 153.

44. *Freese v Lemon,* 210 NW2d 576 (1973).

45. *Kaiser v Suburban Transportation Systems,* 65 Wash 2d 461, 398 P2d 14 (1965).

46. *Gooden v Tips,* 651 SW2d 364 (1983).

47. *Wharton Transport Corp. v Bridges,* 606 SW2d 521 (1980).

48. *Simmons v Aldi-Brenner Company,* 162 Ill App 3d 238, 515 NE2d 403 (1987).

49. *Grant v Joseph J. Duffy Co.,* 20 Ill App 3d 669, 314 NE2d 478 (1974).

Inspire me with love for my art (medicine)
and for thy creatures. In the sufferer
let me see only the human being...

-*Maimonides*
"Oath for the Physician"
1200 C.E.

The good physician knows his patients through and through,
and his knowledge is bought dearly. Time, sympathy,
and understanding must be lavishly dispensed, but the reward
is to be found in that personal bond which forms the greatest
satisfaction of the practice of medicine. One of the essential
qualities of the clinician is interest in humanity, for the secret
of the care of the patient is in caring for the patient.

-*Dr Francis Weld Peabody*
Lecture to the Harvard Medical Students
1927 C.E.

Index

Page numbers in *italic* indicate figures. Page numbers followed by "t" indicate tables.

Abdominal pain, with syncopal spell, 34, 40
Absence seizures, 236
Absent pulses, syncope and, 40
Adams-Stokes syndrome, as cause of syncope, 20
Adenosine receptor blocker, for elderly patient with syncope, 352
Adolescent, syncope in, 305–15
  cardiovascular, 309–10
  classification, 305–14, 306t
  dysautonomic, 309
  dysrhythmias
    normal heart, 311
    palliated structural disease, 311–13
    repaired heart, 311–13
  neurally mediated, 306–7
  neurocardiogenic, 307–8
  noncardiovascular, 313–14
Age-related physiological changes, 337–41
Aging. *See* Elderly
Agoraphobia, panic disorder without, criteria for, 256t
Alabama, syncope, driving regulations regarding, 374
Alaska, syncope, driving regulations regarding, 374
Alcohol, syncope relationship to, 36, 257, 258
Alcoholic neuropathy, 231–32
Algorithm
  for evaluation
    of athlete, *331*
    of elderly, *350*
  for management, *33, 62*
Allgrove's syndrome, 241
Alpha agonists, for elderly patient with syncope, 352
Amiodarone, sinus node function and, 149
Amyloidosis, 231
Analbuminemia, 243

Anand's syndrome, 234
Angina pectoris, as cause of syncope, 20
Angiography, for syncope in athlete, 329–30
Antiarrhythmic drugs, sinus node function and, 149
Antihypertensives, sinus node function and, 149
Anxiety disorder
  as cause of syncope, 258
  generalized, 255, 255t, 258
  criteria for, 255t
Aortic stenosis, as cause of syncope, 20
Arizona, syncope, driving regulations regarding, 374
Arkansas, syncope, driving regulations regarding, 374
Arrhythmias
  as cause of syncope, 22–24
  state driving regulations regarding, 390
Atenolol, 93. *See also* Beta blockers
Atherosclerosis, 235
  as cause of AV block, 141
Athlete, syncope in, 317–35
  algorithm, for evaluation, *331*
  coronary angiography, 329–30
  echocardiography, 320–21
  electrocardiography, 318–20, *319*
  electrophysiological testing, 327–28, *328*
  exercise testing, 326–27
    stress, 321–26, *322–26*
  head-upright tilt test, 326–27
  legal issues, 391–95
  myocardial biopsy, 329–30
  physical examination, 318
Athletic participation, standards for, legal issues, 393–95
Atonic seizures, 236–37
Atrial fibrillation, syncope and, 43
Atrial natriuretic peptide, tachyarrhythmias, 174–75
Atrioventricular conduction disease, 130–48

Atrioventricular conduction disease,
(*Continued*)
  bradyarrhythmia with, 142–47
    extrinsic disturbances, sinus node
      function, AV conduction, 148–50,
      149t
    first-degree AV block, 143
    Mobitz type I AV block, with recur-
      rent dizziness, *144*
    Mobitz type II AV block, with AV
      block, *144*
    second-degree AV block, 143–44,
      144
    sinus node function, drugs affect-
      ing, 149t
    third-degree AV block, *145*,
      145–47, 148t
    treatment, 147
    2:1 AV block, 145
Aura, as symptom related to syncopal
  spell, 34
Autonomic alterations, during tachy-
  cardia, 171–74
Autonomic epilepsy, 237–38
Autonomic failure, idiopathic, 229–30
Awakening, symptoms upon, 37

Bárány syndrome, 245
Back pain, as symptom related to syncopal spell, 34
Baroreflex
  failure, 238
  sensitivity, changes in, with aging, 339
Baseline laboratory tests, 4
Benign positional vertigo. *See* Bárány
  syndrome
Beta-blockers
  for elderly patient with syncope, 352
  for neurocardiogenic syncope, 93
  sinus node function and, 149
Bezold-Jarisch reflex activation, 239
Blood pressure. *See also* Hemodynam-
  ics; Hypotension
  syncope and, 40
Bouveret's syndrome, 243–44
Bradbury-Eggleston syndrome, 229–30
Bradyarrhythmia, 127–66
  with AV conduction disease, 128,
    129t, 130–48
  AV block
    causes of, 141t
    2:1, 145
    etiology, 140–42, 141t

    extrinsic disturbances, sinus node
      function, AV conduction, 148–50,
      149t
    first-degree AV block, 143
    Mobitz
      type I AV block, with recurrent
        dizziness, *144*
      type II AV block, with AV block,
        144
    second-degree AV block, 143–44, *144*
    sinus node function, drugs affect-
      ing, 149t
    third-degree AV block, *145*,
      145–47, 148t
    treatment, 147
  classification of, 128–30
  diagnostic techniques, 156–59
  drug-induced, 128
  extrinsic disturbances of AV conduc-
    tion, 149–50
  intrinsic sinus node, 128, 129t, 130–48
  neurally mediated reflex, 128, 129t,
    150–56, *151*
    clinical presentation, 150–56
      incidence, 153–54
      investigation, 154–55
      pathophysiological mechanisms,
        152–53
      prognosis, 153–54
      treatment, 155–56
  sinus node dysfunction, 130–40,
    131–33, 134t, *135–36*, 148–50
    causes of, 129t
    etiology of, 129t, 132–33
    pacing in, 139t
    treatment, 138–40, 139t
Breath-holding spells, 240
  cyanotic, 240–41
  pallid, 241
Bretylium, sinus node function and, 149
Bruns' syndrome, 237
Bundle branch block, syncope and, 43

Caffeine, elderly patient with syncope
  and, 352
Calcification infiltration, as cause of AV
  block, 141
Calcium channel blockers
  for elderly patient with syncope, 352
  sinus node function and, 149
California
  arrhythmias, driving regulations re-
    garding, 390

syncope, driving regulations regarding, 374
Cardiac arrest, premonitory sign of, syncope as, 16
Cardiac history, obtaining from patient, 38
Cardiac pacing, permanent, for neurocardiogenic support, 93
Cardiac relaxation, changes in, with aging, 339–40
Cardiomyopathy, as cause of AV block, 141
Cardiovascular syncope, in child, adolescent, 309–10
Cardiovascular testing, 4–8
Carotid bruits, syncope and, 40
Carotid massage, 6
  syncope and, 40
Carotid sinus hypersensitivity, 20, 281–95
  afferent, efferent neural connections, neurally mediated syncopy, 282
  anatomy, 282, 282–83
  cardiovascular diseases, electrophysiological abnormalities, 282, 288–89
  clinical syndromes, 285–88, 286, 288
  in elderly, 344–45
  incidence, 285–88, 286, 288
  management, 289–91, 290t
  permanent pacing in, indications for, 290t
  physiology, 282, 282–83
  technique, 283–85, 284
Carotid sinus massage, 39–40
Carotid sinus syncope, 239
Cataplexy, 245
Causes of syncope, 2t, 19–27, 30t
  arrhythmic, 22–24
  autonomic causes, 25–26
  common causes, 19t
  endocrine disorders, 301
  hypoadrenalism, 301
  metabolic, 27, 301t
  micturition, 25–26
  myocardium
    infarction, 26–27
    ischemia, 26–27
  neurocardiogenic syncope, 19–21
  neurological causes, 27
  orthostatic hypotension, 20, 21–22
  psychiatric causes, 27
  seizures, 24–25
  uncommon causes, 20t, 26–28
  unknown etiology, 27–28

Central dysregulation, disorders of, 237–39
  autonomic epilepsy, 237–38
  baroreflex failure, 238
  Bruns' syndrome, 237
  Penfield's syndrome, 238
  Wallenberg's syndrome, 238
  Williams-Bashore syndrome, 239
Cerebral ischemia, conditions leading to, 235–36
  atherosclerosis, 235
  innominate artery syndrome, 236
  isolated, 227
  subclavian steal syndrome, 236
  Takayasu's disease, 235
Cerebrovascular disease, as cause of syncope, 20, 26
Chest pain, as symptom related to syncopal spell, 34
Child, syncope in, 305–15
  approach, 305–14, 306t
  cardiovascular syncope, 309–10
  causes of, 306t
  classification, 305–14, 306t
  dysautonomic syncope, 309
  dysrhythmias
    normal heart, 311
    palliated structural disease, 311–13
    repaired heart, 311–13
  neurally mediated syncopes, 306–7
  neurocardiogenic syncope, 307–8
  noncardiovascular syncope, 313–14
Chronic fatigue syndrome, 266–67
  evaluation, 274–76
  neurally mediated hypotension, relationship, 269–74, 271t
  pathophysiological basis for, 272–74
  treatment, 274–76
  upright tilt, healthy controls, compared, 271t
Classification of syncope, 28–32, 30t
Clonidine, dysautonomic syncope, 118
Collagen-vascular diseases, as cause of AV block, 141
Color of skin, as symptom related to syncopal spell, 34
Colorado
  arrhythmias, driving regulations regarding, 390
  syncope, driving regulations regarding, 374
Complete heart block, syncope and, 43

Confusion
    seizures *vs.* hypotension, differential
        diagnosis, 224
    as symptom related to syncopal
        spell, 34
Congenital AV block, as cause of AV
    block, 141
Connecticut, syncope, driving regula-
    tions regarding, 374
Consult, with specialist, 48–49
Coronary angiography, syncope in ath-
    lete, 329–30
Cost, of syncope, 17
Coughing, as symptom related to syn-
    copal spell, 34, 240
Cyanotic breath-holding spells, 240–41

DBH deficiency. *See* Dopamine-beta-
    hydroxylase deficiency
Death
    family history of, in patient history, 38
    of third party, physician liability for,
        397–99
Defecation syncope, 34, 240
Defining of episodes, in patient history,
    35
Degenerative disease, neurological dis-
    eases associated with, 227
Delaware, syncope, driving regulations
    regarding, 374
Delta waves, syncope and, 43
Depression, major, 255–57, 256t
    as cause of syncope, 258
    criteria for, 256t
Desmopressin, dysautonomic syncope, 118
Diabetes mellitus, 230–31
Diagnostic testing, 4–9, 41–43
    12-lead ECG, 4
    approach to, 8–9, *9*
    baseline laboratory tests, 4
    cardiovascular, 4–8
    carotid massage, 6
    echocardiogram, 6–7
    electrocardiogram, 42–43, 43t
        prolonged, 4–5
            ambulatory loop event monitor-
                ing, 5
    electrophysiological studies, 5–6
    exercise testing, 7
    neurological testing, 8
    patient history, 4
    physical examination, 4
    psychiatric assessment, 8

signal-averaged ECG, 6
    upright tilt testing, 7
Diaphoresis, as symptom related to syn-
    copal spell, 34
Diarrhea, as symptom related to synco-
    pal spell, 34
Diet, for dysautonomic syncope, 118
Diltiazem, sinus node function and, 149
Disopyramide
    for elderly patient with syncope, 352
    for neurocardiogenic syncope, 93
    sinus node function and, 149
Dopamine agonist, for elderly patient
    with syncope, 352
Dopamine-beta-hydroxylase deficiency,
    233
Driving, 240, 371–85, *372*, 374–75t
    epidemiology, 373–78, 374–75t, *376*
    pathophysiology of, *376*, 379–81
    restrictions to, 378–79
    risks, *376*
    state recommendations, 374t
    syncope, 395–97
Drugs
    abuse of, as cause of syncope, 258
    affecting sinus node function, 149t
    as cause of AV block, 141
    causing orthostatic hypotension, 114t
    in patient history, 38
    syncope, relationship to, 36, 299
Dysautonomic syncope, 107–26
    autonomic disorders, investigation
        of, 115–17
    orthostatic hypotension, causes of,
        110–15, 111t
        autonomic disorders, classification
            of, 111t
        clinical features, 113–15
        drugs causing, 114t
        primary causes, 110–13
            acute, 112–13
            chronic, 110–12
        secondary causes, 111t, 113, 114t
        postural normotension, maintenance
            of, 108–10
        therapeutic measures, 117–22, 118–19t
Dyspnea, as symptom related to synco-
    pal spell, 34
Dysregulation, central, disorders of,
    237–39

Eating, as symptom related to syncopal
    spell, 34

ECG. *See* Electrocardiogram
Echocardiogram, 6–7
Ectopic beats, syncope and, 43
EEG. *See* Electroencephalogram
Elastic support hose
    dysautonomic syncope, 118
    neurocardiogenic syncope, 93
Elderly, syncope in, 337–58
    baroreflex sensitivity, changes in, 339
    cardiac relaxation, changes in, 339–40
    causes of, 341–46
        cardiovascular syncope, 343–44
        endocrine diseases, 346
        hypotensive syndromes, 341
        neurological diseases, 344
            autonomic dysfunction, 344
            cerebrovascular disease, 344
            orthostatic hypotension, 341–42
            postprandial hypotension, 342
            reflex mechanisms, 344–46
            carotid sinus hypersensitivity,
                344–45
            cough syncope, 345
            defecation syncope, 345
            micturition, 345
            neurally mediated, 345–46
            neurocardiogenic syncope, 345–46
            vasovagal syncope, 345–46
    cerebral circulation, changes in, 337–38
    evaluation, 346–49
        algorithm, *350*
    heart rate, changes in, 339
    hypertension, effect of, 341
    management, 346–49
    nervous system
        parasympathetic, changes in, 338–39
        sympathetic, changes in, 338
    patient history, 346–47
    physical examination, 347–49, *350*
    physiological changes, age-related,
        337–41
    treatment, 349–53, 351–52t
    vascular tone, changes in, 340–41
Electrocardiogram
    12-lead, 4
    prolonged monitoring, 4–5
        ambulatory loop event monitor-
            ing, 5
    signal-averaged, 6
    syncope in athlete, 318–20, *319*
Electroencephalogram, seizures *vs.* hy-
        potension, differential diagnosis,
        224

Electrophysiological studies, 5–6,
        52–57, 53–56t, *54*, 54t, 55t, 179–221
    abnormality
        borderline, 191t
        definite, 191t
        variables associated with, 211t
    background, 180–82
    data acquired during, 183t
    directing therapy, 190–93, 191–92t
    expected yield, 183t, 183–85, 192t
    frequent recurrent syncope, role in,
        210–12, 211t
    indications for, 211t
    unusual, 212–13
    interpretation of, 193–210, *194–210*
        goals, 186
        prognosis and, 189–90
        uncertainty level, 186–89, *187*
    nondiagnostic findings, 191t
    protocols, 182–83, 192
    in recurrent unexplained syncope,
        359–61, 360t
    therapy, value of, 56t
    timing of, 53t
    twelve-lead ECG, *194, 197*
Embolism, pulmonary, 300
Endless-loop recorders, 51–52, 52t
    event recorders, 51–52, 52t
    Holter monitor, choice between, 52t
Endocrine disorders, syncope and,
        300–302, 301t
    in elderly, 346
Ephedrine sulfate, dysautonomic syn-
        cope, 118
Epidemic fainting, 257–58
Epidemiology, of syncope, 17–18
Epilepsy
    autonomic, 237–38
    as cause of syncope, 20
Epsilon waves, syncope and, 43
Evaluation of syncope, 33t
Event recorders, 51–52, 52t
Exercise
    syncope and, 34, 36
        dysautonomic, 118
    testing, 7
        in athlete, 321–26, *322–26*
Expense, of syncope, 17
Extrinsic disturbances, AV conduction,
        149–50
Eye deviation, seizures *vs.* hypotension,
        differential diagnosis, 224

Fainting, epidemic, 257–58
Family history, of death, syncope, 38
Fatigue
  chronic fatigue syndrome, 266–67
  neurally mediated hypotension, relationship between, 267–68
Fear, as symptom related to syncopal spell, 34
First-degree heart block, syncope and, 43
Flecainide, sinus node function and, 149
Florida
  arrhythmias, driving regulations regarding, 390
  syncope, driving regulations regarding, 374
Fludrocortisone
  dysautonomic syncope, 118
  neurocardiogenic syncope, 93
Fluoxetine
  dysautonomic syncope, 118
  elderly patient with syncope, 352
  neurocardiogenic syncope, 93
Flushing, as symptom related to syncopal spell, 34
Frequency of episodes, 38

Gélineau's syndrome, 245–46
GAD. See Generalized anxiety disorder
Generalized anxiety disorder. See Anxiety disorder
Georgia, syncope, driving regulations regarding, 374
Glossopharyngeal neuralgia. See Weisenburg's syndrome
Guillain-Barre syndrome, 232
Gut peptide release inhibitor, for elderly patient with syncope, 352

Hair-grooming syncope seizures, 299
Hawaii
  arrhythmias, driving regulations regarding, 390
  syncope, driving regulations regarding, 374
Head-up, tilt of bed, for dysautonomic syncope, 118
Headache
  seizures vs. hypotension, differential diagnosis, 224
  as symptom related to syncopal spell, 34
Heart block
  complete, syncope and, 43

first-degree, syncope and, 43
second-degree, syncope and, 43
Heart murmur, syncope and, 40
Heart rate
  changes in, with aging, 339
  syncope and, 40
Hemodynamic disorders, 243
  analbuminemia, 243
  Bouveret's syndrome, 243–44
  diagnosis of, 228
  McKittrick-Wheelock syndrome, 244
  Roenheld's syndrome, 244
  Schroeder's syndrome, 244
  Short's syndrome, 244
  supine hypotension syndrome, 244
Holter monitor, 51, 52
  endless loop recorders, distinguished, 52t
Hospitalization
  after initial evaluation, 44t, 44–48
  criteria for, 44t
  routine evaluation after, 49t
Hyperbradykininism, 241–42
Hyperepinephrinemia, 243
Hypersensitive carotid sinus, as cause of syncope, 20
Hypertension, effect of, in elderly, 341
Hypertensive encephalopathy, as cause of syncope, 20
Hyperventilation, as cause of syncope, 20
Hypoadrenalism, syncope due to, 301
Hypotension
  neurally mediated, 265–66
  chronic fatigue syndrome, relationship between, 269–74, 271t
  evaluation, 274–76
  fatigue, relationship between, 267–68
  response to treatment, 271t
  treatment, 274–76
  neurological diseases associated with, 227
  seizures, differential diagnosis, 224t
  vs. seizures, differential diagnosis, 224
Hysteria, as cause of syncope, 20

Idaho, syncope, driving regulations regarding, 374
Idiopathic fibrosis Lev's disease, as cause of AV block, 141
Idiopathic orthostatic hypotension, 229–30
  idiopathic autonomic failure, 229–30

Illinois
  arrhythmias, driving regulations regarding, 390
  syncope, driving regulations regarding, 374
Implantable syncope monitor, in recurrent unexplained syncope, 360–64, *362–64*
Indiana
  arrhythmias, driving regulations regarding, 390
  syncope, driving regulations regarding, 374
Indomethacin, for elderly patient with syncope, 352
Infiltrative diseases, as cause of AV block, 141
Inflammatory diseases, as cause of AV block, 141
Initial approach, patient with syncope, 32
Injury
  caused by syncope, 17
  as symptom related to syncopal spell, 34
Innominate artery syndrome, 236
Intolerance, orthostatic, diagnostic categories describing, 225t
Intrathoracic pressure, increased, syncope due to, 298–99
Iowa
  arrhythmias, driving regulations regarding, 390
  syncope, driving regulations regarding, 374

Jerks, seizures *vs.* hypotension, differential diagnosis, 224

Kansas
  arrhythmias, driving regulations regarding, 390
  syncope, driving regulations regarding, 374
Kentucky, syncope, driving regulations regarding, 374
Keratoconjunctivitis sicca. *See* Sjögren's syndrome

Laboratory tests, baseline, 4
Laws, restricting driving, 378–79
Left ventricular lift, syncope and, 40
Legal issues, 387–401. *See also* Driving
  administrative proceedings, 389–91, 390t

athlete, with syncope, 391–93
athletic participation, standards for, 393–95
physician liability, for injury, death of third party, 397–99
standard of care, medical, 388–89
statutes, 389–91, 390t
Length of episodes, in patient history, 35
Liability, of physician. *See also* Legal issues
  for injury, death of third party, 397–99
Lidocaine, sinus node function and, 149
Lifestyle, impact of syncope, 16–17
Lisker's syndrome, 234
Location, of syncope evaluation, 32, *33*
Loop recorders, in recurrent unexplained syncope, 361–64
Louisiana
  arrhythmias, driving regulations regarding, 390
  syncope, driving regulations regarding, 374

Maine
  arrhythmias, driving regulations regarding, 390
  syncope, driving regulations regarding, 374
Major depression. *See* Depression
"Malignant" episode, neurocardiogenic syncope, *95*
Maryland
  arrhythmias, driving regulations regarding, 390
  syncope, driving regulations regarding, 374
Massachusetts
  arrhythmias, driving regulations regarding, 390
  syncope, driving regulations regarding, 374
Massage, carotid, 6
Mastocytosis, 242
McKittrick-Wheelock syndrome, 244
MDD. *See* Depressive disorder
Meals, syncope relationship to, 36
Melena, as symptom related to syncopal spell, 34
Metabolism, abnormalities, syncope and, 27, 300–302, 301t
Methylphenidate
  dysautonomic syncope, 118
  neurocardiogenic syncope, 93

Mexiletine, sinus node function and, 149
Michigan, syncope, driving regulations regarding, 374
Micturition, as cause of syncope, 25–26
Midodrine
dysautonomic syncope, 118
elderly patient with syncope, 352
Midodrine for neurocardiogenic support, 93
Migraine, as cause of syncope, 20
Millikan-Siekert syndrome. *See* Subclavian steal syndrome
Minnesota, syncope, driving regulations regarding, 374
Mississippi, syncope, driving regulations regarding, 374
Missouri, syncope, driving regulations regarding, 374
Monoamine oxidase deficiency, 233–34
Montana, syncope, driving regulations regarding, 374
Myocardial infarction, syncope and, 20, 43
Myocardial ischemia, as cause of syncope, 26–27

Narcolepsy. *See* Gélineau's syndrome
Natriuretic peptide, atrial, tachyarrhythmias, 174–75
Nausea, as symptom related to syncopal spell, 34
Nebraska, syncope, driving regulations regarding, 374
Neck vein distension, syncope and, 40
Nefazadone for neurocardiogenic syncope, 93
Nervous system
parasympathetic, changes in, 338–39
sympathetic, changes in, 338
Neurally mediated AV block, as cause of AV block, 141
Neurally mediated hypotension, 265–66
chronic fatigue syndrome, relationship between, 269–74, 271t
evaluation, 274–76
fatigue, relationship between, 267–68
response to treatment, 271t
treatment, 274–76
Neurally mediated reflex origin, 150–56
Neurocardiogenic syncope, 19–21, 73–106
agents exacerbating, 92t
in child, adolescent, 307–8
clinical aspects of, 79–82
"malignant" episode, 95

pathophysiology of, 74–79
prognosis, 98–99
therapeutic approaches, 91–98, 95
therapies for, 93t
tilt table test, 85
head-upright, 82–88, 85–87, 95
indications for, 88, 89, 90–91
contraindicated, 91
not indicated, 91
Neurohumoral disorders, 241–43
Allgrove's syndrome, 241
hyperbradykininism, 241–42
hyperepinephrinemia, 243
mastocytosis, 242
pheochromocytoma, 242–43
Ulick's syndrome, 241
Verner-Morrison syndrome, 241
Neurological causes of syncope, 27, 34, 223–51
Neurological diseases, 226–35, 227–28t
differential diagnosis, 227–28t
multiple system atrophy, 226–29, 229t
Shy-Drager syndrome, 226–29, 229t
Neurological findings, syncope and, 8, 40
Neuropathy
alcohol, 231–32
peripheral, 230–34
Nevada
arrhythmias, driving regulations regarding, 390
syncope, driving regulations regarding, 374
New Jersey
arrhythmias, driving regulations regarding, 390
syncope, driving regulations regarding, 374
New Mexico, syncope, driving regulations regarding, 374
New York
arrhythmias, driving regulations regarding, 390
syncope, driving regulations regarding, 374
Normotension, postural, maintenance of, with dysautonomic syncope, 108–10
North Carolina
arrhythmias, driving regulations regarding, 390
syncope, driving regulations regarding, 374

North Dakota
  arrhythmias, driving regulations regarding, 390
  syncope, driving regulations regarding, 374
Number of episodes, diagnosis and, 38

Octreotide, for elderly patient with syncope, 352
Ohio
  arrhythmias, driving regulations regarding, 390
  syncope, driving regulations regarding, 374
Oklahoma
  arrhythmias, driving regulations regarding, 390
  syncope, driving regulations regarding, 374
Oregon
  arrhythmias, driving regulations regarding, 390
  syncope, driving regulations regarding, 374
Orthostatic hypotension
  as cause of syncope, 20, *20,* 21–22
  causes of, 110–15, 111t
    autonomic disorders, classification of, 111t
    clinical features, 113–15
    drugs causing, 114t
    primary causes, 110–13
      acute, 112–13
      chronic, 110–12
    secondary causes, 111t, 113, 114t
Orthostatic intolerance, diagnostic categories describing, 225t
Orthostatic syncope. *See* Dysautonomic syncope
Orthostatic vital signs, 39

Paced rhythm, syncope and, 43
Pacemaker patients, syncope in, 299–300
Pain
  back, as symptom related to syncopal spell, 34
  chest, as symptom related to syncopal spell, 34
Pallid breath-holding spells, 241
Palpitations, as symptom related to syncopal spell, 34

Panic disorder, 255, 256t
  as cause of syncope, 258
  without agoraphobia, criteria for, 256t
Parkinson's disease, 230
Paroxymal seizures, 227, 236–41
  absence, 236
  akinetic, 237
  atonic, 236–37
Paroxysmal reflex activation, 239–41
  Bezold-Jarisch reflex activation, 239
  breath holding spells, 240
  carotid sinus syncope, 239
  cough syncope, 240
  cyanotic breath-holding spells, 240–41
  defecation syncope, 240
  diver's syncope, 240
  pallid breath-holding spells, 241
  syncope and, 227
  Weisenburg's syndrome, 240
Paroxysmal tachycardia, as cause of syncope, 20
Partial-complex seizures, 237
Patient history, 4, 32–39, 33–35t, 34t
Penfield's syndrome, 238
Pennsylvania
  arrhythmias, driving regulations regarding, 390
  syncope, driving regulations regarding, 374
Peripheral neuropathy, 230–34
  alcohol neuropathy, 231–32
  amyloidosis, 231
  Anand's syndrome, 234
  diabetes mellitus, 230–31
  dopamine-beta-hydroxylase deficiency, 233
  Guillain-Barre syndrome, 232
  hypotension and, 227
  Lisker's syndrome, 234
  monoamine oxidase deficiency, 233–34
  porphyria, 232
Permanent cardiac pacing for neurocardiogenic support, 93
Pheochromocytoma, 242–43
Physical examination, 4, 39, 40t
  anemia, complexion and, 41
  cardiovascular examination, 40
  carotid sinus massage, 39–40
  complexion, 41
  orthostatic vital signs, 39
  physical findings, 40t

Physical examination, (*Continued*)
 respiratory rate, pattern, 39
 shift in blood flow, complexion and, 41
Physician liability, for injury, death of
 third party, 397–99
Physiological changes, age-related,
 337–41
Pindolol, dysautonomic syncope, 118
Polyradiculopathy, demyelinating,
 acute, idiopathic. *See* Guillain-
 Barre syndrome
Porphyria, 232
Position, syncope and, 36
Postmicturition, as cause of syncope, 20
Postsyncopal symptoms, 37
Posture
 normotension, maintenance of, with
  dysautonomic syncope, 108–10
 syncope and, 34, 36
Preceding syncope, situations involved,
 in patient history, 36
Premonitory sign of cardiac arrest, syn-
 cope as, 16
Procainamide, sinus node function
 and, 149
Prodrome
 seizures *vs.* hypotension, differential
  diagnosis, 224
 symptoms, 37
Prognosis, after syncope, 3–4
Prolonged weakness, as symptom related to syncopal spell, 34
Propafenone, sinus node function and,
 149
Propanolol, for elderly patient with
 syncope, 352
Prostaglandin synthetase inhibitors, for
 elderly patient with syncope, 352
Protocol, evaluation of syncope, 60–61,
 62
Psychiatric assessment, 8
Psychiatric disorders, 253–63
 alcohol abuse, 257
 anxiety disorder, generalized, 255, 255t
  criteria for, 255t
 depressive disorder, major, 255–57,
  256t
 depressive episode, major, criteria
  for, 256t
 epidemic fainting, 257–58
 mechanism of syncope in, 259–60
 outcomes, 259

panic attack, 255, 256t
panic disorder without agoraphobia,
 criteria for, 256t
patient evaluation, 261–62
somatization disorder, 254, 254t
 criteria for, 254t
stress, syncope and, 257
substance abuse disorders, 257
testing for, 260–61
Pulmonary embolism, 300
Pulmonary hypertension, as cause of
 syncope, 20
Pulseless disease. *See* Takayasu's disease

QT prolongation, syncope and, 43
Quinidine, sinus node function and, 149

Rash, syncope and, 40
Recovery, slow, as symptom related to
 syncopal spell, 34
Recreational drugs, syncope due to use
 of, 299
Recurrent unexplained syncope,
 359–69
 cost, 364–65
 electrophysiological testing, 359–61,
  360t
  negative, recurrent risk for syncope after, 360t
 final measures, 365–67, *367*
 implantable syncope monitor,
  360–64, *362–64*
 loop recorders, 361–64
 rhythm strip, during episode, *364*
Regulations, restricting driving, 378–79
Respiration rate, 40
 pattern of, 39
Rhode Island
 arrhythmias, driving regulations regarding, 390
 syncope, driving regulations regarding, 374
Rhythm, paced, syncope and, 43
Roenheld's syndrome, 244

S3 gallop, syncope and, 40
Schroeder's syndrome, 244
Second-degree heart block, syncope
 and, 43
Seizures, 236–37
 absence, 236
 akinetic, 237
 atonic, 236–37

as cause of syncope, 24–25
hypotension, differential diagnosis, 224t
vs. hypotension, differential diagnosis, 224
Serotonin reuptake inhibitors, for elderly patient with syncope, 352
Sertraline for neurocardiogenic syncope, 93
Sexual activity, syncope during, 300
Short's syndrome, 244
Signal-averaged ECG, 6
Sinus bradycardia, syncope and, 43
Sinus node
  function, extrinsic disturbance of, 148–50
  intrinsic, 130–48
Situational syncope, 297–98, 298t
  causes of, 298t
Sjögren's syndrome, 233
Skin color, syncope and, 34, 40
Slow recovery, as symptom related to syncopal spell, 34
Somatization disorder, 254, 254t
  criteria for, 254t
Sotalol, sinus node function and, 149
South Carolina, syncope, driving regulations regarding, 374
South Dakota, syncope, driving regulations regarding, 374
Specialist, consult with, 48–49
Sphincter control, loss of, seizures *vs.* hypotension, differential diagnosis, 224
Spinal cord, lesions, 234–35
  degeneration. *See* Vitamin B_{12} deficiency
  hypotension and, 227
  syringomyelia, 235
Stool guaiac, syncope and, 40
Streeten's syndrome. *See* Hyperbradykininism
Stress, syncope and, 257
Subclavian steal syndrome, 236
Substance abuse, syncope and, 257
SUO. *See* Unexplained syncope
Supine hypotension syndrome, 244
Supraventricular tachycardia, 43, 168–69
  autonomic alterations, 173–74
  hemodynamic changes during, 171
  rate, effect of, 169–70
  syncope and, 43

Sympatholytic antihypertensives. *See* Antihypertensives
Symptoms, related to syncopal spell, 34t
Syringomyelia, 235

Tachyarrhythmias, 167–78
  atrial natriuretic peptide, 174–75
  autonomic alterations, during tachycardia, 171–74
    supraventricular tachycardia, 173–74
    ventricular tachycardia, 171–73
  cerebrovascular contribution, 174
  clinical features, syncope due to, 167–69
    supraventricular tachycardia, 168–69
    ventricular tachycardia, 167–68
  hemodynamic changes, during tachycardia, 170–71
    supraventricular tachycardia, 171
    ventricular tachycardia, 170–71
  rate of tachycardia, effect of, 169–70
    supraventricular, 169–70
    ventricular, 169
Tachycardia
  paroxysmal, as cause of syncope, 20
  rate of, effect, 169–70
    supraventricular, 169–70
    ventricular tachycardia, 169
  supraventricular, 43, 168–69
  ventricular, 43, 167–68
Takayasu's disease, 235
Temporally related symptoms, in patient history, 38
Tennessee, syncope, driving regulations regarding, 375
Texas
  arrhythmias, driving regulations regarding, 390
  syncope, driving regulations regarding, 375
Theophylline for neurocardiogenic syncope, 93
Therapeutic drugs, syncope due to use of, 299
Tilt table testing, 50–51. *See also* Upright tilt testing
  for neurocardiogenic syncope, *85*
    contraindication, 91
    head-upright, 82–88, *85–87, 95*
    indications for, 88, *89,* 90–91
    not indicated, 91

Tongue biting, seizures *vs.* hypotension, differential diagnosis, 224
Trauma, as cause of AV block, 141
Triggering events, to episodes, in patient history, 36
Tumors, as cause of AV block, 141
Tussive cause of syncope, 20
Twelve-lead electrocardiogram, 4

Ulick's syndrome, 241
Undiagnosed syncope, 59–60
Unexplained syncope, recurrent, 359–69
cost, 364–65
electrophysiological testing, 359–61, 360t
negative, recurrent risk for syncope after, 360t
final measures, 365–67, *367*
implantable syncope monitor, 360–64, *362–64*
loop recorders, 361–64
management of recurrent syncope with, 59–60
rhythm strip, during episode, *364*
syncope of, 20, 27–28
Upright tilt testing, 7
chronic fatigue syndrome, healthy controls, compared, 271t
Urination, as symptom related to syncopal spell, 34
Utah
arrhythmias, driving regulations regarding, 390
syncope, driving regulations regarding, 375

Vascular tone, changes in, with aging, 340–41
Vasovagal cause of syncope, 20
Ventricular tachycardia, 43, 167–68
autonomic alterations, 171–73
hemodynamic changes during, 170–71
rate, effect of, 169
syncope and, 43

Verapamil, sinus node function and, 149
Vermont
arrhythmias, driving regulations regarding, 390
syncope, driving regulations regarding, 375
Verner-Morrison syndrome, 241
Virginia
arrhythmias, driving regulations regarding, 390
syncope, driving regulations regarding, 375
Visual change, as symptom related to syncopal spell, 34
Vital signs, orthostatic, 39
Vitamin B_{12} deficiency, 234–35
Vomiting, as symptom related to syncopal spell, 34

Wallenberg's syndrome, 238
Washington D.C.
arrhythmias, driving regulations regarding, 390
syncope, driving regulations regarding, 375
Weakness, prolonged, as symptom related to syncopal spell, 34
Weisenburg's syndrome, 240
West Virginia
arrhythmias, driving regulations regarding, 390
syncope, driving regulations regarding, 375
Williams–Bashore syndrome, 239
Wisconsin
arrhythmias, driving regulations regarding, 390
syncope, driving regulations regarding, 375
Wyoming, syncope, driving regulations regarding, 375

Yohimbine, dysautonomic syncope, 118